Behavior

Editor

MARION R. DESMARCHELIER

VETERINARY CLINICS OF NORTH AMERICA: EXOTIC ANIMAL PRACTICE

www.vetexotic.theclinics.com

Consulting Editor
JÖRG MAYER

January 2021 • Volume 24 • Number 1

ELSEVIER

1600 John F. Kennedy Boulevard • Suite 1800 • Philadelphia, Pennsylvania, 19103-2899
http://www.vetexotic.theclinics.com

VETERINARY CLINICS OF NORTH AMERICA: EXOTIC ANIMAL PRACTICE Volume 24, Number 1
January 2021 ISSN 1094-9194, ISBN-13: 978-0-323-73347-2

Editor: Stacy Eastman
Developmental Editor: Nicole Congleton

Veterinary Clinics of North America: Exotic Animal Practice (ISSN 1094-9194) is published in January, May, and September by Elsevier, Inc., 360 Park Avenue South, New York, NY 10010-1710. Subscription prices are $290.00 per year for US individuals, $687.00 per year for US institutions, $100.00 per year for US students and residents, $338.00 per year for Canadian individuals, $735.00 per year for Canadian institutions, $352.00 per year for international individuals, $735.00 per year for international institutions, $100.00 per year Canadian students/residents, and $165.00 per year for international students/residents. To receive student/resident rate, orders must be accompanied by name of affiliated institution, date of term, and the *signature* of program/residency coordinator on institution letterhead. Orders will be billed at individual rate until proof of status is received. Foreign air speed delivery is included in all *Clinics* subscription prices. All prices are subject to change without notice. **POSTMASTER:** Send address changes to *Veterinary Clinics of North America: Exotic Animal Practice*, Elsevier Health Sciences Division, Subscription Customer Service, 3251 Riverport Lane, Maryland Heights, MO 63043. **Customer Service: Telephone: 1-800-654-2452** (U.S. and Canada); **1-314-447-8871** (outside U.S. and Canada). **Fax: 1-314-447-8029. E-mail: journalscustomerservice-usa@elsevier.com (for print support); journalsonlinesupport-usa@elsevier.com (for online support)**.

Reprints. For copies of 100 or more of articles in this publication, please contact the Commercial Reprints Department, Elsevier Inc., 360 Park Avenue South, New York, New York 10010-1710. Tel.: 212-633-3874; Fax: 212-633-3820; E-mail: reprints@elsevier.com.

Veterinary Clinics of North America: Exotic Animal Practice is covered in *MEDLINE/PubMed (Index Medicus)*.

Contributors

CONSULTING EDITOR

JÖRG MAYER, Dr med vet, MSc
Diplomate, American Board of Veterinary Practitioners (Exotic Companion Mammals); Diplomate, European College of Zoological Medicine (Small Mammals); Diplomate, American College of Zoological Medicine; Associate Professor of Zoological Medicine, Department of Small Animal Medicine and Surgery, University of Georgia College of Veterinary Medicine, Athens, Georgia, USA

EDITOR

MARION R. DESMARCHELIER, DVM
Diplomate, American College of Zoological Medicine; Diplomate, European College of Zoological Medicine (Zoo Health Management); Diplomate, American College of Veterinary Behaviorists; Assistant Professor, Department of Clinical Sciences, Faculté de Médecine Vétérinaire, Université de Montréal, Saint-Hyacinthe, QC, Canada

AUTHORS

LAURIE BERGMANN, VMD
Diplomate, American College of Veterinary Behavior; NorthStar VETS, Robbinsville, New Jersey, USA

LEIGH ANN CLAYTON, DVM
Diplomate, American Board of Veterinary Practitioners (Avian, Reptile/Amphibian); Vice President of Animal Care, New England Aquarium, Boston, Massachusetts, USA

SHARON CROWELL-DAVIS, DVM, PhD
Diplomate, American College of Veterinary Behaviorists; Professor, Department of Veterinary Biosciences and Diagnostic Imaging, College of Veterinary Medicine, University of Georgia, Athens, Georgia, USA

MARION R. DESMARCHELIER, DVM
Diplomate, American College of Zoological Medicine; Diplomate, European College of Zoological Medicine (Zoo Health Management); Diplomate, American College of Veterinary Behaviorists; Assistant Professor, Department of Clinical Sciences, Faculté de Médecine Vétérinaire, Université de Montréal, Saint-Hyacinthe, QC, Canada

SHANNON T. FERRELL, DVM
Diplomate, American Board of Veterinary Practitioners (Avian); Diplomate, American College of Zoological Medicine; Zoo de Granby, Granby, Quebec, Canada

SUSAN G. FRIEDMAN, PhD
Emeritus Professor, Psychology, Utah State University, Behavior Works, LLC, Logan, Utah, USA

BARBARA HEIDENREICH, BSc (Zoology)
Animal Training Consultant, Barbara's Force Free Animal Training, Austin, Texas, USA

MICHAEL P. JONES, DVM
Diplomate, American Board of Veterinary Practitioners (Avian); Avian and Zoological Medicine, Director of Student Services, Diversity, and Recruitment, Department of Small Animal Clinical Sciences, The University of Tennessee, College of Veterinary Medicine, Knoxville, Tennessee, USA

MAYA KUMMROW, DMV, DVSc, FTA Wildtiere (ZB Zootiere)
Diplomate, American College of Zoological Medicine; Diplomate, European College of Zoological Medicine (ZHM); Senior Lecturer, Clinic for Zoo Animals, Exotic Pets and Wildlife, Vetsuisse Faculty, University of Zurich, Zurich, Switzerland

ISABELLE LANGLOIS, DMV,
Diplomate, American Board of Veterinary Practitioners (Avian); Clinical Teacher, Centre Hospitalier Universitaire Vétérinaire (CHUV), Université de Montréal, Saint-Hyacinthe, Quebec, Canada

SYLVAIN LARRAT, DVM, MSc
Diplôme d'Études Spécialisées (Zoological Medicine); Diplomate, American College of Zoological Medicine; Exotic Pet Department, Clinique Vétérinaire Benjamin Franklin, Brec'h, Bretagne, France

GREGORY A. LEWBART, MS, VMD
Diplomate, American College of Zoological Medicine; Diplomate, European College of Zoological Medicine (ZHM); Professor of Aquatic Animal Medicine, Department of Clinical Sciences, NC State University College of Veterinary Medicine, Raleigh, North Carolina, USA

COLIN McDERMOTT, VMD, CertAqV
Veterinary Surgeon, Zodiac Pet and Exotic Hospital, Fortress Hill, Hong Kong

HÉLÈNE RUEL, Dr Med Vet, MSc, PhD Candidate, Diplomate, American College of Veterinary Internal Medicine (Neurology); Clinical Sciences Department, Université de Montréal, Saint-Hyacinthe, Québec, Canada

LIONEL SCHILLIGER, DVM
Diplomate, European College of Zoological Medicine (Herpetology); Diplomate, American Board of Veterinary Practitioners (Reptile and Amphibian Practice); Clinique Vétérinaire du Village d'Auteuil, Paris, France

ELIZABETH STELOW, DVM,
University of California, Davis, Davis, California, USA

CYNTHIA E. STRINGFIELD, DVM
ZooTampa, Tampa, Florida, USA

NOÉMIE SUMMA, DVM, IPSAV
Diplomate, American College of Zoological Medicine; Clinical Instructor in Zoological Medicine, Département de Sciences Cliniques, Faculté de Médecine Vétérinaire, Université de Montréal, Montreal, Quebec, Canada

VALARIE V. TYNES, DVM,
Diplomate, American College of Veterinary Behaviorists; Diplomate, American College of Animal Welfare; Veterinary Services Specialist, Companion Animal, Ceva Animal Health, Sweetwater, Texas, USA

CLAIRE VERGNEAU-GROSSET, DVM, IPSAV, CES
Diplomate, American College of Zoological Medicine; Assistant Professor, Service de Médecine Zoologique, Department of Clinical Sciences, Université de Montréal, Saint-Hyacinthe, Québec, Canada

Contents

Applied behavior analysis (ABA) is a relevant field for veterinarians helping clients whose animals engage in problem behaviors. In ABA, learning is defined as behavior change due to changes in the environment. Changing behavior then requires changes in conditions. Understanding the importance of control and the difference between emotional behavior and emotional feelings also is informed by ABA. Every behavior intervention should start with a systematic, analytical process called a functional assessment. Behavior change strategies are described, including an ethical procedural hierarchy based on the least intrusive, effective behavior change solution.

 Video content accompanies this article at http://www.vetexotic. theclinics.com.

Literature regarding the clinical use of psychotropic drugs in exotic animals remains scarce. Psychotropic drugs acting on serotonin, dopamine, norepinephrine, and gamma-aminobutyric acid pathways work by decreasing fear and anxiety, reactivity, and hypervigilance, and by improving impulse control. They are indicated for some cases of aggression, self-mutilation, and compulsive and anxiety disorders, including feather-damaging behavior. Side effects are rarely seen when dosages are appropriately adjusted to the individual, starting with a low dose and slowly titrating to effect. Several drug interactions exist between psychotropic drugs and other classes. Psychotropic drugs cannot be used to replace appropriate environmental conditions in exotic animals before "Side effects".

Domestic ferrets (Mustela putorius furo) are common zoologic companion animals and display specific body language and vocalizations. Social interactions, play behavior, and resting periods are important keystone in domestic ferret behavior. Specific housing and environmental enrichment are recommended to preserve the expression of normal behavior and physiology in ferrets. Presence of abnormal behaviors, including aggression, urination and defecation outside the litter box, stereotypies, and absence of play behavior, should be carefully monitored by veterinarians and ferret owners to assess ferret wellness. Specific considerations,

> Feather damaging behavior (FDB), also referred to as feather picking, feather plucking, or pterotillomania, is one of the most common and frustrating clinical presentations in captive psittacines. The clinical approach to identify underlying medical conditions associated with FDB is reviewed. Primary feather or skin diseases as well as systemic diseases may lead to this syndrome. This article focuses on the medical causes of FDB documented in the current avian literature. Medical causes are presented using the VITAMIN D algorithm. Key components of the multifaceted therapeutic approach in managing FDB of medical origin are discussed.

> Birds of prey are highly complex and intelligent species with many of their activities deeply rooted in modal action patterns, such as foraging, courtship and nest building, migration, bathing, or preening. Raptors in managed care are susceptible to presenting undesired behavior when the environment provides antecedents for these behaviors and consequences to maintain them. This article aims to describe concepts of behavior in birds of prey in managed care, with inferences from their wild counterparts, to assist in understanding the etiologies and management of undesired behaviors.

 Video content accompanies this article at http://www.vetexotic. theclinics.com.

> Reptile behavior varies widely among the approximately 11,000 species of this class. The authors' objective is to allow practitioners to discriminate between normal and abnormal behaviors in reptiles. Some of the most common reasons for presentation of behavioral issues are discussed, including hyperactivity, self-mutilation, biting, repetitive behaviors, and postural abnormalities. Medical problems and suboptimal husbandry causing abnormal behaviors should be ruled out by attending veterinarians. Addressing behavior issues involves determining a differential diagnosis through a systematic approach, which then allows implementation of necessary environmental changes including enrichment, developing plans for behavior modification and biomedical training, and medication when appropriate.

> Amphibians represent a diverse group of animals with highly varied behaviors depending on their anatomy, physiology, and ecological niche. Behavioral and welfare issues in amphibians are frequent in captive settings and warrant evaluation. Welfare criteria and clinical diagnostic assays when combined with a comprehension of the natural history of a species are

useful tools to improve both the well-being of the individual animal and the population. Correction of environmental factors that affect behavior and, secondarily, survival and reproduction is important in captivity and for the conservation of wild populations.

Interpreting fish behavior is an important component of providing veterinary care. There are over 28,000 species of fish and while only a handful are commonly encountered by exotic pet and public display veterinarians, there are still hundreds of species to consider. Three models—natural history (species typical modal action patterns), medical (disease state), and learning experience (classical and operant conditioning)—are useful for taking an actionable, holistic approach to interpreting behavior. Models help clinicians formulate appropriate differentials, ensuring they do not exclusively consider disease, particularly in unfamiliar species.

Invertebrate animals comprise more than 95% of the animal kingdom's species and approximately 40 separate phyla. Yet, invertebrates are an artificial taxon, in which all members simply possess a single negative trait: they lack a vertebral column (backbone). In fact, some invertebrates are more closely related to vertebrates than to their "fellow" invertebrates. For the purpose of this veterinary article, we have elected to review a handful of important groups: Coelenterates, Gastropods, Cephalopods, Chelicerates, Crustaceans, Insects, and Echinoderms. We have primarily included behavlors that may have an impact on clinical case outcome, or be of interest to the veterinary clinician.

Abnormal behavior in nonhuman primates is oftentimes prematurely blamed on certain conditions, in the case of captive non-human primates, readily so on their husbandry, largely ignoring the underlying pathophysiological processes in the brain. Each life history shapes an individual's predisposition to develop or resist the development of a psychopathological disorder, which manifests itself in abnormal behavior when triggered by certain situations or conditions. In order to sustainably address the symptoms of psychopathologies, therapeutic approaches must be based on a structured, comprehensive diagnostic procedure, including behavioral and functional analyses, research into life history, and personality assessment.

VETERINARY CLINICS OF NORTH AMERICA: EXOTIC ANIMAL PRACTICE

FORTHCOMING ISSUES

May 2021
Respiratory Medicine
Vladimír Jekl, *Editor*

September 2021
Herd/Flock Health and Medicine for the Exotic Animal Practitioner
Shangzhe Xie, *Editor*

January 2022
Anesthesia
Joao Brandão and Miranda Sadar, *Editors*

RECENT ISSUES

September 2020
Geriatrics
Paul Raiti, *Editor*

May 2020
New and Emerging Diseases: An Update
Nicole R. Wyre and Sue Chen, *Editors*

January 2020
Renal Disease
Christal Pollock, *Editor*

SERIES OF RELATED INTEREST

Veterinary Clinics of North America: Small Animal Practice
Available at: https://www.vetsmall.theclinics.com/

Preface

Behavior Medicine in Exotic Animal Practice

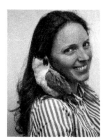

Marion R. Desmarchelier, DVM, DACZM,
DECZM (ZHM), DACVB
Editor

In starting my specialty training in behavior medicine, one of my main objectives was to help develop the field of exotic and wild animal behavior medicine. Therefore, I was elated when presented with this remarkable opportunity to bring together so many highly esteemed colleagues to assemble this issue of *Veterinary Clinics of North America: Exotic Animal Practice* Behavior Medicine issue. Behavior can be defined as the internally coordinated responses (actions or inactions) of living organisms to internal and/or external stimuli. Behavior is about what the animal *does* and how it acts (or not) in response to the environment. Behavior results from the expression of our genes under the influence of the environment. Exotic animals follow the same rules of behavior science. Consequently, when behavior problems occur, veterinarians should be able to use the knowledge acquired from human and domestic animals and apply it to their patients, no matter the species. However, knowing what is normal in every patient, how natural selection has shaped their genome, and how they learn in various natural and captive environments is critical to the approach and management of behavioral issues in various species. This Behavior Medicine issue contains a wealth of information accumulated over the years by attentive observers and presents clinically useful information for veterinarians, as well as for anyone interested in furthering exotic animal welfare. The first article on applied behavior analysis provides the essence of how to approach any behavior problem in all species and the frame to follow to a successful outcome. The second article also applies to all species and offers an insight into the best practices when considering the use of psychotropic drugs. All following articles cover more specific topics in different groups of animals, from various zoological companion animals to nonhuman primates. Understanding the natural behaviors of exotic companion animals is key to appropriately adjust their environmental needs, solving many behavioral issues. Being able to differentiate between

Vet Clin Exot Anim 24 (2021) xiii–xiv
https://doi.org/10.1016/j.cvex.2020.09.013
1094-9194/21/© 2020 Published by Elsevier Inc.

behaviors that are stress related, pain induced, or linked to neurotransmission dysfunction helps us reach a diagnosis and then treat the patient adequately without delay.

I am extremely grateful to all the authors who managed to review the literature, gather together their respective years of clinical experience, and craft this knowledge into a very practical resource that will undoubtedly improve the quality of life of many individuals, including some of the often forgotten species, such as amphibians or invertebrates.

I hope this issue will pave the road for future research efforts as so much remains to be discovered to better manage repetitive behaviors, self-mutilations, and some forms of aggressions. In addition, there are significant gaps in the literature in regard to behavior and welfare of amphibians, fish, and the more than 1.3 million species of invertebrates, which can be improved by diligent scientific investigation. Finally, the links between the brain and other organs (gut, skin, bladder, and so forth) are being better described every day thanks to the newest technologies and offer a very interesting insight to many conditions (inflammatory bowel disease, cystitis, and so forth). Recent advances in evolutionary biology, epigenetics, neuroscience, applied behavior analysis, and psychiatry all come together to offer a better life to many of our exotic and wild patients.

I hope the readers will find these articles useful and as inspiring as I did.

Marion R. Desmarchelier, DVM, DACZM, DECZM (ZHM), DACVB
Department of Clinical Sciences
Faculté de Médecine Vétérinaire
Université de Montréal
3200 Rue Sicotte
Saint-Hyacinthe, QC J2S 2M2, Canada

E-mail address:
marion.desmarchelier@umontreal.ca

Animal Behavior and Learning

Support from Applied Behavior Analysis

Susan G. Friedman, PhD[a],*, Cynthia E. Stringfield, DVM[b],
Marion R. Desmarchelier, DVM, DACZM, DECZM (ZHM), DACVB[c]

KEYWORDS

- Animal • Behavior • Learning • Applied • Behavior analysis • Problem behavior
- Ethical

KEY POINTS

- Applied behavior analysis is essential for assessing and resolving problem behaviors with animals.
- Each behavior intervention should start with a functional assessment of the behavior-environment relations.
- The ethical standard for behavior change should include the most positive, least intrusive effective behavior change procedures.

INTRODUCTION

For the past 20 years, the first two authors of this article have collaborated after first meeting as members of the California Condor Recovery Team. Although it is standard operating procedure for veterinarians to consult with specialists within the larger veterinary field, this partnership between a skilled veterinarian and an experienced applied behavior analyst has led to uniquely successful behavioral solutions much greater than the sum of their parts. Clearly, a behavior problem that is diagnosed as a symptom of an underlying physical dysfunction or disease process requires the specialized training of medical practitioners. Behavior problems resulting from an ill-fit environment and maladaptive learning history, however, are the specialized purview of behavior analysis, the science of behavior change. The authors believe that it takes collaboration among experts from these very different

[a] Psychology, Utah State University, Behavior Works, LLC, Logan, UT, USA; [b] ZooTampa, 1101 West Sligh Avenue, Tampa, FL 33604, USA; [c] Department of Clinical Sciences, Faculté de médecine vétérinaire, Université de Montréal, 3200 rue Sicotte, Saint-Hyacinthe, Québec J2S 2M2, Canada
* Corresponding author. PO Box 331, Millville, UT 84326.
E-mail address: sg.friedman@usu.edu

Vet Clin Exot Anim 24 (2021) 1–16
https://doi.org/10.1016/j.cvex.2020.08.002
1094-9194/21/© 2020 Elsevier Inc. All rights reserved.
vetexotic.theclinics.com

levels of analysis to fully account for the physical and behavioral wellness of the animals in human care.

Of course, there is the human element. As Stanovich[1] boldly wrote in his book, *How to Think Straight About Psychology*, "We must give up the idea that personal recipe knowledge of human behavior is adequate, that this is the only psychology we need." Indeed, the same words must be said for personal recipe knowledge as it relates to nonhuman animal behavior. One mystery that often surrounds problem behavior is its very persistence. Clients may have a litany of failed behavior-change programs by the time they turn to you for help. As they wade through the personal recipes of one Internet charlatan after another, clients do not realize that with each failed attempt at behavior change, the window of opportunity closes a little bit more as animals learn to ignore changes in their environment that otherwise would facilitate behavior change.

Training the next generation of animal care professionals is another consideration. The authors have spent much of their careers teaching their respective science and application to students. These students need teachers who model the interdisciplinary collaboration required to truly facilitate the least intrusive effective behavioral solutions for animals. This article is intended to inspire readers to seek out professionals from different related fields with whom to work shoulder to shoulder, as the authors have done, to improve behavioral outcomes for all animals.

UNDERSTANDING BEHAVIOR

The governing principles revealed by the experimental analysis of behavior has widespread applicability across species and has produced an applied technology for teaching, training, and managing behavior. The technology is called applied behavior analysis (ABA). Within this field, learning is defined as behavior change due to changes in the environment. The ability to learn is itself part of every animal's biological endowment, the result of natural selection. Learning is the mechanism by which individuals cope with the demands of an ever-changing environment during their lifetime. It is evolved modifiability that "takes up where reflexes, fixed action patterns, and general behavior traits leave off."[2]

Common misunderstandings about ABA should be dispelled. The central interest and main contribution of ABA are the behavioral level of analysis, that is, how behavior-environment relations account for the behavior observed. Behavior never is wholly independent of conditions. Therefore, the goal of any behavior intervention is to arrange the environment so that behavior problems are irrelevant, inefficient, and ineffective, and new skills are learned.[3] Behavior analysis does not discount the existence of animals' thoughts or feelings. Thoughts and feelings are private events, however, which makes them difficult to measure directly. More importantly, they too are influenced by environmental events. To clarify, consider this common explanation for biting behavior: The animal bit its caregiver because it was afraid. This causal account of biting is problematic because it is based on circular reasoning. If the question is asked, Why did the animal bite? the answer is, Because it is fearful. If the question is asked, How does one know the animal is fearful? the answer is, Because it bites. The more useful question asked by behavior analysts is, What environmental events account for both the biting and fear behaviors?

For an explanation to qualify as a valid, scientific account of behavior, the physical (measurable) events that reliably produce it must be identified. As Skinner said:

> It is does not help in the solution of a practical problem to be told that some feature of [an individual's] behavior is due to frustration or anxiety; we also need

to be told how the frustration or anxiety has been induced and how it may be altered.[4]

As to the how frustration or anxiety is induced, the environmental conditions for things that can be changed can be looked at, on behalf of the learner. This is a critically important piece of every behavior puzzle.

Contingencies

The concept of contingency is central to understanding, predicting, and changing behavior. A contingency describes a dependency between 2 or more events. Behavior never occurs in a vacuum. It depends on events that precede it, called antecedents, and outcomes, called consequences. The complete unit — antecedents, behavior, and consequences — is the behavior ABCs. No smaller unit of analysis is meaningful.

Antecedents are the stimuli, events, and conditions that precede behavior and set the occasion for the behavior to occur. Antecedents do not cause the behavior; rather, they signal the contingency ahead: When antecedent A is present, if behavior B occurs, then consequence C will follow.

Behavior is a power tool, part of every animal's biology, used to control the environment.

Behavior is defined as what an animal does that can be measured. All analyses start with an unambiguous, measurable description of overt behavior and conditions. Hypothetical, psychological constructs and diagnostic labels do not describe specific behaviors in context and, therefore, are too vague and ambiguous for effective intervention. For example, a dog does not take food gently from a stranger because it is friendly; rather, the dog takes food gently and it is called friendly. Friendliness is not a cause; it is a label for the gentle behavior in the context of a stranger offering food. It can accurately be said that the behavior causes the label.

Consequences are the engine that drives future behavior. Antecedents are the signposts that signal the behavior-consequence (BC) contingency immediately ahead. For example, an offered hand (A), may set the occasion for a parrot to step up (B), which results in caregiver attention (C). Over time, stepping up may increase as a function of attention, in the presence of an offered hand. For another parrot, an offered hand (A), may signal a different BC contingency — stepping up (B), which results in confinement in a cage (C). For this second parrot, stepping up may decrease as a function of confinement in the cage. Behavior is selected by consequences and the value placed on any particular outcome is very individual, truly a study of 1. For any individual, behaviors that produce desired outcomes are repeated; behaviors that produce aversive consequences are modified or suppressed.

Assessing the ABCs also is known as functional assessment. It is key to understanding what environmental events maintain behavior. Then, to change behavior, conditions are changed. Changing an animal's functional behavior is not a casual or cavalier process. If the outcomes of the problem behavior were not important to the animal, it would not behave in this way. Thus, the ultimate goal of any behavior change program is to protect the rate and quality of valued outcomes an animal behaves to get. This is best achieved by replacing the problem behavior with a desirable alternative behavior and teaching new skills, rather than solely suppressing a problem behavior.

Key Questions for Functional Behavior Assessment

Functional assessment requires observation skills that clients can quickly develop. The following key questions help focus their observations on the ABCs[3]:

- What does the problem look like in terms of actual behavior, that is, what is seen?
- Under what conditions does the animal do this behavior, that is, what events predict it?
- What does the animal get, or get away from, by emitting this behavior?
- Under what conditions does the animal not do this behavior, that is, when is it successful?
- What does the client want the animal to do instead?
- What prerequisite skills does the animal need to succeed?
- How will the prerequisite and alternative behaviors be taught to the learner?

CONTROL

It is a small step from observing that behavior is done to achieve functional outcomes and realizing that control over outcomes matters in the lives of all animals. Control is reasonably classified as primary reinforcer, that is, an innate and necessary requirement for survival and behavioral health. As discussed by Leotti and colleagues,[5] "Converging evidence from animal research, clinical studies and neuroimaging work suggest that the *need for control is biological imperative for survival*, and a corticostriatal network is implicated as the neural substrate of this adaptive behavior."

When an animal's control over outcomes is blocked as a lifestyle, maladaptive behaviors often increase,[6] including depression, learning disabilities, emotional problems,[7] and suppressed immune system activity.[8] Restriction of behaviors, in particular those that are highly valued by a species, produces behavioral and physiologic stress.[9] The restriction of motion (ie, restraint) results in increased heart rate, increased norepinephrine and cortisol release, and the production of gastric ulcers.[10] Additional research evidence suggests lack of control is a major cause of abnormal stereotypic behaviors, failure to thrive, and impaired reproduction commonly observed in animals raised in captivity.[11]

In a study of 90-day-old babies, the group that controlled the onset of the mobiles over their cribs (by raising their heads and closing a switch under their pillows) were more active and happier than the group of babies with the same amount of moving mobile time but no control over the onset of their devices.[12,13] Furthermore, the contra-freeloading research, which has been replicated with dozens of species and shows that animals, in general, prefer contingent access to commodities, such as food, water, and lighting rather than free access, that is, they prefer to work for outcomes.[14–17] Alternatively, when control is provided, animals make effective use of it.[18,19]

Of course, control is a continuum, not a dichotomy. It is unnecessary and counterproductive to work in the extremes (no control vs total control). No cat should be allowed to scratch a keeper and no alligator should be allowed to eat a bucket. If an error is to be made in either direction, however, it is better to fall on the side of providing more control. This can be achieved by arranging stimulus-rich environments that foster many more choices than restrictions.

Least Intrusive Ethical Standard

Just because behavior can be changed does not mean it should be. And, when it is decided that it is necessary, it is the process by which behavior is changed that is most critical from a welfare point of view. Effectiveness is not enough when it comes to choosing and applying behavior-change interventions.[20] Borrowing from the field of ABA with human learners, an expanded hierarchy of procedures[21] is proposed that adds a second criterion to effectiveness: relative intrusiveness. Intrusiveness refers to both the social acceptability of a procedure and, most importantly, the degree to which a learner controls its own outcomes.[22] Without this ethical standard, interventions likely are selected on the basis of convenience, familiarity, speed, or blind authority and inadvertently may produce the detrimental side effects of punishment and learned helplessness in animals (discussed later). The commitment to using the most positive, least intrusive, effective interventions allows thinking before acting, so that choices are made about the means by which behavior goals are accomplished. In this way, actions can be both effective and humane. This is the minimum standard of care that should be stretched to meet on behalf of the welfare of learners and caregivers alike. **Fig. 1** depicts the suggested hierarchy of behavior change procedures.

Veterinarians note that the first stop on the hierarchy is to assure "Wellness: Nutritional and Physical." Medical problems are not solved with learning solutions (and vice versa). For example, a problem, such as a ferret urinating in inappropriate places, may well be a medical issue. It is unethical and ineffective to proceed with a learning solution before determining if the behavior is symptomatic of an underlying medical problem. Likewise, intervening with a medical solution is neither ethical nor effective in the long run, when the cause of the behavior problem is ill-fit environment or skill deficit. And then there are those behavior challenges in which both the medical and behavioral models must join forces to provide an ethical, effective intervention, requiring the collaboration described in this article.

EMOTIONS

It is useful to differentiate between the emotional behavior that is done and the emotional feelings that are perceived. Emotional behavior (eg, tail wagging, ears

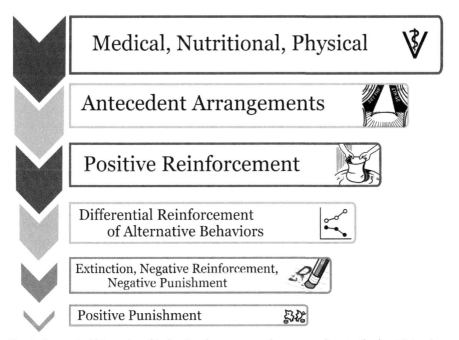

Fig. 1. Suggested hierarchy of behavior change procedures according to the least intrusive, effective intervention guideline.

back, and fleeing) easily is accounted for by both classical and operant learning processes. Respectively, new elicitors of innate responses are learned through the process of classical conditioning (eg, raised hackles elicited by a passing vehicle); and new behaviors are selected by consequences via the process of operant learning (eg, hiding in a kennel during a thunderstorm [ie, negative reinforcement]).

Private emotions, however, are a different matter. A behavior analysis perspective on emotions can be empowering. As Layng[23] explains, "emotions neither cause behavior nor are caused by behavior; they are instead part of consequential contingencies." In other words, as with overt behavior, emotions are not independent of environmental influence. It is the BC contingency that emotions closely reflect. Said another way, happy is a function of a positive reinforcement contingency, fear is a function of an escape contingency, anxiety is a function of an avoidance contingency, and frustration is a function of an extinction contingency.

To further make this point, consider the 20 different kinds of aggression listed in Barrows,[24] "Animal Behavior Desk Reference: A Dictionary of Animal Behavior, Ecology, and Evolution." They are antipredatory, aversion induced, behavioral, defensive, direct, displaced, dominance, ecological, frustration-induced, intrasexual, intraspecific, moralistic, parental, parental disciplinary, predatory, redirected, sexual, territorial, and weaning. On closer inspection, however, notice that it is actually different conditions, not different behaviors, that are described by this list. For any given species and individual, the behavior pattern (topography) described as "aggressive" is fairly consistent.

Lewon and Hayes[25] contend, "When we conceive of emotions and hunger not as *things* but as verbal descriptions of environment-behavior relations, we are able to see important similarities between humans and nonhumans." The empowering bottom line then is to change emotions, change conditions (antecedent events and consequences). Changing the conditions in which animal live often is in the caregivers' control.

Trust

One emotion often evoked as a key to successful relationships is trust. A critical thinker asks, What does this construct really mean? What does trust look like? and How can it be built? Trust can be operationalized as the level of sureness that approaching and interacting with another individual (human or conspecific) will produce safe and reinforcing outcomes. With this description, both the measures of trust and the path to create it can be generated. When caregivers provide a preponderance of safe and positively reinforcing outcomes, animals approach and interact more. The label trust is the emotion that reflects those experiences (contingencies) for both parties.

A great metaphor to make this point to clients is to describe a trust account at the bank of relationships. To build big trust accounts, it is important to provide animals with control through choice situations and to ensure that the frequency of positive interactions far exceed the frequency of negative interactions. Resilient animals bounce back after an occasional aversive event, but keeping the overall ratio of positive interactions to negative interactions really big must be ensured. That is the way to keep trust accounts in the black.

BEHAVIOR CHANGE STRATEGIES

ABA offers a practical model of behavioral support to help clients prevent and resolve behavior problems with their animals. It often is helpful to think of behavior problems as falling into 1 of 2 general categories—either not enough of the "right" behavior or too much of the "wrong" behavior. Depending on which of the 2 problems are faced, the goal will be to teach caregivers how to work with their animals to increase desirable behaviors and replace undesirable behaviors. Most often both are done. Understanding the functional relations between behavior and environmental events is key to accomplishing these goals. Behavior never is independent of the strong influence of conditions and in cases of animals in human care, where so many of the conditions (antecedents and consequences) are provided, this is good news for knowledgeable caregivers.

Reducing problem behaviors is not the only goal when planning an intervention. A good plan is one in which the physical and social contexts of the environment are redesigned to provide the animal with an opportunity to preserve the function served by the problem behavior with an acceptable alternative behavior and to allow an animal to learn new skills that make the problem less likely to occur.[3] The focus on preserving the function of a problem behavior with an appropriate alternative is fundamental to understanding behavior and respecting behaving organisms: if the behavior did not matter to the animal, it would not keep doing it. For example, the function typically served by biting is to remove someone's hand—that is, to say no. Because all animals have a right to say no, the first goal should be to replace biting with an acceptable way to say no—for example, moving away. The second goal is teaching the learner that saying yes, by approaching calmly, yields even better outcomes (**Tables 1** and **2**).

Changing Behavior with Antecedent Strategies

Antecedents are the signposts that give order to behavior in the sense that they tell what to do when. There are 3 general types of antecedents: cues, setting events, and motivating operations. Each type of antecedent can be an important tool for changing problem behavior.

Add or remove the cue

When clients report a behavior problem, ask, What cues the behavior? A stimulus becomes a cue (discriminative stimulus) for a particular behavior if it is repeatedly present when the behavior is reinforced. A ringing telephone can become a cue for raucous vocalizations if raucous vocalizations result in attention when the phone rings. An offered hand can become a cue for lunging if lunging removes the hand when the hand is offered. The strength of a stimulus to cue a particular behavior is related to the strength of the reinforcer that follows the behavior. To build strong cues, deliver strong reinforcers in the presence of the cues.

Removing the stimulus that cues a problem behavior is one way to reduce it. For example, with companion parrots, buttons and jewelry often cue chewing because chewing results in social and sensory reinforcers in the presence of those buttons and jewelry. By removing the cues (wearing T-shirts and removing jewelry), chewing necessarily decreases. Adding a cue for an alternate behavior is another way to reduce the frequency of a problem behavior. For example, opening the food door may cue lunging because lunging has been reinforced with the delivery of food. Teaching an animal to station on a distant perch when cued prevents lunging.

Increase or decrease effort with setting events

When clients report a problem behavior, ask, How can the setting be changed to make the right behavior easier than the wrong behavior? Setting events are the context, conditions, or situational influences that affect behavior. For example, coming out of the cage

Table 1
Applying behavior analysis: rainbow lorikeet presented for a biting behavior

Signalment	A 5-month-old flighted rainbow lorikeet, unknown sex
Background	One owner is blind and one has limited mobility.
Target behavior	Biting caregiver's hand, puncturing the skin

	Functional Assessment	**Suggested Changes**
Context 1	Setting: the bird is out of her cage. It is time to be removed from an activity (appropriate or deemed inappropriate by owner [pulling on buttons, destroying remote control, etc.]) and/or return to her cage.	To preempt the behavior: Provide and encourage appropriate activities. Prevent the bird from accessing unwanted activities (put away objects before getting her out of the cage, cover ears, remove earrings, pin hair up, etc.)
	Antecedent (A): hand approaches for step up.	Use a perch instead of a hand. Stepping up on perch should first be trained outside of problem situations, with positive reinforcement. Reduce rapid hand movements in Sunshine's presence. Present step up hand with fingers wrapped around thumb until confidence is restored in bird and caregivers.
	Behavior (B): the bird bites hand.	Carefully observe the bird's body language and vocalizations that predict a bite and do not offer hands at those times. To reinforce alternate behaviors: Teach the bird with an alternate appropriate behavior to say "No, thanks".
	Consequence (C): hand is removed (R−), attention and sensory stimulation is delivered (R+), activity on cage top resumes (R+), and going inside cage is avoided (R−). Prediction of future behavior if nothing changes: the bird will continue biting.	Reinforce stepping up with strong reinforcers, such as praise, food treats, and favorite items. Vary the outcome of stepping up. Do not always follow Sunshine's stepping up with returning her to her cage. Offer reinforcers not available any other time to increase Sunshine's motivation to step up and/or to return to her cage. Move preferred toys and foraging activities in the cage to provide wanted sensory delivery. Offer attention and do a training session after stepping up on the perch and/or in the cage.

(continued on next page)

	Functional Assessment	Suggested Changes
Table 1 **(*continued*)**		
Context 2	• Setting: the bird is in her cage. A caregiver comes to replenish the food and bowls. • Antecedent (A): hand approaches food door. • Behavior (B): the bird bites.	To preempt the behavior: 　Take the bird out of the cage 　before replenishing the bowls. • Train the bird to station in one 　spot of the cage (eg, skewer) 　when food door is approached. Carefully observe the bird's body 　language and vocalizations that 　predict a bite and do not offer 　hands at those times.
	• Consequence (C): hand is removed from inside cage (R−), attention and sensory stimulation are delivered (R+); replenished bowls are installed (R+). • Prediction of future behavior if nothing changes: the bird will continue biting.	To reinforce alternate behaviors: 　Reinforce the bird for perching 　on cage skewer for longer 　durations while bowls are 　replenished.
New skills and teaching strategies	• Teach the bird that she can make choices by not forcing her to step up. Increase her choice to step up with strong reinforcers, including occasionally allowing her to immediately step back down again. • Begin target training to teach her more acceptable ways of interacting with the caregivers and increase the overall level of available positive reinforcement. • Practice stepping up under many different conditions and contexts frequently throughout the day. • Training in protected contact through the cage bars until confidence is restored between bird and caregivers. • Train the bird to use vocal communication to allow easier interactions with the blind caregiver.	
Environmental adjustments	Change the location of the sleep cage to provide quiet, restful sleep. Ensure that the bird gets adequate exercise daily; provide a new play stand and offer a larger variety of toys and foraging items.	

can be made easier by selecting cages with large doors, which ultimately may reduce biting. Chewing the window frame can be made harder by locating the play-tree in the middle of the room. The relations between setting events and problem behavior should be considered carefully because the setting often is one of the easiest things to change.

Strengthen or weaken motivation

When clients report a problem behavior, ask, What is the motivation? (ie, What consequence does the behavior produce?)Motivating operations (also known as establishing operations) temporarily alter the effectiveness of consequences. For example, a few carrots may be a highly motivating consequence to an animal that rarely has access to them but not motivating at all to an animal that has unlimited access to them every day. An iguana may be more motivated to go to a warm rock on a cool day and chasing a conspecific may be less reinforcing after an energetic training session.

Antecedent behavior-change strategies often are preventative management solutions rather than learning solutions. As a result, antecedent strategies can be the most positive, least intrusive, effective behavior-change procedures.

Table 2
Applying behavior analysis: ferret presented for a biting behavior

Signalment	A 3-year-old neutered male ferret
Background	Adopted from a shelter by a veterinary technician student
Target behavior	Biting caregiver's hand, puncturing the skin

	Functional Assessment	Suggested Changes
Context 1	Setting: the ferret is free in the house. An object falls on the floor (pen, utensil, etc.). Antecedent (A): hand approaches to pick up the fallen object. Behavior (B): the ferret bites hand. Consequence (C): hand is removed (R−), attention and sensory stimulation are delivered (R+). Prediction of future behavior if nothing changes: the ferret will continue biting.	To preempt the behavior: Keep the ferret in a ferret-proof pen (also useful to prevent gastrointestinal foreign bodies). Carefully observe the ferret's body language (ex. lunging) and that predict a bite and do not pick up objects at those times. Avoid rapid hand movements close to the ferret, especially if coming from above him. To reinforce alternate behaviors: Choose an alternate incompatible behavior, such as touching a target or stationing away from the objects, and reinforce the behavior while slowly picking up the object.
Context 2	• Setting: the ferret is free in the house, with access to his cage. A caregiver comes to clean the litter box. • Antecedent (A): hand enters the cage to pick up the litter box. • Behavior (B): the ferret runs back to the cage and bites the caregiver's hand. • Consequence (C): hand is removed from inside cage (R−), attention and sensory stimulation are delivered (R+). • Prediction of future behavior if nothing changes: the ferret will continue biting.	To preempt the behavior: Prevent access to the cage room during the litter box cleaning. • Train the ferret to station in one spot during the litter cleaning. Carefully observe the ferret's body language that predict a bite and do not approach hand at those times. To reinforce alternate behaviors: Reinforce the ferret for entering his transport cage before cleaning session. Offer a treat that requires time to be eaten (Kong with food in it, peanut butter, coconut oil spread on a toy, etc.) in the transport cage during the cleaning.

(continued on next page)

Table 2 (continued)		
	Functional Assessment	**Suggested Changes**
New skills and teaching strategies	• Teach the ferret that he can make choices by not forcing him to get in or out of the cage. Increase his choice to station in the wanted area (eg, transport cage) with strong reinforcers, including occasionally allowing him to immediately get out of the cage again.	
	• Begin target training to teach him more acceptable ways of interacting with the caregiver and increase the overall level of available positive reinforcement.	
	• Practice stationing under many different conditions and contexts frequently throughout the day.	
	• Training in protected contact through the cage bars until confidence is restored between the ferret and the caregiver	
Environmental adjustments	Ensure that the ferret gets adequate exercise daily by encouraging play. Provide an environment encouraging natural behaviors, such as tunneling, climbing, hiding, etc. Provide daily ferret-proof enrichment items.	

Decreasing Behavior with Consequences

When clients report a problem behavior, ask, What purpose does it serve the animal? (ie, What does the animal get, or get away from, by doing the behavior?) Reinforcement is the process by which behavior is maintained and increased. It is a natural process that, like gravity, is in effect whether realized or not. Behavior is repeated because it results in reinforcement—even problem behavior. Clients often look in the wrong place, inside the animal, for answers to why animals do what they do (eg, the animal lunges because it is hormonal, dominant, or neurotic). By focusing on the functional relations between observable behavior and consequences, clients consider the actual causes for behavior that they can do something about, namely changing the antecedent conditions and consequences they provide.

Extinction

Once the reinforcer for a problem behavior is identified from a functional assessment, the maintaining reinforcer can be withheld permanently to reduce the behavior. When the contingency between a behavior and its consequence (if B then C) is removed, the behavior serves no function and eventually diminishes. This process is called extinction. There really are few problem behaviors that are well suited to extinction due to the problems with the procedure (described later). Extinction is most effective the very first time a problem behavior occurs, that is, do not give the behavior function in the first place.

- Extinction can be a slow process, especially with behaviors maintained on an intermittent reinforcement history (usually the case with problem behaviors).
- There often is an intolerably sharp increase in the frequency and intensity of the problem behavior before it eventually decreases (extinction burst) that may result in clients reinforcing even less desirable behavior.
- Extinction can result in frustration-elicited aggression.
- Uncontrolled or inadvertent reinforcement can undermine the procedure (bootleg reinforcement).
- Behaviors that previously were extinguished in the past can resurge when a new extinction procedure is started.

- Over time, the problem behavior can recover, and the extinction procedure will need to be implemented again.
- Other animals may imitate the problem behavior.

All told, extinction as a sole procedure for reducing problem behaviors usually is insufficient. It is a difficult strategy to implement well, and, more importantly, animals should have the opportunity to learn new skills to replace undesirable behavior.

Punishment

Punishment is the process by which consequences decrease and suppress behavior. It rarely is necessary to use this approach because (1) there are less intrusive, effective alternative teaching approaches, and (2) punishment occasions detrimental side effects (discussed later).

Behavior can be punished by contingently adding an aversive stimulus, called positive punishment (or discipline or corrections, in lay terms), or by contingently removing positive reinforcers, called negative punishment (fines or penalties, in lay terms). For example, while the handler arranges the jesses with her ungloved hand (A), if the raptor throws a foot at the handler (B), then the handler shakes her arm sharply (C). In this scenario footing may decrease (punishment), given the addition (positive) of the sharp shake of the arm. Alternatively, as a handler raises the food hand (A), if the raptor lunges at the hand (B), then the handler intentionally drops the food back into his pouch. (C). Lunging at the handler may decrease (punishment), given the removal (negative) of the food (the reinforcer).

Decades of scientific studies have demonstrated the problems with positive punishment that are listed. As a result of these problems, and the efficacy with which alternate strategies can be used, positive punishment should be used only to solve behavior problems when more positive, less intrusive procedures have failed (indeed, an uncommon occurrence among experienced practitioners).

- Punishment is associated with 4 detrimental side effects
  - Increased aggression
  - Generalized fear
  - Apathy
  - Escape avoidance behaviors
- Additional considerations before using punishment
  - Punishment does not teach learners what to do instead of the problem behavior.
  - Punishment does not teach caregivers how to teach alternate behaviors.
  - Punishment is really 2 aversive events—the onset of a punishing stimulus and the forfeiture of the reinforcer that has maintained the problem behavior in the past.
  - Punishment requires an increase in aversive stimulation to maintain initial levels of behavior reduction.
  - Effective punishment reinforces the punisher, who, therefore, is more likely to punish again in the future, even when antecedent arrangements and positive reinforcement would be effective.

Time out from positive reinforcement

Time out from positive reinforcement (time out) is a negative punishment procedure that can effectively reduce problem behavior with fewer detriments than positive punishment but, like extinction, it is a difficult procedure to effectively implement. Time out is the temporary reduction of access to positive reinforcers contingent on a problem behavior. For example, when a client installs a food cup through a cage door (A), if the animal swipes at the cage bars (B), then the client temporarily removes food cup (C). Swiping cage bars likely will decrease due the process of negative punishment in which the food cup, a positive reinforcer, was removed. Time out can be a relatively unintrusive behavior-change procedure if it is implemented correctly. It should be implemented consistently, with close contiguity (immediacy) between the behavior and the consequence; it should be short (only a few seconds usually is effective with many individuals); the animal should be brought back quickly into the situation to do it again better and earn positive reinforcement; and the client should let the procedure do the job (no emotional responses necessary).

A New Standard of Best Practices

The use of any behavior reduction technique should be rare in the course of a caregiver's work. By strengthening alternative desirable behaviors and teaching new skills, punishment rarely, if ever, is necessary. When an animal does not behave according to expectations, their "missed behavior" is important data that something needs to change in the training program and/or the environment in which the animal behaves.[26,27] The environment is changed, and, the animal changes its behavior.

This is not an easy call to action. Many use punishment reflexively because it most assuredly is a society-wide legacy. Laying down the old tools of force and coercion and replacing them with tools of choice and cooperation will require learning new information and building different skills. It is a commitment that must be made for the animals (human and nonhuman alike) that are cared for. Doing so will pay big dividends for animal welfare.

Increasing Behavior with Consequences

Without question the 2 sharpest behavior change tools are variations of differential reinforcement. Differential reinforcement is the process of reinforcing 1 class of behaviors and not others. Differential reinforcement of alternate behavior (DRA) is used to replace problem behavior with a more appropriate behavior. Differential reinforcement of successive approximations (shaping) is used to teach new skills. Both procedures avert the problems and side effects of positive punishment and also result in the high rates of positive reinforcement vital to behavioral health. This is why both procedures are preferred, that is, less intrusive, on the ethical hierarchy of effective behavior-change procedures.

A crux training move is selecting the goal behavior to replace problem behavior with or the new skill to teach a learner. Lindsley[28] wrote that goal behavior should pass the dead man's test: if a dead man can do it (eg, be still and be quiet), it is not going to make a good target behavior. This amusing (or shocking) criterion is important to consider. Behavior targets should specify active over measurable behavior to the greatest possible extent. Animals are built to behave.

Differential reinforcement of alternative behavior

When clients report a behavior problem, ask, What behavior does the animal already know that the client would like it to do instead? With DRA, a desirable replacement behavior is reinforced (increased) while the problem behavior is extinguished (not reinforced). For example, vocalizing for attention can be replaced with chewing an enrichment item for attention. To use DRA, a functional assessment is necessary to identify the reinforcer that has been maintaining the problem behavior in the past, in order to withhold it. There are 3 things to consider when selecting an alternate behavior. First, although the behavior targeted for reduction is a problem to people, it serves a legitimate function for the animal or it would not continue to exhibit the behavior. The function is either to gain something of value, for example, vocalizing to gain attention (positive reinforcement); or, the function is to remove something aversive, for example, lunging to remove intruding hands (negative reinforcement). An alternative or incompatible behavior should be selected that replaces the function served by the problem behavior but in a more appropriate way. If the alternative behavior is incompatible with the problem behavior (ie, if both behaviors cannot physically be performed at the same time), the behavior change program can proceed more quickly. This variation of DRA is called differential reinforcement of an incompatible behavior (DRI). For example, chewing is incompatible with vocalizing, and standing on a far perch is incompatible with lunging at the food door.

Second, the alternate behavior should produce even more reinforcement than the problem behavior in order to successfully compete with and replace it. According to the principle called the matching law, "the distribution of behavior between alternative sources of reinforcement is equal to the distribution of reinforcement for these alternatives."[1] Thus, given a choice between 2 alternative behaviors, animals tend to exhibit the behavior that results in the greater reinforcement. The matching law is itself a powerful tool for managing behavior. For example, if staying on a perch produces double the reinforcement as flying off, birds tend to stay on the perch. Third, the alternative behavior should be one the animal already knows how to do. During extinction of the problem behavior, a well-established alternative behavior more likely is to be performed than one that is newly acquired. When alternative behaviors are strengthened and maintained, differential reinforcement can provide long-lasting results. Because this method relies on both positive reinforcement (to teach animals what to do), in addition to extinction of the undesirable behavior, DRA and DRI offer a less intrusive and practical approach to managing an animal's problem behavior than do punishment strategies or extinction alone.

Shaping

When clients report a behavior problem, ask, What skill does the animal need to learn? Differential reinforcement of successive approximations, also known as shaping, is another type of differential reinforcement procedure. Shaping is used to teach new behaviors by the process of successively reinforcing subtle variations in responses (approximations) along a continuum that leads to the final goal behavior.

Shaping starts by reinforcing the closest approximation the animal already does. Next, an even closer approximation is reinforced, at which time reinforcement for the first approximation is withheld. Once the second approximation is performed without hesitation, an even closer approximation is reinforced while withholding reinforcement for all previous approximations. In this way, the criterion for reinforcement gradually is shifted incrementally closer and closer to the goal behavior. Finally, every instance of the final behavior is reinforced. For example, to teach an animal to interact with an enrichment item, the following approximations can be reinforced in turn: looking at toy, leaning toward toy, moving a foot in the direction of toy, taking 1 step toward toy, taking several steps to arrive beside toy, touching toy with foot, holding toy with foot while manipulating it in mouth, and reinforcing longer durations of engagement with the item. If the learner experiences difficulty at any approximation, the teacher can back up and repeat the previous successful step or reinforce even smaller approximations. Ultimately, it is the learner who determines the pace, number of repetitions, and size of the approximations in a shaping procedure.

Implementing a shaping procedure requires keen observation of the subtle, natural variation in the way behaviors are performed repeatedly. For example, each time an animal lifts its foot, it is naturally done differently from the last time (left or right, high or low, fast or slow, with toe movement or without, and so forth.). In daily life, these variations are unimportant and simply classified as 1 behavior, or operant class, called "lifting a foot." This subtle variation in foot lifting, however, is exactly what allows shaping new behaviors, such as offering a steady foot for nail trims.

With shaping, theoretically any behavior can be taught within the biological constraints of the learner. Husbandry and medical and enrichment behaviors can be shaped to reduce stress and increase physical and mental stimulation. Animals can learn behaviors, such as going in and out of crates, staying calm wrapped in towels, flying to designated perches, and even playing basketball. Shaping also can be used to change different dimensions of existing behaviors, such as duration, rate, intensity, topography (specifically what the behavior looks like), and latency (response time).

A FINAL WORD

Each behavior intervention should start with a careful functional assessment and the intervention should be designed to meet the needs of the individual learner using the most positive, least intrusive effective methods. The plan also should be feasible for the client to implement. The greater the knowledge of the scientific principles and procedures of learning and behavior, the more effectively these goals will be met and improve the welfare of the animals in care improved.

Far from carrot-and-stick strategies or mechanistic reflex arc stuff, ABA harnesses animals' innate, biological flexibility to change their behavior based on experience, that is, the past outcomes of behaving. If not for this extraordinary, inherent adaptability, animals would not survive this ever-changing world. It is the nature of all animals to learn. Together with other behavior sciences and technologies, such as ethology and medicine, connecting the dots from science to practice provides patients and clients with a much better future. It is the authors' earnest hope that the information provided here will help forge such a path.

DISCLOSURE

The authors have nothing to disclose.

REFERENCES

1. Stanovich K. How to think straight about psychology. Needham Heights (MA): Allyn & Bacon; 2001.
2. Chance P. Learning and behavior. Belmont (CA): Thomson/Wadsworth; 2003. p. 24.
3. O'Neill RE, Horner RH, Albin RW, et al. Functional assessment and program development for problem behavior: a practical handbook. Pacific Grove (CA): Brooks/Cole; 1997.
4. Skinner BF. Science and human behavior. New York: The Free Press; 1953. p. 167.
5. Leotti LA, Iyengar SS, Ochsner KN. Born to choose: the origins and value of the need for control. Trends Cogn Sci 2010;14(10):457–63.
6. Brown GE, Hughes GD, Jones AA. Effects of shock controllability on subsequent aggressive and defensive behaviors in the cockroach (Periplaneta americana). Psychol Rep 1988;63:563–9.

7. Maier SF, Seligman MEP. Learned helplessness: theory and evidence. J Exp Psychol Gen 1976;105:3–46.
8. Laudenslager ML, Ryan SM, Drugan RC, et al. Coping and immunosupression: inescapable but not escapable shock suppresses lymphocyte proliferation. Science 1983;221:568–70.
9. Friend TH. Recognizing behavioral needs. Appl Anim Behav Sci 1989;22:151–8.
10. Glavin GB, Paré WP, Sandbak T, et al. Restraint stress in biomedical research: an update. Neurosci Biobehav Rev 1994;18:223–49.
11. Clubb R, Mason G. Animal welfare: captivity effects on wide-ranging carnivores. Nature 2003;425:473–4.
12. Watson JS. Memory and "contingency analysis" in infant learning. Merrill Palmer Q 1967;13:55–76.
13. Watson JS. Cognitive-perceptual development in infancy: setting for the seventies. Merrill Palmer Q 1971;12:139–52.
14. Coulton LE, Warren NK, Young RJ. Effects of foraging enrichment on the behavior of parrots. Anim Welf 1997;6:357–63.
15. Gilbert-Norton L. Captive birds and freeloading: the choice to work. Research News 2003;4(1).
16. Inglis IR, Ferguson NJK. Starlings search for food rather than eat freely available food. Anim Behav 1986;34:614–6.
17. Osborne SR. The free food (contrafreeloading) phenomenon: a review and analysis. Anim Learn Behav 1977;5(8):221–35.
18. Cerutti D, Catania AC. Pigeons' preference for free choice: number of keys versus key area. J Exp Anal Behav 1997;68:349–56.
19. Carlstead K, Seidensticker J, Baldwin R. Environmental enrichment for zoo bears. Zoo 1991;10:3–16.
20. Friedman SG. What's wrong with this picture? Effectiveness is not enough. Good Bird Magazine 2008;4(4):12–8.
21. Alberto PA, Troutman AC. Applied behavior analysis for teachers. NJ: Merrill Prentice Hall; 1999.
22. Carter SL, Wheeler JJ. Considering the intrusiveness of interventions. Int J Spec Educ 2005;20:132–42.
23. Layng TVJ. Private emotions as contingency descriptors: emotions, emotional behavior, and their evolution. Eur J Behav Anal 2017. https://doi.org/10.1080/15021149.2017.1304875.
24. Barrows EM. Animal behavior desk reference: a dictionary of animal behavior, ecology, and evolution. Boca Raton (FL): CRC Press; 2001.
25. Lewon M, Hayes L. Toward an analysis of emotions as products of motivating operations. Psychol Rec 2014;64:813–25.
26. Rosales-Ruiz J. Teaching dogs the clicker way. 2007. Available at: http://stalecheerios.com/blog/wp-content/uploads/2011/07/Teaching-Dogs-the-Clicker-Way-JRR.pdf.
27. Friedman SG. Tsk, No, Eh-eh: Clearing the Path to Reinforcement with an Errorless Learning Mindset. Paper Presented at the Annual Conference of the Animal Behavior Management Alliance 2016, Tampa, FL.
28. Lindsley OR. From technical jargon to plain English for application. J Appl Behav Anal 1991;24(3):449–58.

Clinical Psychopharmacology for the Exotic Animal Practitioner

Marion R. Desmarchelier, DVM, DACZM, DECZM (ZHM), DACVB

KEYWORDS

- Behavior • Exotic animals • Psychopharmacology • SSRI • Psychotropic drug
- Anxiety • Avian • Fluoxetine

KEY POINTS

- Psychotropic drugs can be useful adjuncts to behavior modification therapy and environmental adjustments to address behavioral issues, and therefore improve animal welfare and human-animal bond.
- Psychotropic drugs cannot be used to replace appropriate environmental conditions in exotic animals. They can be important to allow fearful and anxious animals to use their environmental enrichment and participate in their behavior modification therapeutic plan.
- Psychotropic drugs work by decreasing fear and anxiety, reducing reactivity and hypervigilance, and improving impulse control.
- Side effects are rarely seen when dosages are appropriately adjusted to the individual by starting with a low dose and slowly titrating to effect.
- Several drug interactions exist between psychotropic drugs and other classes and should always be verified before prescription. Combination or overdose of serotoninergic agents, such as selective serotonin reuptake inhibitors, tricyclic agents, tramadol, and inhibitors of monoamine oxidase can lead to serotonin syndrome.

 Video content accompanies this article at http://www.vetexotic.theclinics.com.

INTRODUCTION

Psychotropic drugs by definition include any medication that can be prescribed to affect emotions and behavior. Many drugs indirectly affect animals' behavior by treating pain or medical conditions, modifying hormonal status, or inducing neurotransmitter imbalances as side effects (ie, corticosteroids).[1] However, these have been excluded from the 5 recognized classes of psychotropic medications: stimulants,

---

Conflict of interest: The author has no commercial or financial conflict of interest.
Department of Clinical Sciences, Faculté de médecine vétérinaire, Université de Montréal, 3200 rue Sicotte, Saint-Hyacinthe, Québec J2S 2M2, Canada
E-mail address: marion.desmarchelier@umontreal.ca

antidepressants, antipsychotic, mood stabilizers, and antianxiety agents. Literature on the clinical use of these agents in exotic animals is limited. Behavior medicine is a recent discipline in veterinary medicine. Evidence regarding the clinical usefulness of antidepressants and antianxiety medications in dogs and cats has been steadily growing over the last decade. As knowledge on how to properly use these drugs in domestic animals with behavior problems improves, appropriate extrapolation to new species becomes reasonable. Basic understanding of the neurochemical processes underlying behavioral disorders is useful to comprehend how psychotropic medications could help with clinical cases. This knowledge will also allow clinicians to understand when they are truly indicated or not. Potential side effects, contraindications, and drug interactions are also discussed to ensure maximum safety when prescribing these extralabel drugs in practice. This article presents practitioners with a clinically useful guide on how to include psychotropic drugs into their practices. For a more comprehensive review of empiric use of psychotropic drugs in exotic animals and detailed mechanisms of action, the reader is referred to other previously published review articles.[2–4]

HOW DO PSYCHOTROPIC DRUGS WORK?

Mechanisms of action of psychotropic drugs are still poorly understood. Behavior can be studied at many different levels, from what can be observed from any living being, to which proteins are activating the genes coding for these visible behaviors. This complex system involves neurotransmitters as diverse as amino acids, hormones, opioids, and even gas, such as nitric oxide.[5] More than 50 neurotransmitters are known and new ones are regularly discovered. These agents allow neurons in the central nervous system to communicate with each other and then create new synapses and eventually new pathways, as new behaviors emerge and the learning process occurs. The level of interrelationship between all these messengers, how they upregulate or downregulate each other's receptors on various sites of the neuron, is highly intricate. For example, norepinephrine turns off serotonin release by interacting with presynaptic alpha-2 noradrenergic receptors on serotoninergic neurons, whereas stimulation of postsynaptic alpha-1 receptors induces the release of more serotonin.[5] Any attempt to oversimplify this reality by assuming one drug increases the levels of one neurotransmitter in the brain unfortunately results in inaccuracy. However, even if most practitioners will never get to fully appreciate what is happening in the brains of their patients with abnormal behaviors, a basic understanding of the major neurotransmitters and the pathways influenced by common psychotropic drugs can be very useful.

Basic Principles of Neurotransmission

Among the multitude of neurotransmitters, 4 are known to be of clinical importance in veterinary medicine: serotonin, dopamine, norepinephrine, and gamma-aminobutyric acid (GABA). Serotonin pathways originate from the raphe nuclei in the brain stem and send axons to almost every part of the brain.[6] Serotonin is involved in every important function of the brain, such as appetite regulation, pain, reproduction, sleep, memory and cognition, aggression, emotions, and response to stress.[6] Dysfunction of the serotonin system has therefore been implicated in multiple conditions, including anxiety, pathologic fear, abnormal aggression, and impulse control disorders. Stimulation of some serotonin receptors also directly affects other neurotransmitter pathways, such as dopamine or norepinephrine. Several dopaminergic pathways have been associated with a particular function, such as the nigrostriatal pathway involved in motor function, reward-related cognition, and associative learning.[7] Dysfunction of the dopaminergic system has been associated with abnormal motor activity, including hyperactivity and restlessness, addiction, and compulsive/stereotypic behaviors.[8] Norepinephrine is a catecholamine and the major neurotransmitter for the sympathetic system throughout the body. The central noradrenergic system has several projections in the brain, involved in sexual and feeding behaviors, as well as cognitive functions. Norepinephrine pathway dysfunction is thought to be associated with increased reactivity, high level of arousal and vigilance, aggression with loss of impulse control, and cognitive dysfunction.[9] In addition, GABA is the main inhibitory neurotransmitter in the adult mammalian brain. Therefore, GABA pathways have direct inhibitory effects on many others. GABAergic neurons and interneurons are at the center of multiple functions, including memory, cognition, and fear conditioning.[10,11] GABA reduces the activity of neurons in the amygdala (brain center for fear and other emotions) and in the corticostriatothalamocortical (CSTC) loops, also called loops of worry.[5] Molecules acting on GABA receptors have been shown to help with abnormal fear, anxiety, phobia, and panic disorders.[11] Receptors for these 4 neurotransmitters are the targets of most drugs used in veterinary psychopharmacology. As previously stated, there are multiple intricate pathways in the central nervous system that cannot be ignored to bridge the gap between what happens at the molecular level and the observed behavior.[10] Although knowledge of the mechanism of action of each molecule can help make the initial drug choice, every case is unique and several trials can be necessary to find a drug and dose that best fits the patient. Side effects most commonly observed vary between species. It can therefore be assumed that behavioral effects are also species dependent. Future research will help with better species-specific decision-making processes when choosing a drug.

Selective Serotonin Reuptake Inhibitors

Selective serotonin reuptake inhibitors (SSRIs) are antidepressant drugs sharing the pharmacologic property of inhibiting the serotonin transporter (SERT). It has long been thought that the action of these drugs consisted in increasing levels of serotonin in the brain, mainly through keeping this neurotransmitter in the synapse for a longer period of time. However, this hypothesis did not explain why drugs in this category take weeks to provide some significant antidepressant effects, whereas the synaptic increase of serotonin levels occurs much more rapidly. Newer research has shown that SSRIs start a cascade of events from the initial increase of serotonin level in the synapse to downregulation of presynaptic and postsynaptic receptors, through desensitization of these receptors, to eventually activate new neuronal genes and stimulate synaptogenesis and neurogenesis in specific areas such as the hippocampus.[12] Side effects observed in the first days of SSRI use are most likely related to an acute action of excess serotonin at nontargeted receptors on undesirable pathways.[5] Although a lot is still to be discovered about SSRI's mechanism of action, the selectivity of each drug can be used for a variety of receptors to target specific clinical effects. In addition to its SERT inhibition, fluoxetine also inhibits the norepinephrine transporter and acts as an antagonist on the serotonin 2C receptors ($5HT_{2C}$). Antagonism at the $5HT_{2C}$ receptors may be linked to side effects such as increased anxiety and agitation, and loss of appetite.[5] In parallel, this action leads to an enhanced release of dopamine and norepinephrine, responsible for an energizing effect in withdrawn patients, as well as improved concentration and attention, helping the behavior modification plan to take place.[5] Paroxetine is another SSRI that is used in avian medicine.[13] In addition to SERT inhibition, paroxetine also has mild anticholinergic actions on muscarinic receptors, which can be calming, in contrast with the energizing effects of fluoxetine.[5] In our experience in various species, paroxetine is also beneficial in anxious patients with associated gastrointestinal signs.

Tricyclic Agents

Most tricyclic agents (TCAs) block both serotonin and norepinephrine reuptake to some extent.[5] They also share other pharmacologic actions that might lead to additional and sometimes unwanted effects, by blockade of the following receptors: muscarinic cholinergic receptors, creating a calming effect but also possible urinary retention and constipation; H1-histaminic receptors, causing sedation and increased appetite; alpha-1-adrenergic receptors, potentially decreasing blood pressure; and voltage-sensitive sodium channels, which could be a problem in patients with cardiac arrhythmias.[5] Clomipramine has anticompulsive effects that have been shown to be more effective than 3 SSRIs in humans, and is used in cases of trichotillomania (people pulling out their own hair), for which parrot feather picking is a research model.[14,15] Many TCAs, such as amitriptyline, are also used for neuropathic pain.[5] However, their margin of safety being lower than SSRIs and other newer molecules, they are generally not recommended as first-line agents in avian and exotic species.

Benzodiazepines

Benzodiazepines are anxiolytic drugs enhancing the action of GABA at the level of the amygdala and in the prefrontal cortex within the CSTC worry loops.[5] They are positive allosteric modulators at the $GABA_A$ receptors, which means that they have no effect on their own but can increase the frequency of opening of inhibitory channels in the presence of GABA.[5] $GABA_A$ receptors are also the targets of alcohol. For this reason, parallels exist between side effects of benzodiazepine use and alcohol consumption: high risk of dependence with chronic use, sedation, amnesia, disinhibition of certain behavior (ie, aggression), and impaired psychomotor capacities.[16] Although powerful anxiolytics, their impact on memory and sedative effects negatively affects the learning process. Increased risk of aggression is also a common concern when considering benzodiazepines with exotic animals. In veterinary medicine, these adverse effects limit the use of benzodiazepines to short-term treatment when other options are not available to help with a quality-of-life emergency.

Gabapentin

Gabapentin has grown in popularity in veterinary medicine over the last decade for pain management but also more recently for its antianxiety properties.[17] Gabapentin is an $\alpha_2\delta$ ligand binding to the $\alpha_2\delta$ subunit of presynaptic voltage-sensitive calcium channels, which results in decreased release of excitatory neurotransmitters, such as glutamate, both in the amygdala and in the CSTC circuits (loops of worry).[5] Balance between glutamate, the main excitatory neurotransmitter in the brain, and GABA is thought to be a key to solving many behavior problems. Gabapentin acts on the opposite end of the benzodiazepine spectrum by inhibiting the pathways competing with the ones enhanced by the benzodiazepines. Mechanism of action of gabapentin is still not fully understood, but side effects seem to be minimal, especially compared with benzodiazepines, in veterinary medicine.

Alpha-2 Agonists

Alpha-2 agonists, such as clonidine, bind to the α_2-adrenoreceptors in the central nervous system, decreasing sympathetic outflow in specific regions of the brain, such as the prefrontal cortex.[18] These drugs cause a dose-dependent sedation and decrease hyperarousal.[18] Patients with high reactivity, with self-injurious behaviors, or with sleep disorders can sometimes benefit from including clonidine in a combination of drugs.[19]

Other Miscellaneous Psychoactive Molecules

Trazodone is classified as a serotonin antagonist/reuptake inhibitor (SARI) because it inhibits SERT like SSRIs but also blocks 2 other serotonin receptors ($5HT_{2A}$ and $5HT_{2C}$), preventing the extra serotonin released in the synapse to act on these receptors.[20] Because stimulation of $5HT_{2A}$ and $5HT_{2C}$ receptors has been associated with side effects such as anxiety, insomnia, and sexual dysfunction, trazodone presents a great advantage over SSRIs.[20] Trazodone is also an antagonist of the α_1-adrenergic and the H_1-histaminic receptors, and therefore causes sedation at low doses. Its effects are rapidly observable, within an hour in dogs.[21] Trazodone is a useful adjunct to long-term drug combination or can be used for short-term stressful situations such as hospitalization or postoperative periods.[22]

Buspirone is a serotonin 1A partial agonist, and is considered anxioselective with no sedative effect. It is generally used in combination with SSRIs or TCAs when patients do not respond well to a single molecule. Buspirone is also thought to increase confidence in fearful animals and is commonly used in cats that are victims of intercat aggression.[23]

Among the large variety of natural products containing psychoactive substances, a few have been used in veterinary medicine and could be of interest for exotic animals. Alpha-casozepine originates from the cow's milk protein S1 casein and has an activity on GABA receptors creating antianxiety effects through a mechanism comparable with benzodiazepines.[24] However, no side effects have been reported. It has been shown to be useful for various stressful situations in cats and dogs.[24–26] *Valeriana officinalis* extract is also used to decrease stress in veterinary medicine. Mechanism of action is thought to be mainly binding to the β subunit of the $GABA_A$ receptors causing an effect similar to benzodiazepines.[27] However, studies have shown that valerian is also a partial serotonin 5HT2A agonist.[28] L-Theanine (green tea extract) is another molecule known to have antianxiety effects in multiple species.[29] Although its mechanism of action has not been completely elucidated, it is thought to act mainly on glutamate receptors.[29] Because all these molecules have been tested on laboratory animals, their effects are well documented in several exotic pet species.

Antipsychotic Agents

Older antipsychotic agents (eg, haloperidol) have been used to manage behavioral conditions in exotic pets. However, these agents mainly act on dopaminergic receptors and have no antianxiety effects.[30] Therefore, their apparent efficacy is based on the fact that they inhibit movement and cause sedation, which could reduce compulsive disorder such as feather picking. However, they do not treat the underlying condition leading the animals to self-mutilation and do not improve the quality of life. They do not promote normal behavior and they do not decrease fear, stress, or anxiety.[31] They are also associated with serious side effects.[30] For all these reasons, their use should no longer be recommended. Newer atypical antipsychotic agents could be investigated in the future to help with some rare refractory cases, but they still cause significant side effects in humans and their efficacy has not yet been documented in veterinary medicine.[31]

HOW TO APPROPRIATELY PRESCRIBE PSYCHOTROPIC DRUGS?

The choice to use or not to use psychotropic drugs is not an easy one. Many myths are associated with these drugs and still affect the capacity to prescribe them well.

Personal experiences of clients or veterinarians also influence their prescribing. Too often are antidepressants only considered as the last-resort option, when everything else has failed. In addition, trying a medication when the animal has been performing an inappropriate behavior for years, when the owners are close to the euthanasia decision, or when they have been discouraged by the lack of results of behavior modification therapy or environmental enrichment is most likely to result in additional failure and potential dramatic consequences for the patient. Although the use of antipsychotic drugs is not required in all exotic pets presented for behavioral problems, they should be considered, even on the first consultation if they are indicated in a particular case.

Box 1 summarizes the main indications for the use of psychoactive molecules as a part of the treatment plan for exotic patients. Antidepressants are important to consider in the rare situations where behavior modification and/or environmental adjustments cannot take place without them. Such situations include separation anxiety, because clinicians cannot perform exercises when they are not there, and not every owner can avoid leaving a parrot alone at home, for example. In these cases, medication helps break the vicious circle of separation anxiety by placing the animal's brain in a status where it can learn that being alone is not life threatening and that there is no need to anticipate any danger. By breaking the loops of worry and decreasing anxiety, the animal is able to learn to perform normal behavior in the absence of the owner and therefore benefits from the enrichment that is usually not experienced by these anxious patients. Once the patient is comfortable when left alone and is observed on video recordings displaying normal relaxed behavior consistently for 3 months, the medication can be tapered down and discontinued. Separation anxiety is probably an underestimated anxiety disorder in parrots, which are not expected to relax when separated from their group in the wild. Working on a more natural environment is obviously key, but some birds have to be kept isolated for medical reasons (virus carriers, and so forth) and could benefit from psychotropic drugs.

Another situation when the use of antidepressants is essential is when the animal is so fearful that communication with the human required for the behavior modification techniques is not possible. Examples include when a ferret is so fearful that it does not take any treat but attacks humans as soon as they approach, or when a rabbit's stress is so intense that it freezes and does not offer any behavior, including eating, in the presence of humans. Most patients respond to positive reinforcement, especially if offered in protected contact (to protect the patient and not only the handler),

---

Box 1
Indications to use psychotropic medications

- Separation anxiety
- Fear preventing the animal from using environmental enrichment
- Fear preventing the animal from participating in the behavior modification therapeutic plan
- Compulsive disorders and stereotypic behaviors
- Generalized anxiety
- Phobia
- Redirected aggression and severe impulse control disorders
- Any neurotransmitter disease
- Short-term stress relief in exceptional situations (postoperative period, transport)

but rare patients require medication for the behavior modification process to start. In some cases, medications can also dramatically increase the ease of this process and get faster results, leading to a more rapid improvement in quality of life. Not all owners are born great trainers and they can easily get discouraged if minor results take weeks to be visible. They also often think that they are responsible for the failure and are unaware that their pet's fearful emotional status prevents it from being capable of learning new, appropriate behaviors. Inform the owner on first consultation that there are some other therapeutic options if the pet is not amenable to behavior modification despite all the efforts or if the animal is fearful of all environmental enrichment. Clients are often blamed for not using enough enrichment. However, many have tried and observed fearful reactions in their pets, leading them to believe that enrichment was just not for them. No animal is able to enjoy its environment when in an overwhelming state of fear or anxiety. Clinicians should not hesitate to prescribe antidepressant agents in such cases, because relieving fear is a first important step in improving these animals' quality of life and allowing any positive learning process to take place.

Other indications of psychotropic drugs include compulsive and stereotypic behaviors that have been going on long enough to involve modifications of both dopaminergic and serotoninergic pathways. These behaviors are often challenging to treat, and a multimodal approach including medication to help rebuild normal brain pathways is often required. Some of these behaviors also involve the endogenous opioid system (feather plucking, self-mutilations) and addressing pain and potential habituation to opioid release, as with human drug addictions, is necessary.

Patients with high arousal and high reactivity, such as birds suddenly flying to bite their owners' face, can also benefit from medication. Antidepressants help these patients with improving their impulse control. Completely unpredictable behaviors are rare but difficult to manage with behavior modification techniques alone. Redirected aggression occurs when an animal attacks another one that was not originally the target of the aggression or fear. For example, when a noise-phobic parrot bites its mate when hearing a specific sound. Not being able to recognize the target of aggression is considered a sign of abnormal neurotransmission and is an indication that psychotropic drugs could be helpful.

In addition, when an animal is placed in a stressful situation that cannot be avoided, all should be done to reduce its fear during that time. Then using drugs to reduce fear and anxiety in hospitalized patients or during long transport can not only improve the animal's experience but also avoid self-induced trauma, excessive release of endogenous corticosteroids, and all their negative effects. In all cases, the use of psychotropic drugs cannot replace appropriate behavior modification and environmental changes. Drugs can only help to reduce fear and anxiety, allowing neurogenesis and synaptogenesis to occur, building foundations for the patient to learn to better adjust to its environment.

Expectations should be well explained to the owners (**Box 2**). It is critical for them to understand that each patient has unique requirement in terms of molecule and dose, and that clinicians can only adjust it appropriately based on response to behavior and environmental modifications. They need to comprehend that the medication will not solve the problem on its own, but will help and allow the other part of the treatment plan to take place.

Starting medication at the lowest dose of the range is usually the safest option, especially in species in which data are limited or inexistent. After 10 to 14 days at a low dose, if no significant change is observed, the dose can be increased (usually doubled; ie, for fluoxetine, from 0.5 mg/kg to 1 mg/kg) for another 2 weeks. The patient can then be reassessed. This method allows avoiding major side effects by detecting

---

Box 2
Expectations from the use of psychotropic medication

- Reduce fear and anxiety
- Allow the patient to use its enrichment
- Allow the patient to participate in the behavior modification plan and training
- Allow the patient to be distracted from compulsive behaviors
- Allow the patient to rest when appropriate
- Decrease hyperarousal and abnormal reactivity to the environment
- Allow the patient to communicate appropriately with conspecifics
- Allow the patient to learn new appropriate behavior
- Allow the patient to learn to be left alone if appropriate
- Decrease unpredictable aggression
- Place the patient in a physiologic status favorable to learning

---

highly sensitive individuals at low doses that are unlikely to be associated with significant issues. It also allows patients to adjust smoothly to the changes in their brain chemistry. Full effects of antidepressants are generally visible in 6 to 8 weeks but improvement is usually rapidly obvious when the molecule is the right choice for a patient. Once good effects are starting to be seen, waiting 6 weeks at the same dose is recommended, at which point, if the effects are still considered incomplete (ie, if many situations remain in which the patient cannot be made to participate in behavior modification exercises, if unpredictable aggression still occurs frequently, or if self-mutilation intensity is still too high), the dose can be increased again. If the patient worsens after a dose increase and remains consistently worse after 2 weeks of that new dose, it is likely that the optimal dose for that individual has been exceeded. If sufficient effects are not obtained when the optimal dose has been reached and continued for 8 weeks, a change of molecule or combination with another one should be considered. **Fig. 1** shows an algorithm for how to adjust the dose of a psychotropic drug. This algorithm is one method of adjusting doses of psychoactive agents that has worked well in the author's practice, but there are multiple other appropriate ways to do it. Although adverse effects of SSRIs and TCAs are generally minimal with long-term use, slow weaning is recommended after a minimum of 3 months of what is considered an appropriate behavior in a patient with a good quality of life. Should the animal recur during the weaning process, a review of the entire therapeutic plan should be done, including drug-dosing adjustments.

Side effects are uncommon but can be seen at the beginning of the treatment or after each dosage increase. They are usually self-limiting after 2 weeks or reversible once the treatment is discontinued. **Table 1** presents the most common side effects reported with psychotropic drugs in various species.

Antidepressants and anxiolytic medications should be used carefully in combination with other drugs for 2 main reasons. They often involve the cytochrome P450 system in the liver either as inducers or metabolites. In addition, they could lead to excess effects on their target receptors, such as serotoninergic and dopaminergic receptors, creating neurologic signs in cases of overload. **Table 2** summarizes some of the possible problematic drug interactions, and **Table 3** presents the main contraindications for the most common psychotropic drugs used.

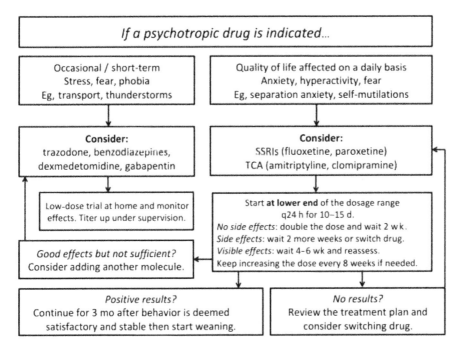

Fig. 1. Simplified algorithm to guide psychotropic drug prescription. q, every.

In addition, it is important to emphasize cases that do not require and would not benefit from psychotropic medication. When most animals of the same species can be expected to behave similarly in the same situation, the behavior is most likely normal and not the result of any neurochemical imbalances. For example, a rabbit eats the electrical wires or a ferret takes treats from the box left in a cabinet. Inappropriate behaviors that have been inadvertently reinforced but do not involve anxiety or fear are most likely to respond to appropriate behavior modification. For example, a pot-bellied pig can learn that screaming when handled gets it released. Unless the pig is truly fearful of humans, this behavior can be changed without the use of medication. Normal inappropriate behavior, such as birds screaming in the early morning, should not be managed with medication either. In addition, when a suboptimal environment is the primary cause for the abnormal behavior, improvement must be made in order to solve the problem before considering a medication. For example, a chinchilla removing its fur in the presence of several cats in its environment will benefit from having its own room without any predator staring at it and might not require any medication if the problem has been addressed soon enough in the process.

WHICH PSYCHOTROPIC AGENT TO CHOOSE?

The choice of the molecule to use is still difficult in exotic pets because quality research data are severely lacking. There are few pharmacokinetic studies available, and very few efficacy studies. Therefore, extrapolation from other species (domestic animals, humans) is still necessary. Readers are referred to veterinary psychopharmacology textbooks for details about how each drug should be prescribed in each situation.[30] Consulting a veterinary behaviorist can be useful to guide the choice of drug

Table 1
Suggested empirical oral dosages for psychotropic drugs in exotic pets

Drug Class	Drugs	Small Mammals		Birds		Notes
		Starting Dosage	Therapeutic Range	Starting Dosage	Therapeutic Range	
SSRI	Fluoxetine	0.5 mg/kg q24 h	1–5 mg/kg q12–24 h	0.5–1 mg/kg q24 h	1–5 mg/kg q12–24 h	Increased anxiety and agitation occurs when the dose is too high for an individual
	Paroxetine	?	?	1 mg/kg q24 h[a]	1–4 mg/kg q12–24 h[a]	
TCA	Amitriptyline	1 mg/kg q12 h	1–4 mg/kg q12 h	1 mg/kg q12 h[a]	1–5 mg/kg q12 h[a]	Low margin of safety in some individuals
	Clomipramine	1 mg/kg q12 h	1–4 mg/kg q12 h	1 mg/kg q12 h	1–5 mg/kg q12 h	
Anticonvulsants	Gabapentin	5–10 mg/kg q12 h[a]	15–30 mg/kg q8–12 h[a]	15 mg/kg q8–12 h[a]	15–50 mg/kg q8–12 h[a]	Useful adjunct for chronic pain
SARI	Trazodone	3 mg/kg q12 h	?	5–10 mg/kg q12 h[a]	15–30 mg/kg q12 h[a]	Based on PK data in birds but no efficacy study
Benzodiazepines	Lorazepam	0.5 mg/kg q6–12 h	0.5–1 mg/kg q6–12 h	0.05 mg/kg q12 h	0.1 mg/kg q12 h	Side effects and dependency with long-term use
	Diazepam	0.25 mg/kg q12 h	0.5–2 mg/kg q6–12 h	0.25 mg/kg q12 h	0.5–4 mg/kg q6–12 h	

Abbreviations: PK, pharmacokinetic; q, every.
[a] Pharmacokinetic data are available in some species.
Data from Refs.[3,4,13,32,44–46,51]

Table 2				
Potential side effects of most commonly used psychotropic agents				
Drug Class	**Drugs**	**Small Mammals**	**Birds**	**Notes**
SSRI	Fluoxetine Paroxetine	Decreased appetite Increased anxiety Irritability Agitation Lower seizure threshold May alter blood glucose levels	Increased anxiety Irritability Agitation Diarrhea May alter blood glucose levels	Paroxetine has fewer gastrointestinal side effects than fluoxetine Fluoxetine has a long half-life in most studied species
TCA	Amitriptyline Clomipramine	Sedation Vomiting Constipation or diarrhea Urinary retention Increased appetite Cardiac arrhythmias Changes in blood pressure Weight gain	Sedation Regurgitation Diarrhea Increased appetite Increased agitation Weight gain	Toxicity has been observed at low dosages
Anticonvulsants	Gabapentin	Sedation Hyperphagia Agitation Irritability	Sedation Hyperphagia Agitation Irritability	Rare side effects in exotic pets
SARI	Trazodone	Sedation Increased thirst	Sedation Agitation Increased thirst	Wide margin of safety in all studied species
Benzodiazepines	Lorazepam Diazepam	Sedation Ataxia Impaired learning Loss of memory Increased appetite Increased aggression	Sedation Ataxia Impaired learning Loss of memory Increased appetite Increased aggression	Liver toxicity and dependency when use long term

Data from van Zeeland Y. Medication for Behavior Modification in Birds. *Veterinary Clinics of NA: Exotic Pet.* 2018;21(1):115-149 and Crowell-Davis SL, Murray T, *Veterinary Psychopharmacology.* Ames, IA: Blackwell Publishing; 2006.

Table 3
Potential drug interactions and contraindications for psychotropic drugs

Drug Class	Drugs	Potential Drug Interactions	Contraindications/Caution Warranted
SSRI	Fluoxetine Paroxetine	Tramadol IMAO Buprenorphine Fentanyl Other SSRIs TCA Trazodone Warfarin Propranolol Benzodiazepines Antipsychotics Tryptophan Ketoconazole Metoclopramide Cimetidine Clarithromycin and other macrolides All drugs metabolized by cytochrome P450	IMAO Patients with seizures Diabetic patients
TCA	Amitriptyline Clomipramine	Tramadol IMAO Barbiturates SSRI Other TCAs Benzodiazepines Ketoconazole Enrofloxacin/ciprofloxacin Clarithromycin and other macrolides Omeprazole Dexamethasone Propranolol Cimetidine All drugs metabolized by cytochrome P450	Liver disease IMAO Patients with seizures Glaucoma Preexisting cardiac arrhythmias Nursing and pregnant women

Anticonvulsants	Gabapentin	Low profile of interaction with other drugs	Severe liver and renal diseases
SARI	Trazodone	SSRI TCA Antipsychotics Ketoconazole All drugs metabolized by cytochrome P450	IMAO Hypertensive patients Nursing and pregnant women Liver and renal diseases Severe cardiac disease Glaucoma
Benzodiazepines	Lorazepam Diazepam	Organophosphates Ketoconazole/itraconazole All drugs metabolized by cytochrome P450	Liver or renal disease Glaucoma Nursing and pregnant women

Abbreviation: IMAO, inhibitor of monoamine oxidase.
Data from Crowell-Davis SL, Murray T, *Veterinary Psychopharmacology.* Ames, IA: Blackwell Publishing; 2006.

for particular cases. Information regarding what is known about the use of psychotropic drugs in various groups of exotic pets is presented next.

Rabbits and Rodents

Doses reported for antidepressants in various exotic pet textbooks are much higher than the ones used for all other species and do not seem to be based on peer-reviewed literature.[32] These doses might come from laboratory animal research and might not apply to clinical situations. For example, clomipramine is generally used at 2 mg/kg every 12 hours in dogs and suggested doses for rodents are between 16 and 32 mg/kg. Fluoxetine doses found in the literature for pet rodents range from 1 to 10 mg/kg. Galeano and colleagues[33] attempted to reduce fur chewing in chinchillas with 10 mg/kg/d of fluoxetine for 3 months, but less than 50% of severely affected chinchillas showed some response to treatment. This condition is mostly environmental in fur-bearing farmed chinchillas, which is why clinicians should not expect a good response to medication without significant environmental modifications. Buspirone has been used in rabbits to attenuate novelty-elicited head bobs and has been suggested for timid, anxious rabbits.[30]

Pharmacokinetic study of gabapentin in rabbits shows plasma levels that would be considered therapeutic for humans at 25 mg/kg by mouth.[34] Benzodiazepines have been extensively tested in rabbits and rodents. Diazepam has been shown to decrease cat avoidance and neophobia in rats.[35] Lorazepam decreased conflict behavior in rats and mice.[36]

Rabbits, rats, and guinea pigs have been diagnosed with mild anxiety disorders by the author. These cases responded well to behavior modification, environmental adjustments, and, in a few cases, to psychoactive supplements. Alpha-casozepine has been shown to be anxiolytic in rats and mice.[37,38] An empiric dose of 30 mg/kg has been used with no adverse effects in several cases. Green tea extract, L-theanine, at 0.4 mg/kg/d has been shown to decrease anxiety in laboratory rats.[29] Valerian has also proved anxiolytic in rats and mice, without causing any sedation.[39,40]

Without better data, it seems reasonable to start rabbits and rodents on similar dosages to the ones used in cats and dogs and to titrate the dosages to effect. The lack of data in the exotic pet literature also suggests that behavior problems in small mammals do not often require the use of medication. Self-mutilation, fur chewing, and fur plucking are frequently secondary to pain, hormonal problems, and/or environmental problems. Interspecific aggression toward humans is common in pet rabbits and is usually easily managed with behavior modification, including positive reinforcement training and environmental management to decrease fear. House soiling is rarely secondary to anxiety in small mammals.

Although almost no use of psychotropic drugs has been reported for pet rabbits and rodents, they have been extensively used as laboratory animals to test psychotropic drugs. Toxicity studies indicate that fluoxetine did not cause any adverse effects in rats at 5 mg/kg, but decreased appetite was seen at higher doses. However, rabbits started losing weight at doses of 2.5 mg/kg.[41] No developmental toxicity was seen at dosages that were safe for the females, which suggests that fluoxetine is safe to use at therapeutic doses in pregnant female rats or rabbits.[41]

Ferrets

To our knowledge, there are no peer-reviewed reports on the use of psychoactive drugs to treat behavior problems in pet ferrets. Most behavior problems seen in ferrets can be managed through behavior and environmental modifications. The author has consulted for several ferrets that were diagnosed with anxiety disorders. One with aggression toward familiar and unfamiliar humans was treated with behavior modification only. Another ferret had concomitant gastrointestinal disease and severe fear and aggression issues that were successfully managed with appropriate inflammatory bowel disease treatment, behavior and environmental modification, and oral alphacasozepine. A third ferret with increased motor activity, intraspecific aggression, hyperarousal, and noise reactivity responded well to fluoxetine but only when the dosage was increased to 3 mg/kg every 24 hours. Although behavior modifications were partially implemented by the ferret's owner, fluoxetine therapy appeared to allow the ferret to sleep normally during the day, including with the other ferrets, which was never the case before, and reduced the frequency of intraspecific aggression and the intensity of motor activity. Because ferrets are small carnivores, extrapolating dosages from cats and dogs and titrating up to effect seems a reasonable choice pending more research.

Sugar Gliders

Several resources report dosages of fluoxetine of 1 to 5 mg/kg by mouth every 8 hours in sugar gliders, especially for self-mutilation.[32,42] However, the authors could not find any evidence of its efficacy for this specific purpose. Most self-mutilations in sugar gliders are induced by pain, especially surgical pain. Adapting surgical technique and postoperative care is likely to be more efficient than fluoxetine.[43] Stress-induced overgrooming seems to be common in sugar gliders. Social issues are often manageable without fluoxetine, but some patients could benefit from a medication, especially if the abnormal behaviors have been ongoing for a long period of time before initiating treatment.

Birds

Extensive reviews of psychopharmacology in pet birds are available in the literature.[2,3] Therefore, the focus here is on presenting only the most common and newer psychotropic agents used in avian behavioral medicine. Pharmacokinetic studies are available for amitriptyline, paroxetine, and trazodone in avian species.[13,44,45] Large interindividual variations were observed for paroxetine and amitriptyline, which reinforces the idea to start at a low dose and titrate to effect. SSRIs such as fluoxetine and paroxetine are among the most commonly used drugs to help with behavioral issues in pet birds. However, data on efficacy are still lacking. Two research studies have shown positive effects of the TCA clomipramine in feather-picking parrots.[46,47] Although the low dosage used in 1 study (1 mg/kg once or twice a day by mouth) may explain the partial results obtained, there were some interesting effects on more than half of the birds in these studies, including positive behavioral changes and reduced feather-damaging behavior. However, the durations of the studies were too short (6 weeks) to draw any conclusion on long-term effects, because parrots are known to improve at the beginning of the treatment, then relapse.[46,47] The TCAs clomipramine and amitriptyline have been used for many years in parrots with anxiety disorders and feather-damaging behavior, and have improved the quality of life of many patients. Lessons learned from their empiric use is that individual variations with regard to adequate dosing are very broad and toxic effects can been seen at dosages that could be therapeutic for other patients. Barboza and Beaufrere[48] (2018) reported an acute onset of dystonic reactions (repetitive and abnormal motions as well as head bobbing) and akathisia (restlessness and pacing) a few hours after a single partial dose of amitriptyline (5 mg/kg) orally in a blue and gold macaw (*Ara ararauna*). Another blue and gold macaw showed extrapyramidal signs when treated with a combination of clomipramine (3.9 mg/kg) and haloperidol.[49] The author has witnessed a similar case in another blue and gold macaw on accidental ingestion of a combination of fluoxetine and clomipramine that was intended for a nonhuman primate housed in the same building (Video 1). All birds survived these episodes of serotonin overload with supportive care. Only the bird that received the antipsychotic drug haloperidol responded to diphenhydramine treatment, confirming extrapyramidal signs.[49] Because SSRIs seem to be safer to use, they are now often recommended in parrots with anxiety and compulsive disorders.[3] Seibert[50] reported the successful treatment of a cockatiel with compulsive toe-chewing behavior with fluoxetine (1 mg/kg) and behavior modification. The author has been using fluoxetine and paroxetine at dosages ranging from 1 to 3 mg/kg by mouth every 12 to 24 hours without major side effects in various parrot species. Increased agitation and anxiety have occasionally been observed when doses were increased, but these effects were reversible when the drug was titrated back down to what was then considered the optimal dose for the patient.

Gabapentin is an interesting adjunct in birds with anxiety disorders, especially when chronic pain is present. Pharmacokinetics in Amazon parrots suggest that 15 mg/kg by mouth every 8 hours would be a good starting dosage.[51] No side effects were seen in the 3 parrots administered 30 mg/kg by mouth.[51]

Reptiles

Hormones are the most common drugs that have been used successfully to modify pet reptile behavior.[4,52] Although serotonin pathways are involved in intraspecific and interspecific aggression in reptiles, little is known about clinical use of serotonin-modifying agents in practice. Sertraline at 10 mg/kg has been shown to decrease aggression in an experimental model of aggression in *Anolis carolinensis* (placing 2 males in the same enclosure).[53] Most reptile patients can be managed with environmental changes and an appropriate behavior modification plan and do not require the use of psychoactive medication. The use of trazodone for short-term stressful situations such as transport or relocation warrants further investigation.

SUMMARY

When addressing behavioral problems in exotic pets, quality-of-life assessment should always be prioritized and should be clearly discussed with the owners. Although clients often consult because of concerns for vocalizations, house soiling, or poor esthetics of plucking animals, education about the true reasons behind these observed unpleasant behaviors, including captivity-related issues, chronic stress, and sometimes anxiety, is critical. The first objective should be to improve the patient's welfare by allowing the animal to display normal species-specific behaviors, and gain choice and control over its environment. Medications can play an important role in achieving these goals but can never be sufficient on their own. They should not be seen as the last resort before euthanasia but should be appropriately prescribed only when necessary. When receiving antianxiety medication, many patients with neurotransmission dysfunction show significant improvements and are eventually able to participate in their enrichment programs and interact normally with conspecifics and humans, allowing the foundations of a better life to be built.

SUPPLEMENTARY DATA

Supplementary data to this article can be found online at https://doi.org/10.1016/j.cvex.2020.08.003.

REFERENCES

1. Notari L, Burman O, Mills D. Behavioural changes in dogs treated with corticosteroids. Physiol Behav 2015;151(C):609–16.
2. Seibert LM. Pharmacotherapy for behavioral disorders in pet birds. J Exot Pet Med 2007;16(1):30–7.
3. van Zeeland Y. Medication for behavior modification in birds. Vet Clin North Am Exot Anim Pract 2018;21(1):115–49.
4. Tynes VV. Behavior of exotic pets. Chichester, West Sussex, United Kingdom: John Wlley & Sons; 2010.
5. Stahl SM. Stahl's essential psychopharmacology. Cambridge, United Kingdom: Cambridge University Press; 2013.
6. Charnay Y, Léger L. Brain serotonergic circuitries. Dialogues Clin Neurosci 2010; 12(4):471–87.
7. Luo SX, Huang EJ. Dopaminergic neurons and brain reward pathways from neurogenesis to circuit assembly. Am J Pathol 2016;186(3):478–88.
8. Lewis MH, Presti MF, Lewis JB, et al. The neurobiology of stereotypy I: environmental complexity. In: Mason G, Rushen J, editors. Stereotypic animal behaviour fundamentals and applications to welfare. CABI Publishing: Wallingford, United Kingdom; 2008. p. 190–226.
9. Herrmann N, Lanctôt KL, Khan LR. The role of norepinephrine in the behavioral and psychological symptoms of dementia. J Neuropsychiatry Clin Neurosci 2004;16(3):261–76.
10. Schmidt-Wilcke T, Fuchs E, Funke K, et al. GABA-from inhibition to cognition: emerging concepts. Neuroscientist 2018;24(5):501–15.
11. Lucas EK, Clem RL. GABAergic interneurons: the orchestra or the conductor in fear learning and memory? Brain Res Bull 2018;141:13–9.
12. Zavvari F, Nahavandi A, Goudarzi M. Fluoxetine attenuates stress-induced depressive-like behavior through modulation of hippocampal GAP43 and neurogenesis in male rats. J Chem Neuroanat 2020;103:101711.
13. Van Zeeland YRA, Schomaker NJ, Haritova A, et al. Pharmacokinetics of paroxetine, a selective serotonin reuptake inhibitor, in Grey parrots (*Psittacus erithacus erithacus*): influence of pharmaceutical formulation and length of dosing. J Vet Pharmacol Ther 2013;36(1):51–8.
14. Wilson M, Tripp J. Clomipramine. StatPearls [Internet]. Treasure Island (FL): StatPearls Publishing; 2019-2020.
15. Bordnick PS, Thyer BA, Ritchie BW. Trichotillomania parrot model. J Behav Ther Exp Psychiatry 1994;25:189–90.
16. Shushpanova TV, Bokhan NA, Lebedeva VF, et al. The effect of chronic alcohol abuse on the benzodiazepine receptor system in various areas of the human brain. J Psychiatry 2016;19:365.
17. van Haaften KA, Forsythe LRE, Stelow EA, et al. Effects of a single preappointment dose of gabapentin on signs of stress in cats during transportation and veterinary examination. J Am Vet Med Assoc 2017;251(10):1175–81.
18. Sabus A, Feinstein J, Romani P, et al. Management of self-injurious behaviors in children with neurodevelopmental disorders: a pharmacotherapy overview. Pharmacotherapy 2019;39(6):645–64.
19. John Ciribassi DD, Kelly Ballantyne D. Using clonidine and trazodone for anxiety-based behavior disorders in dogs. Vet Med 2014;109(4):131. Available at: https://www.dvm360.com/view/using-clonidine-and-trazodone-anxiety-based-behavior-disorders-dogs.

20. Stahl SM. Mechanism of action of trazodone: a multifunctional drug. CNS Spectr 2009;14(10):536–46.
21. Jay AR, Krotscheck U, Parsley E, et al. Pharmacokinetics, bioavailability, and hemodynamic effects of trazodone after intravenous and oral administration of a single dose to dogs. Am J Vet Res 2013;74(11):1450–6.
22. Gilbert-Gregory SE, Stull JW, Rice MR, et al. Effects of trazodone on behavioral signs of stress in hospitalized dogs. J Am Vet Med Assoc 2016;249(11):1281–91.
23. Ogata N. Animal behavior case of the month. J Am Vet Med Assoc 2013;243(5):641–3.
24. Landsberg G, Milgram B, Mougeot I, et al. Therapeutic effects of an alpha-casozepine and L-tryptophan supplemented diet on fear and anxiety in the cat. J Feline Med Surg 2017;19(6):594–602.
25. Palestrini C, Minero M, Cannas S, et al. Efficacy of a diet containing caseinate hydrolysate on signs of stress in dogs. J Vet Behav 2010;5:309–17.
26. Naarden B, Corbee RJ. The effect of a therapeutic urinary stress diet on the short-term recurrence of feline idiopathic cystitis. Vet Med Sci 2019;210(1):46.
27. Bent S, Padula A, Moore D, et al. Valerian for sleep: a systematic review and meta-analysis. Am J Med 2006;119(12):1005–12.
28. Dietz BM, Mahady GB, Pauli GF, et al. Valerian extract and valerenic acid are partial agonists of the 5-HT5a receptor in vitro. Brain Res Mol Brain Res 2005;138(2):191–7.
29. Ogawa S, Ota M, Ogura J, et al. Effects of L-theanine on anxiety-like behavior, cerebrospinal fluid amino acid profile, and hippocampal activity in Wistar Kyoto rats. Psychopharmacology (Berl) 2018;235(1):37–45.
30. Crowell-Davis SL, Murray T. Veterinary psychopharmacology. Ames (IA): Blackwell Publishing; 2006.
31. Mead A, Li M, Kapur S. Clozapine and olanzapine exhibit an intrinsic anxiolytic property in two conditioned fear paradigms: contrast with haloperidol and chlordiazepoxide. Pharmacol Biochem Behav 2008;90(4):551–62.
32. Carpenter JW, Marion CJ. Exotic animal formulary. St. Louis, Missouri: Elsevier; 2017.
33. Galeano MG, Ruiz RD, Cuneo MF de, et al. Effectiveness of fluoxetine to control fur-chewing behaviour in the chinchilla (Chinchilla lanigera). Appl Anim Behav Sci 2013;146(1–4):112–7.
34. Kozer E, Levichek Z, Hoshino N, et al. The effect of amitriptyline, gabapentin, and carbamazepine on morphine-induced hypercarbia in rabbits. Anesth Analg 2008;107(4):1216–22.
35. Bulos EM, Pobbe RLH, Zangrossi H Jr. Behavioral consequences of predator stress in the rat elevated T-maze. Physiol Behav 2015;146:28–35.
36. Gluckman MI. Pharmacology of lorazepam. J Clin Psychiatry 1978;39(10 Pt 2):3–10.
37. Violle N, Messaoudi M, Lefranc-Millot C, et al. Ethological comparison of the effects of a bovine αs1-casein tryptic hydrolysate and diazepam on the behaviour of rats in two models of anxiety. Pharmacol Biochem Behav 2006;84(3):517–23.
38. Benoit S, Chaumontet C, Schwarz J, et al. Mapping in mice the brain regions involved in the anxiolytic-like properties of α-casozepine, a tryptic peptide derived from bovine αs1-casein. J Funct Foods 2017;38:464–73.
39. Murphy K, Kubin ZJ, Shepherd JN, et al. Valeriana officinalis root extracts have potent anxiolytic effects in laboratory rats. Phytomedicine 2010;17(8–9):674–8.

40. Hattesohl M, Felstel B, Sievers H, et al. Extracts of *Valeriana officinalis L. sl* show anxiolytic and antidepressant effects but neither sedative nor myorelaxant properties. Phytomedicine 2008;15(1–2):2–15.
41. Byrd RA, Markham JK. Developmental toxicology studies of fluoxetine hydrochloride administered orally to rats and rabbits. Fundam Appl Toxicol 1994;22:511–8.
42. Meredith A, Delaney CJ. BSAVA manual of exotic pets. Chichester, United Kingdom: BSAVA. Wiley; 2010.
43. Cusack L, Cutler D, Mayer J. The use of the ligasure™ device for scrotal ablation in marsupials. J Zoo Wildl Med 2017;48(1):228–31.
44. Visser M, Ragsdale MM, Boothe DM. Pharmacokinetics of amitriptyline HCl and its metabolites in healthy African Grey Parrots (Psittacus erithacus) and Cockatoos (Cacatua Species). J Avian Med Surg 2016;29(4):275–81.
45. Desmarchelier MR, Beaudry F, Ferrell ST, et al. Determination of the pharmacokinetics of a single oral dose of trazodone and its effect on the activity level of domestic pigeons (*Columba livia*). Am J Vet Res 2019;80(1):102–9.
46. Seibert LM, Crowell-Davis SL, Wilson GH, et al. Placebo-controlled clomipramine trial for the treatment of feather picking disorder in cockatoos. J Am Anim Hosp Assoc 2004;40(4):261–9.
47. Ramsay EC, Grindlinger H. Use of clomipramine in the treatment of obsessive behavior in Psittacine birds. Journal of the Association of Avian Veterinarians 1994;8(1):9–15.
48. Barboza T, Beaufrere H. Extrapyramidal side effects in a blue and gold macaw (*Ara ararauna*) treated with amitriptyline. J Vet Behav Clin Appl Res 2017;22: 19–23.
49. Starkey SR, Morrisey JK, Hickam HD, et al. Extrapyramidal side effects in a blue and gold macaw (*Ara ararauna*) treated with haloperidol and clomipramine. J Avian Med Surg 2008;22(3):234–9.
50. Seibert LM. Animal behavior case of the month. J Am Vet Med Assoc 2004; 224(9):1433–5.
51. Baine K, Jones MP, Cox S, et al. Pharmacokinetics of compounded intravenous and oral gabapentin in Hispaniolan Amazon Parrots (*Amazona ventralis*). J Avian Med Surg 2015;29(3):165–73.
52. Kirchgessner M, Mitchell M, Domenzain L, et al. Evaluating the effect of leuprolide acetate on testosterone levels in captive male Green Iguanas (*Iguana Iguana*). Journal of Herpetological Medicine and Surgery 2009;19(4):128–31.
53. Larson ET, Summers CH. Serotonin reverses dominant social status. Behav Brain Res 2001;121(1–2):95–102.

Ferret Behavior Medicine

Sylvain Larrat, DVM, MSc, DES (Zoological Medicine), DACZM[a],
Noémie Summa, DVM, IPSAV, DACZM[b],*

KEYWORDS

• Ferret • *Mustela furo* • Behavior • Physiology • Aggression

KEY POINTS

• Domestic ferrets display specific normal behaviors, such as piloerection of the tail, "dooking," or "weasel war dance."
• Housing and environmental enrichment should fulfill their need to express normal ferret behavior.
• Social and playful activities are essential in ferret welfare.
• Ferrets may display abnormal behavior, such as intraspecific and interspecific aggression, house soiling, stereotypies, and absence of play behavior.

INTRODUCTION

Ferrets (*Mustela furo*) display behavioral characteristics that are very distinct from other pets. An understanding of these characteristics is key to recognizing normal versus abnormal behavior in ferrets. This article aims at describing normal and pathologic ferret behaviors.

DESCRIPTION OF NORMAL BEHAVIOR AND PHYSIOLOGY

• History
  ○ Domestic ferrets belong to the Mustelidae family, in the Carnivora order. They are closely related to wild European polecats (*Mustela putorius putorius*). They also share morphologic features with steppe polecats (*Mustela eversmanii*), but they have a different karyotype.[1,2]
  ○ The history of their domestication is poorly documented.[3,4] Aristotle (approx. 350 BC), Strabo (approximately 63 BC to 24 AD) and Pliny (23–79 AD) mention animals that are shaped and hunt rabbits like ferrets and come from North Africa.[3] However, these first mentions may refer to other species such as

[a] Exotic Pet Department, Clinique Vétérinaire Benjamin Franklin, 38 rue du Danemark, Brech, Bretagne 56400, France; [b] Département de Sciences Cliniques, Faculté de Médecine Vétérinaire, Université de Montréal, 3200, rue Sicotte, PO 5000, Saint-Hyacinthe, Montreal, Quebec J2S 2M2, Canada
* Corresponding author.
E-mail address: noemie.summa@umontreal.ca

Vet Clin Exot Anim 24 (2021) 37–51
https://doi.org/10.1016/j.cvex.2020.09.001
1094-9194/21/© 2020 Elsevier Inc. All rights reserved.

genets.[5] The most ancient role of domestic ferrets was to hunt rabbits and rats. Among other uses, they have also been used in research since the beginning of the 20th century, for example, in influenza studies.[6] The domestication from polecats to ferrets has been accompanied with several genetic bottlenecks, especially outside of continental Europe. It was also accompanied with behavioral changes.[1,4,7] In contrast with wild polecats, ferrets can make suitable pets.[7]

- Body position
  - When awake, healthy young ferrets exhibit constant motor activity.[8] With age, they become calmer and more prone to rest on their owners' lap. During activity bouts, ferrets show a strong inclination toward exploratory and digging behaviors. They usually move with an ambling gait, but can also walk, trot, gallop, and jump. Excitement tends to cause the hair on their tail to rise ("bottle brush" appearance) (**Fig. 1**). When the intensity of excitement increases, especially while playing (discussed elsewhere in this article), ferrets display characteristic body position and movements: they arch their back, hop, open their mouth, and produce characteristic sounds (discussed elsewhere in this article). This is sometimes called the "weasel war dance" or "dance of joy" (see **Fig. 1**).[8] Ferrets, especially old individuals, usually display sudden interruptions in their activity, lay flat on the floor, rest for a few moments, and start again their activity. Although this is a normal behavior, its occurrence and duration can increase when the animal is sick (eg, insulinoma or lymphoma).
  - Ferrets are very flexible. They can enter and investigate small openings. They are able to turn around even in very small spaces and can also go backward.
  - A ferret investigating a noise, smell, or perceived threat can assume an alert posturing: it stops and stands still on its 4 feet, with a semiarched back.[8]

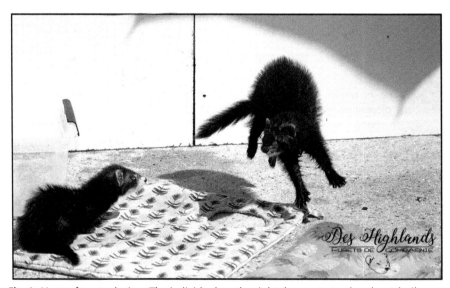

Fig. 1. Young ferrets playing. The individual on the right demonstrates (moderate) piloerection of the tail and is engaged in the "weasel war dance" (arched back and successive jumps). A plastic box with water is visible on the left of the picture. The piece of fabric on the floor is sewn to form a bag with a hole to allow a digging behavior. (*Courtesy of* L. Graslin. Saussay-la-Campagne, France.)

- Vocalization
  - Vocalization in ferrets is rarer than in other domestic carnivores. The most common sound is "dooking," also called "buck-a-buck," which corresponds with series of soft chuckles emitted when the animal is experiencing climactic playful excitation. It is often associated with the playful weasel war-dance and the open-mouth play face (discussed elsewhere in this article).[8]
  - The ferrets are able to produce a hiss, akin to that of cats. It is either a fear-related vocalization or a mark of severe discontentment. It can precede aggression in some instances (although aggression can often occur without any warning).[8]
  - When startled, some ferrets produce a bark, similar to what is described in steppe polecats.[9] The bark can also be emitted in series, after hissing, when the perceived threat increases in intensity.[9]
  - Ferrets may scream, with a prolonged, loud and high-pitched sound emitted when in pain or in distress.[8,9]
- Playing behavior
  - Ferrets engage spontaneously in playful behavior with counterparts, owners and sometimes toys. Ferrets play behavior is rough and chaotic, involves chasing, jumping on other ferrets, inhibited biting at each other's neck, straddling, and wrestling.[8,10] Ferrets often display the weasel war-dance and dooking as an invitation to play. They also wear the open mouth play face, which is characterized by a widely open mouth, and frequently by lateral movements of the head (**Fig. 2**).[11] Males and females display a different playful behavior, with mounting and straddling being more prominent in males, especially intact males.[10]
- Resting–sleep behavior

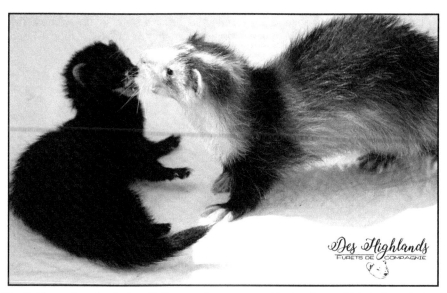

Fig. 2. Young ferrets playing. Both wear the open mouth play face, which is characterized by a widely open mouth and frequently by lateral movements of the head. (*Courtesy of* L. Graslin. Saussay-la-Campagne, France.)

- Ferrets spend a large amount of time sleeping. In a controlled experiment, ferrets under 2.5 years old spend 60% of their time sleeping.[12] They tended to sleep more at night, but nonetheless showed episodes of activity around the clock.[12] Aging ferrets seem to require more rest. Although this may be physiologic, this increase in time spent resting or sleeping may be associated with chronic illness.[8]
  - Ferrets sleep in various positions. They like hidings and hammocks. They are usually curled and may sleep in groups. They have the ability to sleep in strange contorted positions, or on their backs (**Fig. 3**). A ferret in a deep sleep may be so difficult to wake up that their owner thinks them dead or in a coma.[8]
- Reproductive and mating behaviors
  - Ferrets are sexually dimorphic, with males being larger than females. Females, also called jills, are seasonally polyestrous and induced ovulators.[8] During estrus, some females tend to be more vivacious (S. Larrat, personal observation).[13] Intact male ferrets, named hobs, often will "bathe" themselves in a mixture of anal gland secretions and urine in an attempt to attract females.[8]
  - The mating behavior of ferrets is quite aggressive.[14] The male bites the neck of the female. A female that is not in estrus fights back, whereas a female in estrus is more compliant, remains close to the male, and presents her genital area to the head of the male.[14] The male drags the female by the neck for a few minutes. Copulation occurs when the female stops moving. Intromission can last from minutes to hours.[14]

Enrichment

- It is important to try and offer ferrets the most appropriate environmental enrichment to obtain the most positive effects on ferret welfare.[15] Because each individual is different, and because this species appreciates novelty and change, owners of ferrets should be encouraged to get creative, provide varied and changing enrichment items, spend time in observation, and select the enrichment strategies their animals prefer. Interestingly, in a standard unenriched environment, inactivity, eating, and drinking represented 88.7%, 3.6%, and 1.7% of

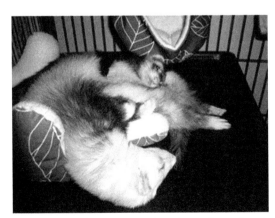

Fig. 3. Ferrets sleeping in group in a contorted position. Some ferrets sleep occasionally with the eyes opened, like the darker female ferret here. This may startle their owner by making them think the ferret is dead. (*Courtesy of* S. Larrat, DVM, Brec'h, France and N. Summa, DVM, Saint-Hyacinthe, Canada.)

the time budget, respectively. Exploration represented only 0.4% of the time budget.[15] In comparison, Blandford[1] reports an average of 4.2 hours (17.5%) and 3 hours (12.5%) spent foraging each day in female and male free-ranging wild polecats, respectively. This represented a typical foraging route of 3 to 4 km/d.[1]

- Housing
  - Ferrets can be housed indoors or outdoors in temperate regions. They do not tolerate well temperatures higher than 30°C (86°F).[16] Their tendency to dig, climb, steal items, and hide them and their ability to escape forces the owners to provide them with a well-designed environment, lest accident or foreign body ingestion occurs.[16] Recommendation of minimal enclosure size in research settings are proposed by the Federation of European Laboratory Animal Science Associations, but not the US Department of Agriculture Animal Welfare Regulations nor the National Research Council's Guide for the Care and Use of Laboratory Animals.[17,18] The recommended minimal size of enclosure ranges from a minimal enclosure size of 0.45 m² (4.8 ft²) for smaller individuals to 0.6 m² (6.5 ft²) for adult males. This should not be considered sufficient a housing for pet ferrets in the long term. Vinke and Shoemaker[19] report a minimal recommended enclosure of 1.5 to 2.0 m² (16–22 ft²) for 1 to 2 ferrets, and an additional 0.5 m² (6 ft²) per additional ferret. They also mention that larger enclosures are better suited to the biological needs of ferrets, especially if one considers the large home range of the polecats, which averaged 12.4 ha (30.6 acres) and 31.3 ha (77.3 acres) for females and males, respectively.[1,19]
  - Ferrets tend to urinate and emit feces in specific spots of their environment. They show a preference for corners, which may be used to litter-train them. However, they are not prone to traveling too far to find a litter and a litter should be placed in every room. They will often eliminate at the beginning and at the end of activity periods.[14] Litter boxes should not be too small as some ferrets need to have their 4 legs in the litter box to defecate (N. Summa, personal observation).
    - Sleeping area
      - Reijgwart and colleagues[20] found that ferrets had a high motivation toward sleeping enrichment, especially hammocks. Ferrets also like to rest in dark boxes (with cloth) or other hiding places. In an enriched environment, ferrets spent most of their inactivity time in their hammocks (17.3 ± 2.0 hours).[15] It is recommended to offer them several resting options and to introduce variability over time in their environment, including their hiding and resting places (**Fig. 4**).[19]
    - Water bowl
      - Ferrets prefer drinking from a bowl opposed to a nipple.[15,20] When offered both option in a study, ferrets mainly chose the water bowl and spent less time drinking overall.[15] Ferrets are also strongly motivated to drink in and play with larger water bowls.[15,20] In addition to drinking, ferrets also like to play with water.[20] Although some ferret owners state their pet like to swim, ferrets can demonstrate an aversion toward being immersed in water or even wetted (S. Larrat and N. Summa, personal observations).
- Activities
  - An interesting list of enrichment activities has been published in a previous article.[21]
    - Social interactions

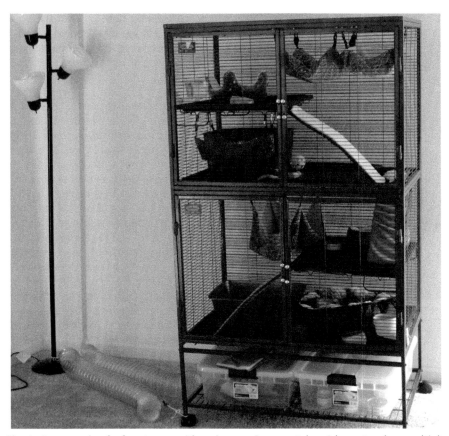

Fig. 4. An example of a ferret cage with various environmental enrichment such as multiple and diverse resting areas, balls, toys, and tunnels. Although ferrets like multilevel cages, it is important to place the different levels and hammocks to prevent an inadvertent fall, especially with younger and older ferrets. Ramp coverts can also prevent them from falling while attempting to get in the lower levels. With a group of ferrets, it is recommended to have a cage that can be easily separated into 2 independent sections, like on this picture, to be able to isolate a ferret from the others when needed. With ferrets with insulinoma, multiple bowls of food should be offered at the different levels of the cage to facilitate food intake. Note the presence of a litterbox at each main level of the cage and the suspended water bowls to prevent water spilling.

- Wild polecats are solitary animals.[1] It thus seems that owning a single ferret can be considered appropriate. However, domestic ferrets demonstrate a strong interest toward social interaction, and benefit from social enrichment.[15,20] Ferrets, in contrast with wild polecats, retain their ability to play when adults, as seen in many domesticated animals.
  - Owner related
    - Owners housing single ferrets are the sole opportunity for social interaction and play of their pets. They should thus be encouraged to spend enough time daily to keep their pet entertained and active. When keeping several ferrets, an extensive daily interaction is less critical. Different ferrets have different personalities and will engage

differently in interactions with humans. Most of them seem to enjoy chasing and catching items such as balls or toys attached to a string. Movement patterns seem to carry more importance than the material itself. Ferrets like to engage in a gentle tug of war and will respond to tickling, usually by wrestling with their owners' hands. Owners should be warned that some ferrets might bite in such circumstances. Another way to play with ferrets and get them very excited is to play hide and seek, for example, by covering and uncovering alternatively them with a piece of cloth.

- Like other animals, ferrets can be trained through positive reinforcement, especially with food treats. For example, training a ferret to come is quite easy and might prove useful when it is hiding in an unidentified part of the house.
  - ○ Intraspecies interaction
    - Reijgwart and colleagues[20] showed that ferrets were strongly inclined toward intraspecific interactions. Ferrets housed in groups often sleep and play with conspecifics. They also easily share water and food.[16] When playing together, ferrets demonstrate extremely active bouts of chasing, wrestling, and inhibited biting at each other's necks.
  - ○ Interspecies engagement
    - Ferrets play rough, which is not always appreciated by other pets. As predators, it is inadvisable to let them play with prey animals. Cats will generally tend to avoid interaction with ferrets. Although some dogs like to play with ferrets, supervision is warranted. Ferrets will chase other pets, and sometimes bite their necks, ears, lips, or other available body parts.
- Water or snow play
  - ○ In addition to drinking water bowls, water-related enrichment can be provided to ferrets (see **Fig. 1**). Even those that dislike being bathed will investigate and scratch running water (tap, fountain). Ferrets can also interact with toys immersed or let floating in large water bowls. Some ferrets might enjoy playing in the snow. Although wild polecats thrive in cold parts of Europe, an indoor ferret should not be carelessly exposed to cold temperatures.
- Olfactory enrichment
  - ○ Ferrets have a keen olfaction. When placed in a new room, ferrets explore by walking along the walls, constantly sniffing the floor. Olfactory enrichment is thus appropriate to this species. Some owners use natural water-based food flavoring (such as lemon extract or vanilla extract) as enrichment.
- Foraging: Food-related enrichment
  - ○ Ferrets establish their food preference between 2 and 4 months, through a process of olfactory imprinting.[14,22] After that period of time, it becomes difficult to change their diet. The animals that have been fed only with dry kibble during this period of time are unlikely to easily accept biologically appropriate raw food or whole prey and vice versa.
  - ○ Ferrets are usually highly motivated by certain types of food, so much so that offering a ferret its preferred treat is a good way to have it stay still during an ultrasound examination or when taking its rectal temperature. Most ferrets will for example, appreciate Nutri-Cal (Vetoquinol, Fort

Worth, TX), Ferretone Skin & Coat Supplement (8 in 1, Melle, Germany), rehydration solutions such as Pedialyte (Abbott, Abbott Park, IL), or fish oil.
- Ferrets like to collect and hide food, as do their wild counterparts.[23] This particular behavior causes hygienic issues when whole preys are offered.
- Dry kibble can be offered in toys that promote foraging such as foraging balls or tumblers. In a motivation study, ferrets worked to gain access to foraging toys, although they also had free access to food, demonstrating contrafreeloading in this species.[20]
- Although the provision of live prey would provide ferrets with the opportunity to express their natural hunting behavior, this is ethically questionable and cannot be recommended.
- Ball and toys
  - Ferrets can engage in play with a number of toys. Reigwart and colleagues[20] observed that ferrets interacted with different kind of ball. Ferret balls were preferred over golf balls. Time spent in interactions with balls with bells was high on average, with a lot of variation.
- Tunnel and maze
  - Ferrets are very interested in exploring burrows, tunnels, and cavities. They also have some digging ability. Providing indoor ferrets with tunnels allows them to express this part of their behavior. Reijgwart and colleagues[20] observed a clear preference toward flexible tunnels over rigid ones. Owners should be aware that ferrets are able to scratch holes in flexible hose of laundry dryers, and escape. Ferrets walked outdoors should be closely watched to prevent them from falling into drainpipes or from having a rest 1 m below the ground in a rabbit hole.
- Digging boxes and ball pits
  - Indoor ferrets express their digging behavior with digging boxes filled with various materials, such as paper cuttings, biodegradable packing peanuts made from starch, or potting soil (**Fig. 5**). Alternatively, they can be offered a ball pit with light filled with plastic balls.
- Outdoor activities

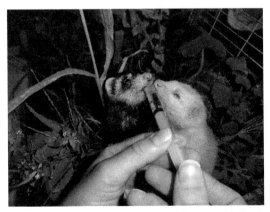

Fig. 5. Ferrets housed in group. They have been trained to come following an auditory cue, they are receiving a rehydrating solution as positive reinforcement. They are standing in their vegetalized digging box.

○ Ferrets can be trained to wear a harness and leash and to be walked outdoors. They might not like to stay in the open, and might prefer the cover of vegetation, walk along hedges and borders, and spend time digging or to enter holes, pipes, and burrows. Unless an extensive work of ferret proofing a garden has been done, it is not advisable to let a ferret roam free outdoors.[16]

COMMON BEHAVIORAL PROBLEM IN FERRETS

- In a survey,[24] the group including 57 ferrets and 2 skunks showed the highest prevalence of behavioral complaints by the owner (52.5%), compared with rabbits and rodents (29.3% and 20.3%, respectively). Aggression toward owners or strangers was higher in mustelids (30.5%) than in rabbits (13.0%) and rodents (5.5%). This finding contrasts with a more recent study based on an online survey,[25] in which overall frequency of undesirable behaviors in ferrets was considered rare to absent according to 466 owners. Online survey studies based on owner subjective appreciations have numerous biases that could explain the overall differences in behavior complaints in these 2 studies. Still, owners' perception of behavioral problems is interesting to evaluate, because it often dictates the outcome of the owner–pet relationship.
- Aggression
  ○ Although most ferrets are usually friendly, aggressive interactions in mustelidae can be violent with a high risk of injuries with other animals[19,26] and humans, especially infants and children.[27]
  ○ The different behavioral displays of aggression in ferrets are described in **Table 1**. Defensive behavior pattern may also reveal aggression behavior from the other ferret during interaction and should be included when assessing social interactions between ferrets.
  ○ Recognition of aggression in ferrets may be difficult for owners and veterinarians. In a large study of 466 owners and 1649 ferrets,[25] strong bites were associated mostly with aggression (46.8%) and fear (45.9%), but could also be associated with play (33.0%) and social interaction (16.5%). It has been observed that social play pattern may escalate under certain circumstances toward a more aggressive display.[14]
  ○ Aggression may be directed toward humans (owners and strangers), others ferrets, and other animal species. Most ferret owners have usually more than 1 ferret,[25] which allows the occurrence of intraspecific aggression and possible issues with the introduction of a new ferret in a household.
  ○ Predisposing and contributing factors
    ■ Familiarity play an important role in the incidence of aggression behavior. In 1 study,[28] none of the 31 pairs of cage mate ferrets placed into direct contact engaged in aggression, whereas 49 of 82 pairs of stranger ferrets did. Some of these fights were stressful enough to have prompted separation of the fighting pairs by the authors for fear of injuries. Contrary to some species, pairs caged next to each other for 2 weeks before introduction were no less likely to fight than were control pairs.
    ■ Previous research has shown that polecats, ferrets, and their hybrids were more likely to show aggressive behavior during the breeding season.[29]
    ■ Older studies of sexually intact in polecats, ferrets, and polecat–ferret hybrids indicated that sex is a factor, with intact males being more aggressive than females.[26]

Table 1
Ethogram of offensive and defensive behavior in ferrets

Main Pattern	Contains	Description
Offensive behavior	Positions for attack	Orientation to reach a position from which an attack may be launched.
	Attack	Movement into a position from which the neck or ear regions of the opponent may be bitten. Attacker crosses over its opponent's back to reach the far side of the neck so that the attack is generally from above.
	Neck bite	Bites opponent in the neck and holds.
	Bite other	Bites to other places (eg, flank, belly, anal).
	Drag	Grips opponent by the neck with teeth and pulls it around (neck bite is implied).
	Shake	Animal bites in a body part of another animal and shakes violently with the head up and down and from right to left (neck bite is implied).
	Oblique attack with physical contact	Approach to the opponent from the side or behind. The attacker's head is turned away from its adversary and its back arched attacker pushes its flank against its adversary and may roll on to it.
	Position for lunge attack	Orientation to a position from which a lunge attack van be launched.
	Lunge attack with contact	Lunges toward the opponent directing the open mouth toward the near side of the opponent's neck and touches opponent's fur, sometimes results in a bite.
Defensive behavior	Ward off	Flank is directed toward an adversary, the head turned away so that the convex side of the neck is presented to the opponent. Generally in response to an attack.
	Extricate	Any movements made by an animal to free itself from its opponent's bite. May include rolling, kicking, scratching with forepaws, and brief attacks.
	Extricate with vocalization	As for extricate, but the animal makes a high pitch vocalization that sound like screaming.
	Defensive	Faces the opponent with back arched.
	Defensive threat	As for defensive but accompanied with vocalizations (vocalizations accompanying different levels of intensity are hiss, scream).
	Snap	Biting movements made without any attempt actually to bite the opponent.
	Passive	The animal that is being bitten makes no attempts to free itself from the opponent grip.
	Scream	Animal vocalizes with high pith tones

From Vinke CM, van Deijk R, Houx BB, et al. The effects of surgical and chemical castration on inter-male aggression, sexual behaviour and play behaviour in the male ferret (*Mustela putorius furo*). Appl Anim Behav Sci. 2008;115(1-2):104-121; with permission.

- Neutering
  - Surgical castration barely decreased aggressive behaviors in ferrets compared with intact males.[28,30] Based on the observation of a limited number of animals, neutered female pet ferrets were not reported to be more or less aggressive than intact or castrated male ferrets.[28]
  - Vinke and colleagues[30] evaluated the effects of chemical castration with a 9.4 mg deslorelin acetate implant on intermale aggression, sexual behavior, and play behavior in male ferrets, compared with a placebo group or surgically castrated males. Intermale confrontation tests and male–female interaction tests were then conducted. Chemically castrated ferrets showed less aggressive interactions, less sexual behavior, more play behavior, and less musky odor than surgically castrated ferrets and control group.[30,31] This shows that a decrease in testosterone levels as described in chemically and surgically castrated ferrets is in itself not enough to decrease aggression or musky odor in ferrets. However, it might affect sexually motivated behaviors and play behavior in male ferrets. Chemical castration with deslorelin acetate implant may act on other hormones levels, such as estradiol and androstenedione, which could have more effect on aggressive behavior in male ferrets. This finding may encourage more chemical sterilization in male ferrets in a near future. This practice is now performed in Europe, but rarely in North America because most ferrets are sterilized at an early age in ferret breeding farms. However, the emergence of a new ferret breeder in Canada offering intact ferrets on the market may change this perspective.
- The inclination to bite seems stronger in (European) hunting ferrets than in ferrets bred for research or pet trade (S. Larrat and N. Summa, personal observations).
- Talbot and colleagues[25] showed a significant interaction between the number of hours ferrets spent confined and the number of enrichment items on the incidence of aggression in ferrets. Size of enclosure had no effect on aggression behavior. Interestingly, ferrets showed less aggression behavior with fewer enrichment items when confined between 19 and 21 hours.[25]
- In polecats, ferrets, and their hybrids, the earlier the animal was introduced in a confrontation test area, the more likely it was to win the fight.[26] On the other side, the weight of males had no influence of aggression behavior, as well as the presence or absence of a receptive female.[26]
  - Identifying the factors associated with the incidence of aggression behavior can be helpful in developing methods for introducing unfamiliar ferrets for owners and shelter workers.[28] All introductions should be monitored carefully. Adopting ferrets in an established pair should be recommended, with the best results being a male–female pair, or a 2-male pair.[19]
  - Decreased aggression may result in a less stressful environment and, hence, in an increase of play behavior.[30] Because opioid systems are involved in the regulation of the rewarding aspects of social play in juveniles rats,[32,33] play behavior could be associated with rewarding properties for ferrets, and an increased incidence of social play behavior could be linked to increased welfare for ferrets.
- House soiling
  - Urination and defecation outside the litter box may frequently occur in litter-trained pet ferrets (S. Larrat and N. Summa, personal observations). This behavior may be related to ferret olfactory communication through scent

marking of their territory.[13] Other scent-marking behaviors in pet ferrets include wiping the preputial sebaceous gland over surfaces, dragging the perianal sebaceous glands on the floor, and defecating on objects.[13]

o Urine and feces soiling may also be owing to inadequate potty training of juvenile ferrets,[14] and possibly stress-induced elimination as in cats.[13]

o Finally, the onset of house soiling in a well litter-trained older ferret may be an early sign of adrenal gland disease. Diagnostic tests, such as abdominal ultrasound examinations and a hormonal panel, should be performed to rule out this disease.

- Stereotypies
  o There are very few publications on stereotypies in ferrets compared with mink. In farmed mink, common stereotypies include pacing along the wall of the cage, compulsive scratching at the cage wire mesh with the front paws, repetitive display stationary behavior in a single spot (whole-body bobbing, head-bobbing, head-twirling, and weaving side to side), repeatedly biting and/or licking the cage mesh, and fur chewing and/or tail biting.[34]
  o Some of these stereotypies have been reported in ferrets, although the literature is scarce on the subject. In 1 study,[25] the incidence of stereotypies according to the owner's perception only was reported as very low. The most common stereotypy reported was compulsive scratching. There was no significant difference between male and female for compulsive scratching or other repetitive behavior, such as pacing in ferrets. However, neutering significantly decreased the incidence of other repetitive behavior in both sexes, but not of compulsive scratching. The number of enrichment items, amount of time spent in confinement, and size of enclosure had no significant effect on compulsive scratching or other repetitive behaviors.[25] It is to be noted that none of these ferrets were evaluated by a specialist in animal behavior medicine. However, an interesting point was that only about one-half of owners considered repetitive behavior as abnormal behavior, showing that owners' perception of their animal behavior pattern may not be accurate.
  o Absence of play behavior
    ▪ Play behavior can be used as a positive welfare indicator because it often disappears when an animal is under stress.[35] However, play behavior can also increase in stressed animals, in response to decreased parental care, or as a rebound after a period of deprivation.[35] Therefore, the presence of play behavior should be not consistently be associated with a positive welfare in animals, and thus in ferrets.

Special Considerations

- Foreign body
  o Special consideration should be taken while providing environmental enrichment in ferrets, as they are especially prone to foreign bodies under 2 years of age, in particular rubber or rubber-like materials.[19] Only ferret-proofed objects should be offered and inspected on a frequent basis. Any damaged toy should be removed immediately.
- Congenital deafness
  o A prevalence of 29% of congenital sensorineural deafness was reported in a population of 152 European pet ferrets, with a strong association between congenital sensorineural deafness and white patterned coat or premature graying.[36] All panda, American panda, and blaze ferrets were deaf. In this

study, although most breeders and owners were unaware of their ferret being deaf based on its behavior, it was occasionally associated with behavioral and training problems, such as abnormal social interactions with other ferrets, biting tendencies, and louder than normal vocalizations.[36]

- Anal gland removal in ferrets
  - Ferret gland scent could provide an olfactory system of sex and individual identity recognition based on its compound analysis.[37] Scent marking occurs as a sex attraction and territorial defense mechanisms. For example, during confrontation tests, male ferrets were more aggressive in the presence of their own rather than their opponent's odor, and less aggressive with their opponent's odor. Although descenting is a very common practice in North America, it is rarely performed in Europe owing to welfare concerns. The effect of the anal gland removal on social interactions in pet ferrets is unknown.
- Ferret and vision
  - Ferrets are near-sighted.[38] They are adapted to see in dim light and to see movement more than details. These characteristics might explain why some ferrets may jump down from inappropriate height (S. Larrat and N. Summa, personal observations), or be easily startled.[8]
  - It may also elicit a predatory response in some individuals confronted with hand moving at the same speed as prey, 25 cm/s to 45 cm/s,[39] which can easily be interpreted as aggression.
- Ferret hybrids
  - In Europe, fertile hybrids between domestic ferret/European polecat (*Mustela putorius putorius*) and ferret/European mink (*Mustela lutreola)* have been produced to obtain darker individuals, owing to a favorable trend for darker coat pattern (S. Larrat and N. Summa, personal observations). Although these hybrids are heavier and bigger (around 2.0–2.5 kg), their training and human interactions may be more challenging compared with domestic ferrets (S. Larrat and N. Summa, personal observations).
- Early socialization in juveniles
  - Although no study has been published on the subject, early socialization is most likely important to reduce stress around humans and other pets in ferrets,[19] as recognized in other species.[40]

SUMMARY

Veterinarians should help ferret owners, breeders, and shelters to provide the best environment and social interaction to fulfill ferrets' normal behavior and prevent behavioral disorders. While assessing behavior in ferrets, specific questions should be asked to the owners to have a complete picture of the behavioral pattern and not relaying on the owner's perception.

DISCLOSURE

The authors have nothing to disclose.

REFERENCES

1. Blandford PRS. Biology of the polecat Mustela-putorius - a literature-review. Mammal Rev 1987;17(4):155–98.
2. Kurose N, Abramov AV, Masuda R. Molecular phylogeny and taxonomy of the genus Mustela (Mustelidae, Carnivora), inferred from mitochondrial DNA

sequences: new perspectives on phylogenetic status of the back-striped weasel and American mink. Mammal Study 2008;33(1):25–33.

3. Thomson APD. A History of the Ferret. J Hist Med Allied Sci 1951;VI:471–80.
4. Gustafson KD, Hawkins MG, Drazenovich TL, et al. Founder events, isolation, and inbreeding: intercontinental genetic structure of the domestic ferret. Evol Appl 2018;11(5):694–704.
5. Amigues S. Les belettes de Tartessos. Anthropozoologica 1999;29:55–64.
6. Oh DY, Hurt AC. Using the Ferret as an Animal Model for Investigating Influenza Antiviral Effectiveness. Front Microbiol 2016;7.
7. Pitt F. Notes on the genetic behaviour of certain characters in the polecat, ferret, and in polecat-ferret hybrids. J Genet 1921;11(2):95–115.
8. Boyce SW, Zingg BM, Lightfoot TL. Behavior of *Mustela putorius furo* (the domestic ferret). Vet Clin North Am Exot Anim Pract 2001;4(3):697–712.
9. Farley SD, Lehner PN, Clark T, et al. Vocalizations of the Siberian ferret (*Mustela eversmanni*) and comparisons with other mustelids. J Mammal 1987;68(2):413–6.
10. Stockman ER, Callaghan RS, Gallagher CA, et al. Sexual-differentiation of play-behavior in the ferret. Behav Neurosci 1986;100(4):563–8.
11. Poole TB. An analysis of social play in polecats (Mustelidae) with comments on the form and evolutionary history of the open mouth play face. Anim Behav 1978;26:36–49.
12. Marks GA, Shaffery JP. A preliminary study of sleep in the ferret, Mustela putorius furo: a carnivore with an extremely high proportion of REM sleep. Sleep 1996; 19(2):83–93.
13. Fisher PG. Ferret behavior. In: Bays TB, Lightfoot T, Mayer J, editors. Exotic pet behavior: birds, reptiles, and small mammals. St-Louis (MO): Elsevier Health Sciences; 2006. p. 163–205.
14. Bulloch M, Tynes V. Ferrets. In: Tynes VV, editor. Behavior of exotic pets. Ames (IA): Blackwell Pub.; 2013. p. 164–92.
15. Reijgwart ML, Vinke CM, Hendriksen CFM, et al. An explorative study on the effect of provision of preferred and non-preferred enrichment on behavioural and physiological parameters in laboratory ferrets (*Mustela putorius furo*). Appl Anim Behav Sci 2018;203:64–72.
16. Lewington J. Ferret husbandry, medicine and surgery. Philadelphia: Elsevier; 2007.
17. Forbes D, Associations Federation of European Laboratory Animal Science Associations. Euroguide: on the accommodation and care of animals used for experimental and other scientific purposes;(based on the revised Appendix A of the European Convention *ETS 123*). Cernobbio, Italy: FELASA; 2007.
18. Garber J, Barbee R, Bielitzki J, et al. Environment, housing, and management. In: National Research Council, editor. Guide for the care and use of laboratory animals. Washington, DC: National Academies Press; 2010. p. 41–104.
19. Vinke CM, Schoemaker NJ. The welfare of ferrets (*Mustela putorius furo*) A review on the housing and management of pet ferrets. Appl Anim Behav Sci 2012; 139(3–4):155–68.
20. Reijgwart ML, Vinke CM, Hendriksen CFM, et al. Ferrets' (*Mustela putorius furo*) enrichment priorities and preferences as determined in a seven-chamber consumer demand study. Appl Anim Behav Sci 2016;180:114–21.
21. Harris LM. Ferret wellness management and environmental enrichment. Vet Clin North Am Exot Anim Pract 2015;18(2):233–44.
22. Apfelbach R. Imprinting on prey odours in ferrets (*Mustela Putorius F. Furo L.*) and its neural correlates. Behav Process 1986;12(4):363–81.

23. Räber H. Versuche zur Ermittlung des Beuteschemas an einem Hausmarder (*Martes foina*) und einem Iltis (*Putorius putorius*). Rev Suisse Zool 1944;51: 293–332.
24. Normando S, Gelli D. Behavioral complaints and owners' satisfaction in rabbits, mustelids, and rodents kept as pets. J Vet Behav 2011;6(6):337–42.
25. Talbot S, Freire R, Wassens S. Effect of captivity and management on behaviour of the domestic ferret (*Mustela putorius furo*). Appl Anim Behav *Sci* 2014;151: 94–101.
26. Poole TB. Aggressive-behavior of individual male Polecats (*Mustela putorius, M. furo* and hybrids) towards familiar and unfamiliar opponents. J Zool 1973;170: 395 414.
27. Applegate JA, Walhout MF. Childhood risks from the ferret. J Emerg Med 1998; 16(3):425–7.
28. Staton VW, Crowell-Davis SL. Factors associated with aggression between pairs of domestic ferrets. J Am Vet Med Assoc 2003;222(12):1709–12.
29. Poole TB. Aspects of aggressive behaviour in polecats. Z Tierpsychol 1967; 24(3):351–69.
30. Vinke CM, van Deijk R, Houx BB, et al. The effects of surgical and chemical castration on intermale aggression, sexual behaviour and play behaviour in the male ferret (*Mustela putorius furo*). Appl Anim Behav Sci 2008;115(1–2):104–21.
31. Schoemaker NJ, van Deijk R, Muijlaert B, et al. Use of a gonadotropin releasing hormone agonist implant as an alternative for surgical castration in male ferrets (*Mustela putorius furo*). Theriogenology 2008;70(2):161–7.
32. Vanderschuren LJ, Spruijt BM, Hol T, et al. Sequential analysis of social play behavior in juvenile rats: effects of morphine. Behav Brain Res 1995;72(1–2): 89–95.
33. Vanderschuren LJ, Stein EA, Wiegant VM, et al. Social play alters regional brain opioid receptor binding in juvenile rats. Brain Res 1995;680(1–2):148–56.
34. Polanco A. The forms of stereotypic behaviour in farmed mink (Neovison vison). PhD dissertation. Guelph (ON): The University of Guelph; 2016.
35. Held SDE, Spinka M. Animal play and animal welfare. Anim Behav 2011;81(5): 891–9.
36. Piazza S, Abitbol M, Gnirs K, et al. Prevalence of deafness and association with coat variations in client-owned ferrets. J Am Vet Med Assoc 2014;244(9): 1047–52.
37. Clapperton BK, Minot EO, Crump DR. An Olfactory Recognition System in the Ferret Mustela-Furo L (Carnivora, Mustelidae). Anim Behav 1988;36:541–53.
38. Ferrets Lewington J. In: O'Malley B, editor. Clinical anatomy and physiology of exotic species: structure and function of mammals, birds, reptiles, and amphibians. New York: W B Saunders Co Ltd; 2005. p. 237–61.
39. Apfelbach R, Wester U. The quantitative effect of visual and tactile stimuli on the prey-catching behaviour of ferrets (Putorius furo L.). Behav Process 1977;2(2): 187–200.
40. Howell TJ, King T, Bennett PC. Puppy parties and beyond: the role of early age socialization practices on adult dog behavior. Vet Med (Auckl) 2015;6:143–53.

Rabbit Behavior

Sharon Crowell-Davis, DVM, PhD, DACVB

KEYWORDS

- Rabbit • Prey animal • Litter box • Dig • Chew

KEY POINTS

- Rabbits (*Oryctolagus cuniculus*) are prey animals that have several behaviors that maximize their chances of survival. Unless they feel very safe, they are alert and reactive. Making a pet rabbit calm and unafraid in a given household takes time.
- They dig warrens. Living as pets does not eliminate their motivation to dig, so rabbits should be provided with objects on substrates to scratch and dig on and in.
- Wild rabbits eliminate in specific latrines. This is the basis for being able to litter box train them.
- Rabbits have open-rooted teeth, which grow throughout their life. In the wild, their teeth are kept constantly worn down by chewing on rough herbage. This makes it essential that they be provided with items that are safe for them to chew on in the domestic environment, in order to prevent their teeth from becoming overgrown.

INTRODUCTION

In order to understand the behavior of the domestic rabbit (*Oryctolagus cuniculus*), the wild ancestor needs to be understood, although the 2 still are the same species and can readily interbreed. The domestic rabbit originated on the Iberian Peninsula, which is modern-day Spain and Portugal.[1] The behavior witnessed in the pet rabbit is driven by the adaptations of the ancestral rabbits to avoid being killed by predators. Wild rabbits live in groups of up to 300 or 400 individuals, although most are smaller. Their long, strong claws are used to dig extensive warrens, that is, tunnels with periodic larger "rooms." The largest warrens may have 50 entrances but again most are smaller.

Wild rabbits are crepuscular, that is, they feed at dawn and dusk.[2] During the daytime and nighttime they rest in the rooms of the warren. They go out to graze in groups, and at least 1 rabbit always is standing watch for predators. If potential danger is spotted, 1 of the hind limbs is slammed forcefully against the ground, creating the characteristic thump that even people who have not been around rabbits usually are acquainted with via books and movies. When a rabbit thumps, all run into the warren as fast as they can. One advantage of being in groups is gaining feeding time. The more rabbits that are outside at 1 time, the more time each rabbit has to graze, and the less time it needs to spend standing watch.[3]

Department of Veterinary Biosciences and Diagnostic Imaging, College of Veterinary Medicine, University of Georgia, 501 DW Brooks Drive, Athens, GA 30602, USA
E-mail address: scrowell@uga.edu

Vet Clin Exot Anim 24 (2021) 53–62
https://doi.org/10.1016/j.cvex.2020.09.002

The Romans, as they conquered Europe, carried rabbits with them in crates as portable sources of meat.[1] Their status as highly social animals made them pre-adapted to survive this. Some escaped and established wild colonies in many parts of Europe. In the middle ages, monks began selectively breeding rabbits for different colors and types. During the industrial revolution, as people moved from the country to the city, some took rabbits with them, because this was a type of livestock that could be kept in the small yards many people had. This was the beginning of the "rabbit fancy." At this point, although many considered their rabbits to be pets, in particular, pets for children, rabbits still typically were kept in hutches. It is only in recent years that keeping rabbits as indoor pets, or house rabbits, has become common.

The rabbits of the American continents, while being members of the family Leporidae, are different species and genuses than the domestic rabbit. The domesticated rabbit is the only surviving member of the genus *Oryctolagus*. Further references to rabbits are specifically about *O cuniculus*.

WHY PET RABBITS?

Rabbits are the third most common mammalian pet in the United States.[4] They have become increasingly popular as house pets for several reasons. First, they are small, a beneficial characteristic for a pet of people living in small apartments. The largest is the Flemish giant, which averages 6.8 kg (15 lb), with the largest of them reaching 10 kg (22 lb). A majority of rabbits kept as pets range from the dwarf breeds, starting at approximately 0.5 kg (1.1 lb), although they can be smaller, to the medium breeds, which range up to 5 kg (11 lb) or a bit larger.

If they are socialized properly to humans while young, they are very friendly. When they are in a household where they feel safe, they play games characteristic of their species, which often are entertaining to their human family. One is to simply run around the house jumping on and off things. Another is to simply "jump for joy," also referred to as a "binky," in which they leap off the ground with all 4 limbs, often going straight up, and not making any significant forward movement. When strongly bonded to their owner, they often sleep with them, cuddling closely, just as many cats and dogs do. Their fur typically is soft and comforting to stroke. They like manipulating things and can provide much entertainment carrying, pushing, pawing, and rearranging their toys. A rabbit the author once had would grab a toy that was made of short dowels organized into a ball-like shape. Then he would stand up on his hind limbs and throw it as far as he could with a rapid twist of his head that ended in release. Their natural instinct to use a specific location as a latrine makes it easy to litter box train them. They also can wear a harness and be leash trained for walks outside, although vigilant watching for loose dogs or other predators is required. They easily are trained to do tricks with the use of various forms of positive reinforcement, including clicker training, Because of their athleticism, they can be trained to do agility and participate in jumping competitions. The heights and lengths that a rabbit, even a lop-eared breed, can jump, is quite impressive to observers.

PREVENTING BEHAVIOR PROBLEMS
Socialization

Socialization is the foundation of a rabbit becoming a good pet. Because they are a social species, it is best to have at least 2 rabbits.[5,6] If someone gets a rabbit kitten and raises it with no contact with its own species, it may be difficult to introduce other rabbits later because the young rabbit was not socialized to its own species when it was at the optimal age to learn social skills. It also is critical to socialize rabbit kittens to people.[7,8] This involves a mixture of pleasant experiences with humans, including gentle petting and handling, and the feeding of various treats that rabbits like. Each rabbit has its own preference for favorite treats, but blueberries, apple slices, broccoli, and bananas all are good options to try. Sweeter treats, such as dried pineapple and yogurt drops, may be the most popular, but should be used sparingly due to the high calorie content. Obesity is a serious problem in rabbits. It is critical that the young rabbit not be subjected to frightening experiences with humans, such as having its ears pulled, being hit, or being dropped. Children should be allowed to be around rabbits only under the direct supervision of an adult. Children should be allowed to handle rabbits only if the supervising adult is confident that they can do so appropriately.

General Activity and Exercise

Rabbits kept in hutches cannot move very much. This historical housing tradition is misleading, because both wild rabbits and pet rabbits that have adequate space are very active. They have only 1 gait, the hop, in which the powerful hind limbs push the rabbit off the ground and forward. The forelimbs function mainly to hold the front part of the body off of the ground when the rabbit is standing on all 4 limbs. The hop can be slow and periodic, such as when they are grazing. They may take only 1 hop, then eat some grass, and then take another hop. These hops also usually only move the rabbit a short distance. At the opposite end of the spectrum, a rabbit "runs" by maximizing both the frequency and distance of hops. A single hop can carry the rabbit more than 2 meters. Depending on the breed, rabbits can run between 40 kilometers per hour and 72 kilometers per hour. Therefore, keeping rabbits in hutches severely limits their normal movement behavior. When a rabbit has access to several rooms of a house or apartment, it moves around the space and varying speeds. It also investigates various items in the house. Allowance for these natural behaviors may help prevent the development of behavior problems, such as excessive self-grooming and self-mutilation, in addition to improving the rabbit's welfare.

Chewing

A rabbit's teeth are open-rooted, erupting and growing throughout their life. In the wild, they chew on a large amount of herbage, some of it very rough. This results in the distal surface of the teeth being steadily worn down. Domestic rabbits typically are fed soft hay and kibble, which does not provide sufficient wear on their teeth. If not addressed, this results in significant dental problems. Rabbits are strongly motivated to chew on things and, in the domestic environment, if they are not provided with items that are acceptable to chew and that provide steady wear on the distal surfaces of the teeth, they chew on whatever is available, for example, furniture, cords, knickknacks, and remote controls. Preventing a rabbit from causing damage to the house and to items within the house, a 2-pronged approach is necessary. Provide the rabbit with items that are acceptable for it to chew, and protect items that are either valuable or dangerous for the rabbit to chew. There is a wide variety of items that are commercially available for rabbits to chew on, usually labeled as toys but sometimes labeled as chewing items. Wood is the most common substrate. It must be nontoxic. Some woods, such as cedar, hemlock, and citrus, are naturally toxic. Nontoxic woods can be made toxic by humans spraying a tree with herbicides, insecticides, and other toxins before it is cut, or by treating it with various preservatives once it is cut. Applewood is a popular wood to offer rabbits, but the wood needs to come from an organic orchard, or from an apple tree that is never sprayed with toxins for other reasons. Many vendors, both large and small, offer packages of small applewood sticks and toys made from applewood. A rabbit owner should query regarding the status of the applewood prior to purchasing it, because some people who are un-aware of this issue may see an opportunity to make money selling applewood over the Internet and collect wood that is toxic for sale in online shops. In addition to the toys that are specifically made for rabbits, toys made for parrots often can be safe and use-ful objects for the pet rabbit.

In addition to simply leaving chewing objects on the floor, it can be enriching, both in terms of psychology and exercise, to hang toys, for example, from the top of the rab-bit's cage. As discussed previously, rabbits in the wild stand up to survey for preda-tors. This action requires use of the epaxial muscles of the spine, which stimulates deposition of calcium in the vertebrae. Insufficient opportunity or motivation to stand up may result in the vertebrae having insufficient calcification and, therefore, being more prone to fracture, just as in humans who get insufficient exercise.

In spite of having several safe objects to chew on, a rabbit may be attracted to household objects that are undesirable for them to chew on. The most serious is cords, in particular electrical cords, because rabbits can electrocute themselves chewing on electrical cords. This can be prevented by various means. One is to wrap the cord in multiple layers of duct tape. Another is to run it through pipes, such as polyvinyl chloride pipe, that can be obtained easily at home building stores. Some creativity may be required if the rabbit is attracted to valuable furniture. The wooden legs of many types of furniture are the most common objects for this type of behavior. They can be wrapped in Saran wrap, aluminum foil, or another material that protects the furniture from duct tape and then thoroughly wrapped in duct tape.

Digging

Underground warrens are important for the survival of rabbits in the wild. Digging war-rens also requires a large amount of effort. To accomplish this, the rabbit claws are long and very strong. They also have a strong, innate motivation to dig, which still ex-ists to some degree in most breeds of domestic rabbits. The best way to prevent a rab-bit from digging in things and locations the owner does not want it to is to provide it with regular access to acceptable opportunities to dig.

Digging boxes can be purchased or made. It is not essential that the substrate be dirt. A thick bed of straw that a rabbit can dig into and make a kind of nest works well for some rabbits. Sisal also is used to make items that a rabbit can make digging and scratching motions toward. Rabbits may make digging motions into a variety of household objects, such as carpets, quilts, and couch pillows. Having items that the rabbit is allowed to dig in and scratch at can address this problem. Gently discourage the rabbit from scratching at things that it is undesirable for the rabbit to scratch at, by picking it up whenever the undesired behavior begins and placing it on the acceptable substrate. Serious problems of digging can be prevented by teach-ing the rabbit to scratch and dig only at acceptable items when it is very young.

The need to dig also brings up the controversial topic of taking a rabbit outside and potentially even housing it outside to some degree. Being outside presents various dangers, including predators and insects, and because of this some people are totally opposed to taking rabbits outside at all. The outdoors, however, also can have advan-tages. If an owner can set up a secure pen, a house rabbit can be taken out to it so as to be able to dig directly into the dirt. Unless the pen is totally secured from potential predators, someone should stay with the rabbit while it is outside. An outside pen also presents an opportunity for enrichment, such as agility training. If a large, predator-proof cage is available, large quantities of hay and/or straw can be placed in it. Some rabbits manipulate and maneuver this material through a mixture of digging motions and pushing and pulling motions. Hay and straw that are to be used in this manner always should be checked for mold and any moldy material discarded.

Litter Box Training

Cats are able to be litter box trained because of their motivation to dig holes and bury their excrement. The motivation is totally different for rabbits. Rabbits have 2 kinds of feces, caecotrophs, which are eaten, and small, firm globe-shaped pellets approximately the size of a small English pea.

Caecotrophs are soft and look somewhat like a cluster of grapes. They are made in the caecum, where bacteria generate nutrients that are not available in grass and the other plants matter that rabbits eat. They often are mistakenly referred to as night feces. The caecotrophs are eaten immediately as they come out of the anus when a rabbit is in a quiet, safe location. In the domestic environment, this typically is at night, after all family members have gone to bed. In the wild, this happens during the night and during the day, when the rabbit is resting in the security of a room in the warren.

The pellets usually are deposited in specific latrines. In the wild, latrines often, although not always, are made on slightly elevated ground. They also may be made near one of the unhidden entrances to the warren. They usually are started by 1 or more rabbits using their strong front claws to dig a shallow bowl. Rabbits that need to defecate go to the latrine to do so.

It is this focus on location that is taken advantage of when litter box training a rabbit. If owners have a specific location in a specific room that they desire to be the location of the litter box, then when they first bring the rabbit home they need to confine it to that area. Some people use a rabbit cage or house as a location for the rabbit to rest, sleep in at night, and do their toileting. If that is the case, the rabbit should be placed in this house when it first arrives home. The owner should watch for which location, usually a corner, of the house the rabbit uses for eliminating and immediately place a litter box there. Triangular litter boxes work well for this situation. If owners are not using a cage or house for the rabbit, or if they want the litter box to not be in the house, then temporary penning needs to be set up to keep the rabbit in the section of the room that the owner wants to be the toileting area. If an owner simply wants the litter box to be in a particular room, then the rabbit can simply be confined to that room. In either case, the owner again watches to see where the rabbit chooses to eliminate and puts a box there. If owners prefer the box to be just a short distance away from what the rabbit initially chose, then they can move the box gradually a little bit, 2 to 6 cm each day, until it is exactly where the owner wants it to be. Once the litter box location is decided on and the rabbit consistently uses the litter box, the owner gradually can allow it access to more and more space.

Once they have had their initial litter box training, most rabbits identify the box as their latrine, allowing for even more flexibility in moving it. Some rabbits also may choose to move their litter box. They can accomplish this by pushing it with their head or grabbing the edge with their mouth and pulling it along. If it is essential that the litter box remain where it is, the owner may have to tie or clamp it in place. Otherwise, it generally is best to let the rabbit place the litter box where it wants it.

Selection of litter is a critical issue, because many of the litters made for cats are unsafe for rabbits. Rabbits often spend long periods of time just resting in their litter box. This is normal and, if owners who are first-time rabbit owners expresses concern about this behavior, a veterinarian can reassure them that it is not, generally, an indicator of illness. Rabbits also commonly eat their litter. Because of this, any litter that clumps is unsafe, because it clumps in the gastrointestinal tract and cause gastrointestinal blockage. Other litters are toxic if consumed. Some are unsafe simply because the fumes that emanate off of them irritate the rabbit's respiratory tract, initiating respiratory disease. **Table 1** shows common examples of safe and unsafe litters.

Just like cats, rabbits exhibit individual preferences for litter, and even litter box. Consistent use of the litter box requires that the owner identify which substrate the rabbit likes best. In some cases, the preferred substrate is a combination, such as peat moss and hay. Rabbits are different from cats in that they do not dig in the litter to bury their excrement. The pea-sized fecal pellets are deposited on the surface and left there, while urine trickles down to the bottom. The location of the urine can make the status of the litter's cleanliness deceptive. The surface may look clean, but if a lot of urine has been deposited in the box, ammonia fumes rise to the surface. Rabbit litter boxes are not cleaned by scooping. Instead, the entire contents of the box are dumped, the box is rinsed, and more litter is placed in the box.

Hiding

As a prey animal, the rabbit's main defense against predators is to hide in a secure, small space deep in the warren. It is important to provide house rabbits with structures that they can hide in. These can be made from cardboard or wood. Ideally, the entrance should be small, just big enough for the rabbit to enter. The interior should have a soft floor for the rabbit to rest on, such as a towel, a flat pillow, or some hay. The pet rabbit then can retreat to this structure to rest and consume its caecotrophs.

TREATING BEHAVIOR PROBLEMS
Human-directed Aggression

Human-directed aggression almost always is due to fear. The frightened rabbit may freeze, run away, or attack. Some rabbits start attacking the hands of anyone who sticks their hands in the rabbit's cage. This situation occurs most commonly if a rabbit is poorly socialized and spends most of its time confined to a cage. Initially, it may try to avoid the hands by hiding in the corner, but if it is grabbed, it may bite as a defensive maneuver. Most people drop the rabbit and remove their hands from the cage if this happens. At this point, the rabbit has learned that biting the scary hands results in the scary hands going away. This is an example of negative reinforcement. The action of biting increases because the rabbit has learned that if it bites, the aversive stimulus goes away. Rabbits that engage in this behavior are often referred to as cage aggressive.

Treatment of the fear aggressive rabbit typically involves a combination of extinction, desensitization, and counter-conditioning. The logistics of how these are done depend on how the rabbit is housed. The first step is to have 1 or more people stay near it much of the time without doing anything to it. They can toss treats gently to

Table 1	
Examples of commonly accessible substrates for a rabbit's litter box that are not safe and that are safe	
Unsafe Litters	**Safe Litters**
Clumping litter	Straw
Pine shavings	Hay
Cedar shavings	Peat moss
All other softwood shavings	Litter made from oats or alfalfa
Clay litter with deodorant crystals	Aspen bark
	Pelleted rabbit food
	Litters specifically made and marketed for rabbits

whatever distance the rabbit approaches in order to get a treat. In this circumstance, an exception may be made to the rule of avoiding the especially sweet treats, such as yogurt drops. Because most rabbits find them highly palatable, this results in an association of humans with something pleasant. Some rabbits adopt a strategy of "the best defense is a good offense." These rabbits charge humans and even bite. A person can deal with this by dressing defensively, for example, sturdy shoes that fully cover their feet; full-length pants made of a thick fabric, such as denim; and leather gloves. Leather gloves that are sold for gardening use can be satisfactory, but those used in falconry, which provide greater coverage of the wrist and arm, are better. Have some treats in a sealed container and sit where the rabbit can attack. With the protective clothing it can be easy to ignore their attacks because their bites do not have as much force as a dog or cat, and they do not have pointed canines. The rabbit, at this point, has learned that charging a person and biting make the person go away. The rabbit is likely to repeat what has worked before several times to drive the scary human away. When it stops, open the treat container and place or gently toss a treat near the rabbit.

A version of this technique can be used for the cage aggressive rabbit. It is easier if 2 people participate, but it is possible for 1 or 2 people to do so. One or both hands are placed through the door of the cage and just stay there, still. Again, if the rabbit charges and bites the gloves, it is easy to ignore this behavior. A treat can be dropped into the cage if there is a solid floor, or tongs can be used to move the treat through the wire if the floor is not solid. Again, only give the treat when the rabbit has stopped attacking.

Once enough progress has been made that the rabbit tolerates a human hand touching it, progress can slowly be made toward normal interaction. Briefly pet the rabbit and then give it a treat. Gradually pet the rabbit more and more extensively. Again, always pair this with a desired treat.

When the rabbit is comfortable being fully petted, begin the process of picking it up. Be sure to pick it up in a way that is secure so that the rabbit feels secure. Do not lift it very high, just 2 or 3 cm. Put it down and give it a treat. Gradually handle and play with the rabbit more and more, always making sure that nothing is done to make the rabbit feel fear or pain.

In the process, it is ideal if the original cause of the fear aggression can be identified. Did someone hit or pinch the rabbit or grab an ear? Did someone pick the rabbit up and drop it or even hold it in an insecure way? For the future, the entire family that the rabbit lives with, and any family friends who have interaction with the rabbit, need to review good practices of rabbit handling and interaction, making sure that no one does something to cause problems again.

Intraspecies Aggression

Rabbits are very social, living in large groups in their warrens. They also are territorial and drive away rabbits from other warrens that attempt to join them. A male rabbit moving from their natal warren to another warren is most likely to be successful outside the breeding season. This has to be taken into account when introducing a new rabbit, because aggression is likely.[9]

The basic principle is to introduce the rabbits gradually without their having the opportunity to fight. This can be done in several ways. One is to have each rabbit in a cage and set the cages down side by side. At first, place the cages far enough apart that neither rabbit exhibits charging or other signs of aggression. Over time, bring the cages closer and closer together but at a pace that does not trigger aggression. Put special foods, such as broccoli, carrots, and slices of apple, on the side of the cage nearest the other rabbit. This, again, associates the object of aggression with something pleasant.[10]

The next step is to expose them to each other without a barrier in between, but in such a way that fighting is difficult or unlikely. One method is to place them both in a bathtub. The insecure footing makes it impossible for either rabbit to leap into an attack. They also are less likely to exhibit even mild aggression, probably because they feel insecure on the slick surface compared with being on, for example, a rug or a grassy lawn. Another technique is to place them in the back seat of a car and take them on a car ride. Again, the insecurity of the situation makes them unlikely to be aggressive. They even may be huddled against each other after a while.[10]

The next step is to allow them to be together with no barrier between them and no insecure situation. For this, a harness and leash on each rabbit is advisable. Ideally, have 1 person holding each separate leash. Allow the rabbits to approach, sniff, and groom each other. One may lower its head while the other puts its head on top of the lowered head. If 1 or both rabbits start to bite, gently pull them apart. They must not be pulled apart with force, because this at minimum frightens them and may injure them. Again, have tasty food available. When they have had several sessions of this and are consistently exhibiting neutral behavior and friendly behavior, such as grooming each other, the leashes and, eventually, the harnesses can be removed.[10]

Sometimes rabbits that have been living together harmoniously develop an aggression problem. This usually is by 1 rabbit against the other. In this case, the harness and leash need to be used, at least on the aggressive rabbit.

Elimination Behavior Problems

A rabbit that is startled or frightened, for example, by children starting to yell in excitement over some game, may release several pellets of feces as it scurries away to a safer locale. These pellets easily are picked up and disposed of with a tissue. In this case, the best treatment is prevention, that is, make sure everyone in the family knows to not cause sudden, unexpected loud noises.[10]

Sometimes rabbits that have been consistently using their litter box start regularly eliminating outside the box. This can happen secondary to various stressors, such as changes in the household, for example, a new baby or a new pet, illness, or a disrupted schedule. If this happens, try to identify the stressor and ameliorate it, if possible. It may be best to keep the rabbit in its own room, where its box is, for a while, assuring that the family changes do not disturb it there. Also, consider if simple changes have happened, such as the rabbit's litter box substrate being abruptly changed. Like dogs and cats, rabbits may be frightened by thunderstorms, and eliminating where it happens to be when a severe storm starts can trigger an elimination problem. If it starts using a specific new location other than the current litter box, it may be easiest to add a second litter box at that site. If that is not an option, block the rabbit's access to the site.

There are many other possibilities for loss of desired elimination behavior, and a detailed behavioral history is necessary to identify these.

Destruction of Household Items

Destruction of household items usually happens because the owners, unaware of the rabbit's need to dig and chew, have not provided the rabbit with an adequate number and variety of items designed for rabbits to dig into and/or chew on. Client education is important. It can be useful to have handouts briefly describing why a pet rabbit would engage in these behaviors and giving examples how to provide the rabbit with its own items to dig in and chew on and how to protect household items while the rabbit learns to use its own items.[10–15] Ideally, a veterinarian visits pet stores that are near the practice to be aware of what is easily available and lets clients know about those. There also are many items for rabbits that are sold over the Internet. Veterinarians should make a list of sites that are currently available. A list is not provided in this article because this information is subject to change, and determination of what are current sites is best.

Overgrooming and Self-mutilation

Just as dogs, cats, parrots, and other species kept in captivity rabbits may overgroom themselves, removing excessive amounts of fur or feathers, and even proceed to self-mutilation. While genetics is a contributing factor,[16] this problem usually begins with some sort of stressor, such as the companion rabbit starting to repeatedly exhibit mild aggression or the regular wailing of a new baby. As with the development of litter box problems due to stressors, a complete history is needed to identify what may be the stressor or stressors. Again, eliminate or at least ameliorate them. Evaluate the rabbit's environment for suitable enrichment in the form of toys and digging sites and suitable safe areas in the form of hiding places.[10]

SUMMARY

The domestic rabbit *O cuniculus* is a prey animal. As well as being domestic, it still lives in wild colonies in much of Europe and the United Kingdom. Its major means of survival is to dig warrens, which comprise tunnels and periodic wider spaces providing rooms. Being small and, generally, nonaggressive, the domestic rabbit makes an excellent pet. It needs to be provided with places to hide when it is frightened, so that it can relax. It is easily trained to use a litter box because the species naturally selects a specific site to be a latrine for defecation. It has open-rooted teeth that grow throughout its life. In the wild, these are worn down constantly by the rabbit chewing on rough forage. The house rabbit needs to be provided with numerous safe, nontoxic, items to chew in order to keep the teeth appropriately worn down. Because digging is critical to survival in the wild, its motivation to dig and scratch is strong, and it needs to be provided with sites in and structures on which to dig and scratch. Staying still all the time, which is what happens when a rabbit is confined to a small hutch, is not natural and leads to weak muscles and bones as well as poor psychological health. Rabbits need the opportunity to run, jump on and over things, and investigate the world with their strong curiosity.

DISCLOSURE

The author has nothing to disclose.

REFERENCES

1. Sandford JC. Notes on the history of the rabbit. J Appl Rabbit Res 1992;15:1–28.
2. Nelissen M. On the diurnal rhythm of activity of *Oryctolagus cuniculus* (Linne, 1758). Acta Zool Pathol Antverp 1975;61:3–18.
3. Monclús R, Rödel HG. Different forms of vigilance in response to the presence of predators and conspecifics in a group-living mammal, the European rabbit. Ethology 2008;114:287–97.
4. United States Department of Agriculture. U.S. Rabbit Industry Profile; 2002. Available at: ttps://naldc.nal.usda.gov/catalog/46311.

5. Cowan DP. Group living in the European rabbit (*Oryctolagus cuniculus*): Mutual benefit or resource localization? J Anim Ecol 1987;56:779–95.
6. Lockley RM. The private life of the rabbit. New York: Macmillan Publishing Co; 1903. p. 27–70.
7. Davis H, Gibson JA. Can rabbits tell humans apart? Discrimination of individual humans and its implications for animal research. Comp Med 2000;5:483–5.
8. Csatádi K, Kustos K, Eiben CS, et al. Even minimal human contact linked to nursing reduces fear responses toward humans in rabbits. Appl Anim Behav Sci 1995;205:123–8.
9. Lockley RM. Social structure and stress in the rabbit warren. J Anim Ecol 1961; 30:385–423.
10. Crowell-Davis SL. Behavior problems in pet rabbits. J Exot Pet Med 2007;16: 38–44.
11. Hulls WL, Brooks DL, Beans-Knudsen D. Response of adult New Zealand white rabbits to enrichment objects and paired housing. Lab Anim Sci 1991;41:609–12.
12. Love JA. Group housing: Meeting the physical and social needs of the laboratory rabbit. Lab Anim Sci 1994;44:5–11.
13. Whary M, Peper R, Borkowski G, et al. The effects of group housing on the research use of the laboratory rabbit. Lab Anim 1993;27:330–41.
14. Baumans V. Environmental enrichment for laboratory rodents and rabbits: Requirements of rodents, rabbits, and research. ILAR J 2005;46:162–70.
15. Hansen LT, Berthelsen H. The effect of environmental enrichment on the behavior of caged rabbits (*Oryctolagus cuniculus*). Appl Anim Behav Sci 2000;68:163–78.
16. Iglauer F, Beig C, Dimigen J, et al. Hereditary Compulsive Self-Mutilating Behavior in Laboratory Rabbits. Lab Anim 1995;29:385–93.

Miniature Pet Pig Behavioral Medicine

Valarie V. Tynes, DVM, DACVB, DACAW*

KEYWORDS

- Miniature pigs • Potbellied pigs • Aggression • House soiling • Exploration
- Destruction • House training • Foraging

KEY POINTS

- Miniature pigs can make excellent pets but their behavioral and environmental needs are unique; if not provided, behavior problems are likely.
- Pigs are highly social animals who readily use overt aggression to establish a social order.
- Pigs are readily house trained because of their naturally discriminating elimination behavior.
- A highly enriched environment (preferably outdoors) that allows the pig to show many of its species' typical behaviors help decrease the incidence of unwanted behaviors.
- Frequent gentle handling, positive reinforcement training, and an avoidance of punishment are most likely to lead to a pig that is an enjoyable pet.

INTRODUCTION

The miniature pig fad began in the United States in the early 1980s with the importation of the Vietnamese potbellied pig. A variety of miniature pet pigs can now be found in the pet trade and they continue to maintain some of the physical and behavioral features typical of the Vietnamese potbellied pig, so they may be referred to as potbellied pigs or simply miniature pigs (**Fig. 1**).

All miniature pigs are simply different breeds or varieties of the domesticated pig, *Sus scrofa domestica*. The first Vietnamese potbellied pigs were typical of the domesticated pigs found across southeastern Asia. They are sway backed and potbellied, often with legs so short that the belly touches, or almost touches, the ground. They have wrinkled, short faces with small upright ears and straight tails. Obesity is a common problem in the miniature pet pig and can lead to a greatly shortened life span (**Fig. 2**). It has been suggested that, with good preventive health care, miniature pigs may live to be 15 to 20 years of age.

A common problem for many pet pig owners is that how 1 individual interprets the meaning of the word miniature and how another individual interprets the meaning of

Companion Animal, Ceva Animal Health, PO Box 1413, Sweetwater, TX 79556, USA
* Corresponding author
E-mail address: pigvet@hughes.net

Vet Clin Exot Anim 24 (2021) 63–86
https://doi.org/10.1016/j.cvex.2020.09.004
1094-9194/21/© 2020 Elsevier Inc. All rights reserved.

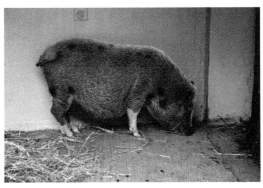

Fig. 1. A miniature pig with several features typical of the Vietnamese potbellied pig: round potbelly, slightly swayed back, straight tail, erect ears, and a short snout. The silver coloring and black spots were not common in the Vietnamese potbellied pigs that were originally bred, shown, and sold in the United States in the 1980s.

the word can be vastly different. Many of the different breeds of miniature pigs average 45 to 57 kg (100–125 pounds) and although that is certainly miniature compared with the average commercial breeding swine that may weigh 225 to 360 kg (500–800 pounds) at maturity, it seems enormous to pet owners who imagined that they were acquiring a pet that would weigh 11 to 23 kg (25–50 pounds) fully grown.

When pet pigs grow significantly larger than their owners expect them to, any and all behavior problems can be perceived as much more insurmountable than they might otherwise be if the owners were more prepared for the fully-grown size of these pets. For this reason, many miniature pet pigs were relinquished to animal shelters and pig sanctuaries in the late 1980s and throughout the 1990s, sometimes because of complaints about their size but often because of complaints regarding their behavior. Because of the small number of veterinarians seeing pet pigs at this time,

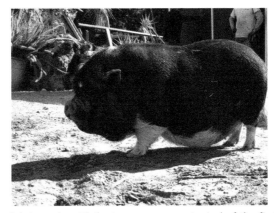

Fig. 2. An obese miniature pig with features even more typical of the first Vietnamese potbellied pigs bred and shown in the United States; the back is shorter and has more sway, and the face is wrinkled with a shorter snout. The obesity is common and, as seen here, often results in a pig that can barely see because of the thick folds of fat around its eyes. In addition, the weight, often combined with overgrown nails, leads to chronic overextension of the carpal joints, and subsequent degenerative joint disease.

treatment was often not attempted so little has been learned regarding the cause, development, and effective treatment of these problems.

SENSES AND COMMUNICATION

A basic understanding of how a particular species perceives the world can help clinicians to better understand their unique responses to stimuli as well as some of their basic behavioral needs.

Domestic pigs evolved from a highly social, forest-dwelling ancestor with largely diurnal activity patterns. Most of their time is spent foraging for food on or under the ground in dimly lit areas while trying to avoid predation. Olfaction and vocalizations by necessity evolved to become their most important sensory modalities, with audition playing a slightly less critical role, and vision and visual cues were least important to their success in this type of environment.

Vision and Visual Cues

Pet owners often believe that the pig has poor eyesight because it startles easily but the visual acuity of the pig is not bad; it is simply not as good as that of humans. They probably startle easily because they see better at a distance than they do at close range, which is common in prey animals whose eyes are located on the sides of their head so as to see approaching predators. They do not need to see well at close range. Good vision and complex visual cues are simply not as useful to the pig as are its other senses.[1] However, pigs can discriminate between people using visual cues, even in dim light (20 lux)[2] and they do have dichromatic color vision.[3] The visual acuity of individual pigs does seem to differ greatly.[4] Obese pet pigs often have poor eyesight, simply because their vision becomes obscured by rolls of fat. This limitation can lead to irritability and increased aggression in some cases.

Olfaction

Olfaction is an important means of communication in many mammals and the pig is no exception. The pig's sense of smell is well developed and research has shown that pigs can recognize other pigs by the odor of their urine.[5,6]

When pigs investigate conspecifics they concentrate on sniffing the facial region, underside of the belly, and the anogenital region.[7] When rendered anosmic by surgical ablation of the olfactory bulbs, pig can still establish a hierarchy but the level of aggression directed toward unacquainted pigs is significantly reduced. These results are similar to those found when pigs were blinded with opaque contact lenses; aggression was reduced but not eradicated. This finding adds further support to the belief that the stimulus for the initiation and continuance of aggression in pigs is multisensory.[8]

Taste

Surprisingly little is known about the sense of taste in the pig. However, research has shown that pigs display a strong preference for glucose, sucrose, fructose, lactose, and saccharin solutions.[9,10] A great deal of individual variation in preferences has been noted, especially with regard to saccharin; some individuals seem to strongly prefer saccharin, whereas others seem to find it strongly aversive.[11]

Pigs show an aversion to quinine, suggesting that they can taste bitter flavors.[11] They also have no preference for salt solutions, as do some other herbivores.[11] They find very strong salt solutions aversive but, if the solution is not too strong, the pig's aversion can be overcome by thirst.

Audition

The hearing range of the pig is similar to that of most other hoofed mammals, with an average range at 60 dB of 42 Hz to 40.5 kHz.[12] Their ability to hear low frequencies is much better than their ability to hear high frequencies, which is also a feature common to hoofed mammals.[12] The pig's ears are relatively immobile, so localizing sound usually requires that they turn the entire head.

Vocalizations

Kiley[1] described the vocalizations of the pig as occurring on a continuum rather than being discreet sounds with a separate meaning for each.[1] Vocalizations are strongly affected by the level of excitement and are generally representative of the pig's motivational state. In general, amplitude, frequency, and pitch of the vocalizations increase as the animal becomes more excited. A low-pitched vocalization, referred to as the common grunt, serves as a contact call for the pig.[1] It indicates the location of the pig for other pigs in the group. It is also frequently used when the pig is foraging, rooting, or eating, and when a familiar noise or change in the environment occurs. The sound of a common grunt from one pig usually leads other nearby pigs to respond in kind.[1]

The staccato grunt is a form of the common grunt. It is shorter and occurs in many of the same situations as the common grunt but is more likely to be heard as the level of excitement grows. For example, a pig that hears food being delivered into the bowl but is unable to get to it will progress from a common grunt to a staccato grunt. The staccato grunt is likely to precede a squeal and often follows a sequence of squeals.[1]

The bark is a short, open-mouthed grunt with a high amplitude initially that occurs when the pig is startled or frightened.[1] It is often followed by the pig freezing. Any of the grunts may be repeated, sometimes with no interval between them, so that they become 1 long, frequently accented call. Repeated grunts are common in situations of frustration, especially if the frustrating situation is prolonged. Repeated staccato grunts are particularly characteristic of greeting and usually elicit a similar response from the pig being greeted. Higher-pitched vocalizations such as squeals and screams increase in rate and length as the pig becomes increasingly excited. Repeated grunts may progress to squeals as pigs become more frustrated or thwarted, such as when a piglet cannot reach the teat.[1]

The most common call made by piglets is the squeal.[1] Squeals are short, repeated calls with constant pitch changes. Once a pig is more than 6 months old, squeals turn to screams.[1] Screams are extremely loud, high-pitched, open-mouthed calls that are longer than squeals. Any unpleasant situation may elicit a scream but they are extremely characteristic of painful or fearful situations.[1] Piglets being castrated without anesthesia produce more high-frequency calls than sham-castrated piglets. These calls are especially pronounced during the severing of the spermatic cord, further suggesting that high rates of higher-frequency calls are a reliable indicator of pain in the pig.[13]

When pigs, especially juveniles, are separated from conspecifics and/or placed in a novel environment, their rate and pitch of vocalization increase.[14] Piglets that are hungry also vocalize more often, at higher pitches and higher rates than piglets that are well fed.[15]

NORMAL BEHAVIOR OF SWINE

Understanding the normal behavior of swine establishes the foundation for understanding the problem behaviors that are common to pet pigs and for differentiating normal behaviors from pathologic behaviors. In the authors experience, pathologic behaviors are uncommon in miniature pet pigs. What is more common is behavior that is best described as maladaptive.[16] These behaviors occur as a result of the pig attempting to adapt to an environment that is unnatural and/or inappropriate; an environment that fails to meet the pig's basic behavioral needs and thus often leaves the pig in a chronic state of frustration or conflict and stress (or more accurately, distress). Another subset of behavior problem arises because of the pet owners lack of knowledge as to how to train the pet appropriately (eg, house soiling). In addition, some behaviors that pet owners complain about are normal pig behaviors that pet owners simply find unacceptable. In these cases, pet owners need to be educated as to how to manage the pet so that these behaviors are less problematic for the owner as opposed to attempting to change the normal behavior of the pig.

Social Behavior

The social behaviors of wild and feral swine are similar and have been well documented. Normal social behavior in most breeds of domesticated swine, including the miniature breeds, shares similar features with their wild counterparts. Most research on the social behavior of the pig has been performed on commercial swine under intensive rearing conditions, because of the many challenges that their normal social behavior poses under these conditions. Minimal research has been performed on the social behavior of miniature swine and even less on pet pigs, so what is known of normal swine social behavior must be extrapolated to a unique situation: a single pig, living in a home with people and other pets.

Swine are highly social species with the ability to make lasting associations with both conspecifics and even humans. Under natural conditions, swine have a matrilineal-type social organization, with the sow and her offspring of the year making up the social group. These groups are called sounders. The animals that make up a sounder seem to be strongly bonded to each other and their behavior is synchronous. Typically, female offspring maintain a close bond with their mother after they mature, whereas male offspring disperse. Other individuals, such as young from the previous year and males, may exist on the periphery of the sounder. Adult males associate more closely with the group whenever a female in the group is showing sexual receptivity.[17,18] Groups of pigs seldom join another strange group of pigs.[19]

Wild and feral swine can have large home ranges (1–25 km^2 [100–2500 ha]) but do not actively defend territory.[18] They do use chemical communication as they move about their territory and have been seen leaving chemical cues by rubbing their faces and their sides on items as they move about the environment. They may also rub their perineal region on the ground in an anogenital rub.[18] These chemical cues may help sounders recognize when groups of unrelated pigs are nearby so they can actively avoid encountering them.

A stable linear hierarchy seems to exist among groups living in natural conditions, and few agonistic interactions are seen except around food. These agonistic interactions are rare when food is abundant.[17] When foraging and feeding, individuals in a group tend to space themselves out and remain several meters apart.[20] This avoidance behavior is just 1 strategy pigs use to avoid conflict.

Pigs are unique among domesticated animals in that they enter the world prepared to use aggression to ensure their own survival, and they are born with the weapons necessary for the job. At birth they possess a fully erupted set of canine teeth, referred to as needle teeth. Neonatal piglets are extremely precocious and can stand, walk, and attempt to nurse within minutes of birth. Piglets begin searching for a teat right away and, once they contact a teat and begin suckling from it, they begin using their needle teeth aggressively against their littermates in order to defend that teat.[18] Within about 24 hours, each piglet has identified a particular teat as its own and continues to defend that teat until weaning. Most piglets more than a day of age have numerous scratches on their faces from competing with their siblings for a teat. After about 24 hours, the teat order is relatively stable and usually remains the same until weaning.[21] As the teat order stabilizes, fighting between piglets declines significantly.[22]

Aggression continues to play an important role in the lives of feral, wild, and domesticated swine[18] because whenever unacquainted pigs are introduced it is likely that there will be vigorous fighting initially in an attempt to establish a hierarchy. This behavior has been studied extensively in commercial swine because of the common practice of mixing multiple litters at weaning. This practice predictably results in injury and decreased weight gain initially, and is considered a welfare issue, so much study has been designed to understand it and develop methods to reduce it. This scenario is rare in swine living in a natural environment.

Fighting in newly mixed swine is most frequent during the first 24 hours and, by 48 hours, a social order is established, after which fighting decreases dramatically.[7] The facial musculature of the pig is less differentiated than in other ungulates so their facial expressions are limited. When pigs encounter unacquainted pigs, their behavior may initially be limited to a broadside display, with hair on the dorsal midline erected and some head-to-tail circling and shoulder-to-shoulder shoving. Another commonly seen agonistic threat is an open-mouthed, lateral toss of the head directed toward the threatened individual. It is often accompanied by a short grunt and rarely seems to include a real attempt to bite. When boars fight, they may also paw the ground and circle shoulder to shoulder while chomping their jaws and producing, thick, white foamy saliva. Although there may be some visual importance attached to the presence of this saliva, the pheromone that it contains is probably sending the more important message.

When fighting among pigs continues, it may include head-to-head or head-to-shoulder butting (head knocks) and progress to both combatants attempting to bite and shove each other about the head and ears. Later, the 2 pigs may stand with their heads to the other pigs' flank and circle while attempting to bite the other's back legs and flanks. They sometimes circle this way until exhausted. Eventually, 1 pig may turn to flee and the other pig chases it, attempting to bite its back legs as it runs away. Sometimes a threatened pig immediately retreats from the aggressor without fighting. In a few instances, 2 pigs simply stare at each other for several seconds before 1 pig retreats, apparently accepting its role as the subordinate.[7] Close examination of the other pig, concentrating on the face, the underside of the belly, and the anogenital region, may also occur when pigs first meet, and, once the initial aggression subsides, this investigative behavior becomes even more intense.[7]

Sometimes submission in the pig can be difficult to recognize because there does not seem to be a clear sign that turns off an attack by a dominant pig. However, subordinate behaviors other than turning or running away from threats and attacks may include standing with drooping ears and tail, with the back arched.[7] A subtle turn of the head away from the threat, or even a turn of the entire body sideways to the threatening individual, has also been described. The benefits of higher status in the hierarchy are clear: dominant pigs have freer access to food, water, and resting places of their choosing. They typically have the ability to displace a subordinate pig from a location that they desire. When 1 pig can be seen to displace another pig at a feeding station or other location, the pig that leaves without a fight can be clearly recognized as a subordinate pig.

Body weight seems to play the most significant role in attaining and maintaining a higher social rank after mixing in commercial swine. Larger pigs typically are the first to begin fighting after mixing and gain higher status.[23] However, attaining higher social status has been shown to be affected by many other additional factors, including age, sex, and experience.[7]

It is the highly social nature of pigs that can make them such appealing pets, but their willingness to use overt aggression under a variety of circumstances can be problematic.

Comfort Behavior and Body Care

Pigs do not sweat[24] and they typically maintain a thick layer of body fat. They are therefore more sensitive to the effects of heat than to cold and they must thermoregulate by changing their behavior. When living outdoors, as temperatures start to increase to more than 14°C to 15°C (59°F), pigs attempt to cool themselves by staying wet or wallowing in mud. Studies have shown that mud provides evaporative cooling that lasts longer than the cooling provided by plain water alone,[24] which may explain why pigs are so quick to make a mud wallow out of any available water. By 26°C to 30°C, most pigs prefer to seek shade if a wallow is not available to them.[25] If a pig is not given shade and some form of wallow at temperatures more than 21°C, they may even use their urine and feces to make a wallow,[25–27] providing further evidence for the importance of a proper environment if the pet owner wants a pet pig to stay clean.

Even in temperatures less than 14°C, pigs spend a certain amount of time in a wallow if one is available, suggesting that wallowing also plays an important role in skin and hair care.[28] As temperatures increase, pigs also spend more time rubbing their trunks and hindquarters against objects in their environment, suggesting that this behavior may also play a role in temperature regulation. Rubbing behavior is also suspected to play a role in ectoparasite control and be a form of comfort behavior.[18]

Pigs spend more time resting than any other domestic animal.[29] When resting, pigs have a clear preference for lying in close contact with conspecifics. Only when temperatures increase do they spread out and avoid skin-to-skin contact. When overly warm, they lie in full lateral recumbency and seek a cooler surface that allows heat transfer from their bodies to the floor.[30] When temperatures decrease (<21°C), pigs seek bedded areas and spend more time lying in sternal recumbency with an increased amount of skin-to-skin contact with their pen mates so as to conserve body heat.[30,31]

Free-living pigs and those living in seminatural conditions show similar shade-seeking and wallow-seeking behaviors during the midday hours when temperatures increase to more than 18°C.[20] These pigs were found to build communal nests each evening. Most older animals in the group participate in nest building by carrying nest materials to the nest or raking materials in and around the nest. Pigs have been seen carrying these nest materials for up to 20 m. These nests average about 3 m in circumference.[20]

Similar nesting behavior is commonly seen in the pet house pig, if given materials such as quilts, blankets, or comforters in which to nest. If not provided with nesting materials, pet pigs may become destructive in their attempt to build a nest for sleeping.

Excretory Behavior

Pigs are known for their discriminating eliminative behavior, and this can make them easy to house train as long as their particular needs are met. When given the appropriate environment, they generally eliminate in 1 location and attempt to keep their resting area clean.[32] Pigs typically drink, urinate, and defecate in close sequence, and studies in commercial swine have shown that wherever the waterer is placed, that is where the dunging area is likely to be.[33] Studies of domestic piglets found that piglets seemed to preferentially defecate near the walls of the pen and that most elimination occurred immediately after feeding and before playing.[34] Some studies have shown a preference for elimination on straw bedding when it is available.[34] All of these preferences can be used to inform the preparation of housing for the pig and the presentation of a litter box that the pig is most likely to use. However, when pigs are allowed outdoors, they seem to prefer eliminating outdoors. The availability of shade also increases the chance that they will eliminate outdoors instead of indoors.[35]

Ingestive Behavior

Swine are omnivores and in the wild spend a significant amount of their waking hours foraging for food. Studies of the activity budgets of wild boars, either captive or free ranging, show that they spend more than 50% of their time resting and 20% to 25% of their time eating or rooting.[17,36] Studies of domestic pigs living in seminatural environments found similar activity budgets, with pigs spending 52% of the daylight period foraging and another 23% moving about exploring the environment.[20] Resting time increases when food is supplied in abundant quantities.[17] In general, the natural behavior of swine is designed to conserve energy and this greatly contributes to the problem of obesity in pet pigs.

Pigs use their specialized noses to root for edible items below the surface of the soil. Feral swine consume whatever plant material is seasonally available but also eat, earthworms, insects, frogs, snakes, turtles, rodents, and eggs of ground-nesting birds. Swine also eat carrion, including carcasses of other pigs, and readily eat garbage, if available.[18]

Domestic swine living in confinement have been shown to have a strongly diurnal pattern of behavior.[31] The amount of food and water consumed is also affected by temperature; pigs eat less and drink more as temperatures increase.[37]

It is normal for captive swine to alternate between eating and drinking until satisfied. **Box 1** provides information on managing this problem in pet pigs. If fed by hand, they consume all of their food and then drink.[38] In general, swine prefer to eat several small

---

Box 1
Managing messy eating and drinking

Pigs commonly alternate between eating and drinking until satisfied, so they can be very messy. This behavior cannot be stopped but it can be managed. Following are some suggestions for managing the problem:

- Place food and water bowls in a mud-boot tray or dog feeding tray that is large enough to contain the mess.
- Some pet owners have found that placing the food and water bowl in a shower stall in a bathroom allows easy clean up.
- Feed the pig outdoors and provide water outdoors from a nipple-type feeder.
- Warn pet owners that, if they provide pigs water in a bowl outdoors, they are likely to turn it over regularly to create a wallow.
- Ideally, pigs should not be offered their food in bowls but instead should have their food offered in food puzzles or other foraging-type devices.
- Pet owners should be warned that they must never restrict water to their pigs because this can result in fatal dehydration and possibly salt toxicity.

meals throughout the day. One study of group-housed swine found that they ate 10 to 12 meals daily and most meals were consumed in less than 2 minutes. With higher temperatures, pigs consumed less by eating the same number of smaller meals each day.

It has also been noted that, when food is restricted to swine, they drink proportionally more water as if to compensate.[39] This tendency can pose a problem for many pet pig owners, who commonly underfeed their pigs in an attempt to keep them small. The subsequent increased water consumption can make house training challenging in these pigs.

Exploratory Behavior

Pigs normally investigate edible and nonedible items by sniffing, rooting, biting, and chewing. Although some of this behavior may be appetitive (searching for food to relieve hunger, also called extrinsic exploration) some of it is apparently caused by curiosity, a strong motivation to gather information about the environment, also known as intrinsic exploration. Pigs clearly have a strong desire to forage and root.[40] Although some studies have shown that restricting food does increase foraging behavior, ad libitum feeding does not completely alleviate the pig's motivation to explore.[41]

Multiple studies have shown that pigs will work to gain access to novel items and materials that they can explore by rooting. Analysis of several studies that examined pig behavior in relation to environmental enrichment clearly shows that pigs prefer items that are changeable by manipulating and destroying them. This changeability is what seems to keep items novel to the pigs, because pigs seem to lose interest in nondestructive items such as tires, chains, bars, and nylon dog bones within a short period of time.[40] Straw and frayed ropes are examples of items that seem to maintain most pigs' interest.

COMMON PROBLEM BEHAVIORS

As is the case with most problem behaviors in pets, behavior problems in the pet pig are much easier to prevent than to treat. In addition, if appropriate methods for solving problems are used quickly, when problems are first noted, they are much easier to change. Following are some guidelines for acquiring a pet pig (**Box 2**) that may help pet owners avoid certain problems, as well as a description of the more common behavior-related complaints associated with pet pigs, and methods for treating them.

Unruly Behavior/Difficulty Handling

Once the new pig is settled into its new home, habituation to handling should begin immediately. Pet owners may need to be educated that, unlike dogs and cats, sows do not pick up their piglets and carry them. The only thing that picks up a baby pig is a predator. Therefore, when grasped and picked up, the pig's first instinct is to panic, scream, and try to escape. The pig owner must be prepared to invest time in repeated gentle handling of the pig in association with food so that the pig learns to associate the person with good things.

Harness and leash training should also begin right away and similarly be combined with a lot of positive reinforcement either with food or scratching. Most pigs seem to enjoy being scratched behind the front legs. Many pigs roll over when scratched in this area. Pigs are not capable of reaching many parts of their bodies with their legs or mouths for the purpose of grooming, as many animals do, so rubbing, scratching, or brushing them can often be highly reinforcing. The key is to note what the pig seems

> **Box 2**
> **Acquiring a pet pig**
>
> *Pet pigs are most easily acquired by adoption from a shelter or sanctuary or by purchasing from a breeder*
>
> If acquiring from a shelter or sanctuary:
> - Be aware that some pigs are there because of problem behaviors, but, just as likely, they were given up because they grew too big or otherwise failed to meet someone's expectations. Others are given up after people discover that pigs are not allowed by their city or property owners association.
> - The pet owner should acquire as much information about the pig's history as possible. In many cases, the pig's behavior improves in a sanctuary setting because they are given a more natural environment and are able to socialize with other pigs.
> - Pet owners should be prepared to adopt 2 pigs because many sanctuaries currently only adopt pigs in pairs because of their strongly held belief that it is in the best interests of the pig and may decrease the incidence of certain behavior problems. There is some evidence to suggest that pigs living in a multipig household are less likely to show human-directed aggression.[42]
> - If given a proper environment, many of these adult pigs still bond to a new owner and make excellent pets.
>
> *Anyone wishing to acquire a baby pig should be certain to purchase from a reputable breeder*
>
> Reputable breeders:
> - Do not sell piglets before 8 weeks of age.
> - Do not guarantee the adult size of the pigs they are selling.
> - Welcome people to visit the site before and after acquiring their pets.
> - Are knowledgeable about pigs and provide the new pet owners with plenty of resources to guide them.
> - Express a willingness to take the pigs back if the owners find they can no longer keep them.
> - Provide health records for the pigs.
>
> Early-life experiences have been shown to play an important role in the development of the behavior of pigs. Under natural, free-range conditions, piglets are not weaned until they are between 8 and 15 weeks of age, and this is a gradual process rather than an abrupt one.[43] Sudden and early (between 3 and 5 weeks) separation from the sow is common in intensively farmed pigs and is unnecessary when raising pigs for pets. This abrupt premature weaning has been proved in studies of commercial swine to be extremely stressful and contributes to decreased play behavior, increased plasma cortisol levels, and increased aggression,[44–46] all of which could be problematic in miniature pet pigs as well. In addition, piglets gain social experience while interacting with their sows and their littermates. This socialization has been shown to help pigs establish stable dominance hierarchies more quickly when they are later regrouped,[47] and multiple studies have reported the positive effects of socialization on agonistic behavior in commercial swine.[48] Well-socialized individuals engage in fewer, shorter, and less intense bouts of fighting than nonsocialized piglets.[48] Although there is no guarantee that this will translate into a pet pig that shows less human-directed aggression, it is highly likely that it will affect the ability of the pet pig to later be introduced safely to another pig if the owner chooses to do so. Fighting will still occur, but any introductions should be much less problematic than they might be if the pig had limited social experience with other pigs.

to prefer and then repeat that behavior when the pig is being exposed to something novel, such as the harness, as a means of making a positive association.

Pigs should never be forcibly held for any procedure or activity. Forcible holding does not teach them to tolerate it; it only increases their fear of the event and may also increases their fear of the person who is forcing the procedure on them. Habituation and classical conditioning are the most effective techniques for preventing unruly behavior in the pig and teaching the pig to be more tolerant of handling.

House Training and Preventing House Soiling

House soiling problems are common in pet pigs when the pet owners, unaware of the pigs' natural behaviors, attempt to house train them using some of the same methods that they would use with a puppy. Many pet owners recognize right away that the pig needs to be confined, but confine it with a litter pan in an area that is so small that the pig is reluctant to eliminate, because of its natural desire to avoid eliminating near where it sleeps (**Box 3**). If allowed out of confinement without close supervision, it will then attempt to establish a latrine site away from its resting area. This site may be in another room or behind a piece of furniture, in an apparent attempt by the pig to avoid being disturbed.

When pet owners wish to house train a pig, the first questions that must be answered are:

- Does the pet owner want the pig to always eliminate indoors and use a litter pan?
- Does the pet owner wish to begin with a litter pan and eventually train the pig to eliminate outside?
- Will the pet owner be home most of the day while the pig is being house trained or must the owner be gone from the home for more than 3 or 4 hours at a time?

If the answer to the first question is yes, the pet owner should be warned right away that this may be the most challenging approach. Even pigs that are litter trained young seem to prefer eliminating outdoors as they get older. Many begin to avoid eliminating until their owners allow them outside and then they eliminate. They seem to have a strong preference for that option and no research has been done to establish why this might be. It may simply be the nature of the pig or it may have something to do with the inability to offer an ideal box or substrate for elimination; something that is so ideal that the pig would prefer to use it as opposed to going outdoors.

The answer to this first question will also allow a determination of whether the pet owner is planning on attempting to make the pig an indoor-only pet. Some people still mistakenly believe that the pig can be a pet that is restricted to the indoors. However, for a variety of reasons that will become more apparent later, when discussed in relation to problem behaviors, this is not recommended. In the author's experience, it is virtually impossible to provide for pet pigs' behavioral needs if they are confined

---

Box 3
Appropriate indoor confinement for the pet pigs

- The space must be small enough that the pig does not choose its own space for elimination but large enough that the pig will eliminate there.
- The litter pan must be able to be placed as far away from the sleeping area as possible.
- If the pan can also be placed far away from food and water, that is ideal.
- If these rules of thumb are followed and the pig still chooses an alternate location to eliminate within the confinement area, then it is too large. It should be made smaller and, if possible, the box placed in the area the pig first chose to eliminate.
- If the pig does not eliminate in the box or the confinement area when left confined for more than a few hours, it may be that the area is too small and crowded for the pig to feel comfortable eliminating there. In these cases, the owner will note that, the minute the pig is released from the confinement, it begins looking for a place to eliminate. If allowed outside immediately after release from confinement, then the pig will likely hurry to a spot and eliminate.

indoors. Pigs not allowed adequate time outdoors show more problem behaviors and have poor welfare.

If the pet owner wants to begin by litter training the pig, but is prepared for it to go outdoors as soon as it is able, this is ideal, especially for young pigs (2–6 months of age). Very young pigs need to urinate frequently, so, if the owner is going to be gone for several hours a day and the pig must be home alone, then confinement with a litter box is necessary in order to successfully house train the pig. **Box 4** provides litter and litter box suggestions for pet pigs. If the owner is going to be home all day with the pig, then litter training is not necessary. The pig can be taken outside at regular intervals and only confined when the owner is not able to supervise closely. As long as the pig can be taken outside hourly for the first few weeks and every 2 to 3 hours for the next couple of months, a litter box may not be required within the pig's crate or confinement area.

Once the plan for house training is chosen (litter box, outdoors, or combination), then the basic rules for house training any pet can be followed:

1. Prevent accidents by confinement, close supervision, and regular outings (if wanting the pig to eliminate outdoors).
2. Feed the pig on a regular schedule and take the pig outside (if not using a box) on a regular schedule, remembering that the pig is likely to need to eliminate after waking up and after eating.
3. Reinforce desired behaviors; if the pig is seen eliminating in the litter box, say quiet words of praise and as soon as the pig finishes eliminating, praise and offer a small food reward. If taking the pig outside, follow the same guidelines; as soon as the pig begins posturing to eliminate, say quiet words of praise. When the pig finishes, praise and offer a small food reward.

Box 4
Guidelines for litter training pet pigs:

- The container chosen for the litter box must be large enough for the pig to turn around in completely.

- The entrance to the box must be low enough that the pig can easily step into it, which requires that most boxes be modified by cutting the entryway down low enough so that the pig can enter without having to jump into the box.

- The litter for the pig should not be traditional clay or clumping cat litter. Pigs like to eat the litter and this can lead to serious health problems if they are given clay. Specialized litters such as wheat-based, alfalfa-based, or recycled paper litters may be used.

- Other safe litters include shredded newspaper, straw or hay, and wood shavings, such as those used for small mammal bedding or horse stalls.

- Most of the litters that are safe for pigs are not very absorbent so waste needs to be removed at least once daily. Leaving some odor associated with the waste is helpful at first so that the pig returns to the box, but, within a few days of regular use, the pig should prefer this location to any other and, if the box is not kept very clean, the pig may choose another location for elimination.

- The box should be located against a wall; if possible, placing it in a corner may also help to make it more attractive to the pig.

Tip: if the weather is bad (eg, rainy, cold), many pigs avoid going outdoors to eliminate and may house soil, so it may be helpful to keep a litter pan available to the pig for use during inclement weather.

4. Never yell at, punish, or do anything that might frighten the pig if caught eliminating in an undesirable location. Doing so only teaches the pig to fear the pet owner and, worse, may teach it to avoid eliminating in the presence of people.

Given time, the right environment, and appropriate training, most pigs eventually prefer to eliminate outside as they mature and they gain more control over their bladders and bowels.

House-training problems in pet pigs are uncommon if pet owners are provided with accurate information regarding training and they are able to spend the time and effort required to supervise the pigs and provide them with an appropriate environment.

When problems do occur, it may be a result of polyurea/polydipsia. In young pigs, this is often caused by underfeeding. Underfeeding is common in pet pigs when people are led to believe that they must underfeed the pig in order to keep it small. Underfed pigs drink excessively and then need to urinate more often, making them difficult to house train. If confronted with a complaint of excessive urination in a young pig, a complete history, including amount and type of food fed and house-training methodology, is the first step, followed by a physical examination and urinalysis.

Another common cause of house-training failure can occur when a young intact female pig reaches puberty and goes into estrus. Females in estrus often urinate more than normal and may begin urinating in alternate locations as well as becoming more active and destructive.

Another problem, not as common but still highly problematic, is the pig that drinks and urinates at the same time. It is not clear why some pet pigs do this, but it is a behavior that has been documented in swine so, again, pet owners need to be informed that this may be normal behavior for some pigs and that watering them somewhere that this behavior will not be so problematic, such as outdoors, is the best solution.

Destructive Behavior

As described earlier, pigs have a strong motivation to explore and this can lead to a great deal of destruction when pet owners attempt to confine pigs to the home. Some pet owners are surprised when they discover just how much damage a pig can do when confined to a yard. If veterinarians are ever able to council pet owners before acquiring a pig, they should be informed that, if having a perfectly groomed yard is important to them, they will not want to own a pig unless they are able and willing to fence off a section of the yard just for the pig's use.

Providing a pet pig with a properly enriched environment is critical to its psychological well-being. What does that mean? It means that the pet pig needs to be able to express as many of its normal species-typical behaviors as possible in order to have the best chance of preventing any and all behavior problems. Pet owners who attempt to confine pet pigs solely to the indoors find this much more difficult, if not impossible. The more time the owner expects the pig to stay indoors, the more critical the enrichment of the home environment will be. If keeping a pig indoors, it needs to be either confined or supervised at all times unless the pet owner does not mind furniture being rearranged, shelves emptied of books, carpet and linoleum uprooted, and dry wall destroyed (**Box 5**).

The confinement area of the pig should be as large as possible. Some people give their pigs a room of its own, empty of furniture and furnished only with items the pig needs, such as a litter box, food and water items, and toys (**Figs. 3** and **4**). In general, because of pigs' interest in using their noses to manipulate their environment, any items that they can push around will be explored and will occupy the pig for some

---

Box 5
Examples of commonly used items for pet pig enrichment

Things that can be pushed or manipulated with the nose:
- Heavy blankets, comforters, or sleeping bags
- Pillows
- Stuffed animals

Most toys that are safe for toddlers are safe for pigs, but pet owners must use their common sense and supervise until they are sure that the item is not so fragile that the pig may break it and swallow small pieces.

Things that can be shredded:
- Newspapers
- Magazines
- Hay or straw

Things that can be chewed:
- Heavy knotted ropes or rope toys, such as those made for dogs
- Heavy rubber dog toys or dog bones, such as Kong toys or Nyla bones
  Just like dogs and children, pigs become bored with toys as they habituate to their presence and the item loses its novelty. Rotation of toys (keeping some put away while leaving only a few for the pig to play with and then switching out the toys every few days) can help keep toys and other items novel. However, most pigs always seem to make use of bedding for manipulating and making a nest for sleeping.

---

period of time (**Box 6**). Pigs also seem to enjoy shredding items such as brown paper bags and old telephone books. They rarely eat these items, but supervision is recommended initially.

One of the most important things that pet pig owners should do to direct the pig's exploratory behavior appropriately is to feed the pig in foraging devices of some type (**Box 7**). The foraging device can take the form of a rooting box (**Figs. 5** and **6**) or homemade toys that drop kibble when manipulated by the pig, and some dog foraging toys also work well for pigs (**Fig. 7**). In the absence of foraging devices, many pet owners just scatter pelleted feed across the yard for their pigs, as long as weather permits. Appropriate environmental enrichment has been shown to play a role in decreasing

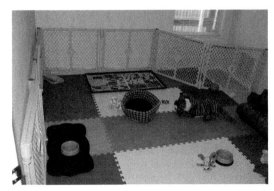

Fig. 3. A well-enriched, pig-proofed room for a young pig. The floor is nonslip, there are several items for manipulation, and the litter pan is simply a tray with newspaper so the piglet can easily step into the pan. The plastic panels have allowed the pig's accessible space to be gradually enlarged as he has learned to use his litter pan reliably.

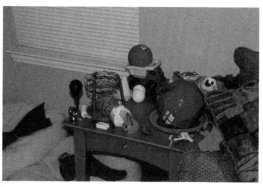

Fig. 4. A variety of toys and novel items for engaging and training the young pig.

aggression in pigs in some instances,[49] so its importance should not be underestimated.

Human-directed Aggression

Aggression directed toward humans seems to be common in pigs but usually appears in the form of threats, such as charging and snapping.[42] However, the threats will escalate to bites, with repeated biting in many cases, if responses by people are

---

Box 6
Examples of foraging devices for pigs

The foraging box

- The box can be made form a large shallow plastic container such as:
- A children's plastic wading pool.
- A large plastic concrete mixing container.
- Any shallow plastic container shallow enough for the pig to step into and large enough for the pig to turn around in.

In the past, some have built shallow wooden boxes, which is fine; they will just not be as easy to keep sanitary as a plastic container.

Once the box is chosen, it needs to have either a single layer of large, smooth river rocks placed in it (large enough that the pig will not be able to eat them but small and smooth enough that the pig can safely and easily walk around on them).

A second choice is to fill the box with many small plastic balls (again, just large enough that the pig cannot eat them) or crumpled balls of paper.

The pig's food can then be scattered in the foraging box twice daily.

Homemade foraging devices

Large plastic juice or soda bottles can easily be converted into foraging toys by cutting appropriately sized holes in them, placing the pigs pelleted feed in them, and then allowing the pig to manipulate the bottle to make the food fall out.

Lengths of PVC (polyvinyl chloride) pipe can have holes drilled in them. With food placed inside and end caps applied, pigs can roll them around to cause the food to fall out.

Commercial food puzzles

Food puzzles for dogs (typically shaped like balls) can work well for pigs as long as they are sturdy.

Box 7
Preventing and managing human-directed aggression in pet pigs

- Pigs should be taught to wear a harness and walk on a leash while still young. Harnesses for pigs are readily available and can be found online.

- Only positive reinforcement training should be used. Pigs are easily food motivated and easy to train by simply reinforcing appropriate and desired behaviors.

- Punishment should never be used in an attempt to stop an unwanted behavior. Punishment, including yelling, squirting with a water bottle, hitting, slapping, or shoving the pig, causes pigs to become afraid of their owners and increases aggression in many cases.

- If a pig does snap at a person, the pig should be calmly removed from the situation, even if this must be done by luring with food. The owner must then consider what could have been done to prevent the situation.

- All pigs should be taught some basic cues, such as to come, sit, or to touch a target. If the pig is to be allowed on the furniture, it can be taught a cue for getting up on furniture and off on request. Pigs can begin learning these things as soon as they are brought into the home.

- Once the pig has learned some cues, the pet owner can frequently ask the pig to perform a cue, such as sit, before being given attention, before being let outside or inside, or before being fed or allowed onto the furniture.

- Positive reinforcement training of cues, and the use of these cues, gives the pig and owner a language with which to communicate. The pig learns how to get what it wants by politely offering a sit, for example, and it never gets anything by being pushy, unruly, or aggressive. If it ever fails to respond to a cue, the worst thing that happens to the pig is that it does not get the good thing that the owner was offering.

- Meetings with strangers should be carefully controlled, especially at first. Having the young pig on a harness and leash and having the visitor give the pig a cue and reward the pig with a special treat can teach the pig that strangers are not to be feared while the leash prevents any inappropriate behaviors. Alternatively, the owner can also just have the pig sit nearby (still being controlled on a leash) and toss it special food treats continuously while the visitor is present, or the visitor could toss the treats. Either way, in this manner classical conditioning can be used to teach the pig to associate good things with the presence of visitors.

- If the pig begins showing aggressive behavior toward anyone, the situations in which these incidents occur must be identified and the initial focus be on preventing those situations. For example, if a pig snaps at people who walk by while it is eating, then it needs to be fed somewhere else so that there is no need for people to pass by while the pig is eating. If the pig snaps at visitors to the home, then it may be easier for the pet owner to always put the pig away somewhere before visitors arrive. Preventing opportunities for unwanted behavior is a crucial part of an overall behavior modification program.

- If the pig is an adult when these problems develop and the pig does not wear a harness and leash and has never been taught any cues, the assistance of a professional may be needed, especially if the owner wishes to do more than just prevent opportunities for unwanted behaviors. In that case, the owner should be encouraged to look to the Web site of the American College of Veterinary Behaviorists (www.dacvb.org) for a behaviorist that will consult regarding a pet pig. If there is none near the pet owner, many will speak with the veterinarian by phone and give what advice they can via telephone consultation.

---

not appropriate (**Box 8**). The threats usually begin when the pig is still young (<1–1.5 years) and are often first directed toward visitors to the home, but in other cases they are directed toward members of the home, including the primary caregiver.

Because it is in the nature of swine to attempt to form a hierarchy with every new individual that they meet, and they typically use overt physical aggression to do so, it has been hypothesized that this behavior might be a form of dominance aggression.

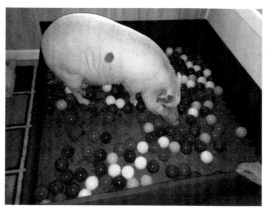

Fig. 5. A rooting box, appropriate for a large pet pig. (Courtesy of L. Seibert, DVM, PhD, DACVB, Lawrenceville, GA.)

However, there is a lack of evidence to suggest that any animal attempts to form hierarchies with individuals of other species, but what should be kept in mind is that artificial selection of the pig has until now been focused more on conformation and reproductive capabilities; features that contribute to its efficiency as a production animal. The ability of the pig to communicate with humans or to respond to human communication has not been selected for. When a pig threatens a new individual, it may simply be using the only tools for communication that it has in its behavioral repertoire. In addition, it has been suggested by some investigators that there may be a limit to how many relationships a pig may be able to remember, especially if those relationships are not regularly reinforced. Again, they did not evolve with a need to meet and remember many new individuals, because normally they are born into small groups and remain in those small groups for most of their lives, unless they are male, in which case they leave their natal groups but are still likely to remain associated with only 1 or 2 other small groups of pigs in their lifetimes. Meeting new individuals frequently results in an unpredictable environment, which can lead to frustration. Frustration can potentially lead to aggression, which may be the reason why many pet pigs first display aggression directed toward visitors to the home.

Once a stable dominance hierarchy exists in a herd, agonistic encounters should be rare, but another of the unique features of pig social structure is that subordinate pigs

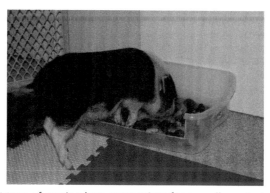

Fig. 6. A different type of rooting box, appropriate for a smaller pet pig.

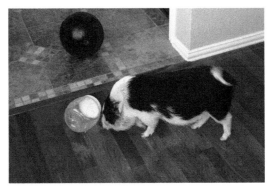

Fig. 7. A pet pig feeding from a homemade foraging toy. The ball in the background is a commercially available foraging toy made for horses and is also regularly used by this pig.

do sometimes direct agonistic behavior toward a high-ranking individual. This behavior does not change the status between the two. However, it has been suggested that this type of retaliatory aggression is more common in situations where pigs are crowded or otherwise stressed. What this suggests is that the response to this type of aggression in the pet pig should not be designed to dominate the pig but to give it a more natural environment where it can express more of its natural behaviors, which is likely to decrease stress and feelings of frustration. **Box 9** provides other possible motivations of human-directed aggression in the pet pig.

Other factors that influence how aggressive an individual pig may be include genetics and the influence of the prenatal and early postnatal environment.[50,51] Several studies support the view that aggressiveness is a stable personality type in pigs and some individuals are simply more aggressive than others.[50,52–55]

Aggression Directed Toward Other Pets

Although it is much less common, pet pigs have been reported to direct aggression toward other pets, particularly cats and dogs. In most of these cases, the aggression

---

Box 8
Other reasons for human-directed aggression in pigs

Fear: if the pet owner does not habituate the pig to gentle handling from a very early age and continue to interact with it in a kind, predictable way, fear aggression may occur. Pigs are prey animals and their initial response to a threat is to attempt to escape. If they are in a situation where they perceive that escape is not possible, they may take a more proactive stance and use aggression to defend themselves. In the authors experience, most cases of fear aggression have occurred in pet pigs that have been punished and/or handled roughly.

Territorial: although free-ranging pigs do not normally defend territory, they may defend a nest. In some cases, pet pigs have shown aggression directed toward people only when people approach their beds, crates, or confinement areas. This behavior is much less common than the other forms of aggression described.

Pain related: a sudden onset of aggression can also be associated with illness or pain in the pet pig just as it can be in other animals. When possible, pigs showing acute-onset aggression should always have a thorough physical examination and radiographs, even if sedation is required, so pain can be ruled out.

> **Box 9**
> **A word about nose rings**
>
> There is no reason to ever place a ring in a pet pigs' nose. Rooting is a natural part of a pig's behavioral repertoire and should be directed appropriately rather than attempting to stop it. Stopping it completely is not possible. Pigs with rings in their noses usually just learn to root with the side of the nose that does not have a ring in it.

is associated with dogs, because most cats seem to recognize when the pig poses a threat to them and simply avoid it. However, in many other cases, if a young pig grows up in the presence of a cat, they seem to tolerate each other well.

What should be kept in mind is that, because pigs use fewer visual cues to communicate and dogs depend greatly on visual cues to communicate with conspecifics, these 2 different species do not seem to be good at reading or responding appropriately to the visual cues of the other species. For example, a dog may stare at a pig and maybe even lift its lip, but this does not always result in a pig walking away. The pig may simply continue with what it was doing. A dog may try to avoid eye contact with a pig and the pig may continue to approach the dog closely, resulting in the dog feeling threatened when that may not have been the pig's intent. In contrast, when a pig wants a dog to leave it alone or a pig wants to defend a resource such as a resting space or food, it usually snaps at the dog, and this is perceived by some dogs as such a severe threat that it provokes a similarly aggressive response in the dog.

Most problems between dogs and pigs occur because pigs can excite the predatory instinct in the dogs. The author knows of many pigs that have been severely injured and even killed by large dogs. In some cases, these were dogs that the pig had lived with for years. These incidents often occur when the owner is not home so no one can be sure of what exactly happened. However, when a pig squeals and runs, dogs will chase, and dogs chasing a pig in a hot climate can cause it to die from heat exhaustion or catch the pig and cause life-threatening damage by attacking it. Most attacks are directed to the neck and shoulders of the pig as if the dog tried to pick the pig up and shake it. In other cases, the pig's rump and hind legs receive numerous deep bite wounds from the dog chasing and biting its rear end. Dogs and pigs can live together companionably, but, when a large dog is in the home, it is recommended that it is never left unattended with the pig.

Conspecific aggression

Aggression between pigs is often a problem for pet owners who wish to add a pig to the family when they already have one. Understanding that pigs fight when introduced is important, but the goal is to try to determine ways to introduce pigs so as to decrease the fighting and thereby decrease the chance of injury associated with the fighting.

In some studies of pigs fighting, it has been noted that sometimes pigs spend more time displaying and on nondamaging pushing and shoving behavior than on actual fighting. It is common for people to believe that the dominant pig in a group is also the more aggressive pig, but this is not always the case. The more aggressive pig is more likely to initiate the biting but not always more likely to win the fight. Most studies of aggression in pigs confirm that heavier pigs are still more likely to win in a contest. If both pigs in a contest are heavy, their fight is more likely to escalate than if both pigs are lighter.[56]

There is some indication that pigs, like most animals, fight less or not as intensely if there is an obvious discrepancy between the size of the pigs in the fight. If the pigs can readily assess the likelihood of winning or losing, then less fighting should be necessary, so there may be some benefit to introducing a smaller or younger pig to the existing pig in a home.

Pet owners may wish to know whether acquiring a pig of the same gender as the existing pig or a different gender would contribute to a more peaceful introduction with less fighting. However, there are no data to suggest which is ideal, especially because most pet pigs of both genders are gonadectomized early and similar studies in commercial swine cannot mimic that situation exactly. However, commercial swine are typically kept in single-gender groups, and studies suggest that there is some preference for social interactions with individuals of the same sex.[57]

When introducing a new pet pig, there similarly are no good data to support a method that results in decreased aggression. However, anecdotally, it has been noted that beginning by allowing the pigs a period of limited introduction, in which they can smell and see each other but not interact, may be helpful to decrease the severity of aggression when the pigs are allowed to interact. The instructions are as follows:

- Use a baby gate, large crate, fencing, or other similar barrier to separate the new pig from the resident initially.
- Allow the pigs to interact freely at the fence or gate as long as they are not acting extremely aggressively (charging the partition repeatedly and forcefully). If this occurs, they may only be allowed in this area periodically, for short periods of time. Feeding them some favored food treats, several meters away from the partition, can help them to associate something good with the presence of the other pig and, it is hoped, decreasing their interest in the other pig.
- Once the pigs can interact at the barrier peacefully, begin observing for signs that 1 pig may be willing to behave submissively. These signs may be subtle, but might include turning away of the head, or even walking away, when the other pig approaches. Once behaviors such as this are witnessed a few times, it is time for the next step.
- If it is possible to introduce the pigs by taking them to a new, novel, neutral environment this can be helpful because introducing the new pig to the resident pig in its home territory may lead to a higher level of fighting.
- If that is not possible, try to introduce the pigs outdoors in as large a space as possible. Ideally, the space should not be empty. It should have some items in it that a pig could use to hide behind because this may decrease aggression in the resident pig.
- There is some indication that introductions at night may result in less fighting.
- The results of 1 study suggests that, if a pleasant odor is used near where the pigs eat and applied it in the area where the pigs will be meeting, it may decrease stress associated with novelty and thus help to decrease fighting.[51]
- If the pigs fight vigorously to the point where they are hurting each other, they can be separated using pieces of plywood that the owner can hold and slide between the pigs. Obviously, it is helpful to have more than 1 person available during this initial meeting.
- The pet owner can try again after a few more days of separation.

Ultimately, pet owners must understand that there will be some fighting between the pigs. Fighting cannot be completely avoided. If they keep separating the pigs, rather than allowing them to establish their hierarchy, then it may take longer and require more fighting before they can live together. This prospect can be difficult for the pet owner

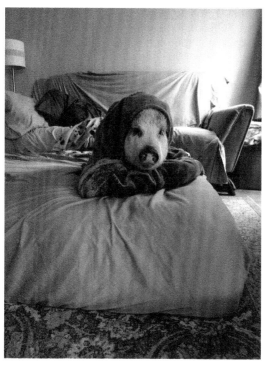

Fig. 8. A beloved pet pig; Pepper, is a 2-year-old male neutered pig, adopted from a minipig rescue after being surrendered at 5 months of age for unknown reasons.

to deal with considering it is difficult to know how much fighting is acceptable and what degree of fighting is normal if the individual does not have some experience with pigs.

PSYCHOPHARMACOLOGY FOR THE PET PIG

Virtually no data exist on the use of psychotropic drugs in pet pigs. In the author's experience, most behavior problems are a result of normal but unwanted behaviors that can be readily managed with owner education, an improved environment for the pig, and some behavior modification. On rare occasions, a pig may show signs of having been so poorly socialized that it truly does not seem to be able to interact normally with other pigs. In these instances, selective serotonin reuptake inhibitors (fluoxetine 1 mg/kg once daily) have been tried and found to be helpful in allowing the pig to be introduced to other pigs.

A few pigs with very fearful behavior have benefited from selective serotonin reuptake inhibitors. Their history was unknown so it was difficult to be certain whether their fearful behavior was primarily caused by genetics or a result of poor socialization or learned behavior. In some cases, the pigs have been able to be weaned off the medication, but others continue to be medicated. There are too few of these cases at this time to be able to say anything with certainty about safety and efficacy.

SUMMARY

Miniature pigs can make excellent pets for people that are willing to educate themselves about the needs of the pig, and then commit themselves to providing the environment that is best for the pig. Pigs are highly social animals and, if not kept in pairs, need even more attention and interaction from owners. They are intelligent and learn readily, but, without appropriate training, they are likely to learn behaviors that owners find unacceptable. With early training, habituation to handling, and the provision of a properly enriched environment, a pig can be a delightful companion (**Fig. 8**). They bond readily to their owners and, with a moderate amount of preventive care (if not allowed to become obese), they can easily live to be 15 to 20 years of age.

DISCLOSURE

The author has nothing to disclose.

REFERENCES

1. Kiley M. The vocalizations of ungulates, their causation and function. Z Tierpsychol 1972;31:171–222.
2. Koba Y, Tanida H. How do miniature pigs discriminate between people? Discrimination between people wearing coveralls of the same color. Appl Anim Behav Sci 2001;73:45–58.
3. Neitz J, Jacobs GH. Spectral sensitivity of cones in an ungulate. Vis Neurosci 1989;2:97–100.
4. Zonderland JJ, Cornelissen L, Wolthius-Fillerup M, et al. Visual acuity of pigs at different light intensities. Appl Anim Behav Sci 2008;111:28–37.
5. Meese GB, Connor DJ, Baldwin BA. Ability of the pig to distinguish between conspecific urine samples using olfaction. Physiol Behav 1975;15:121–5.
6. Mendl M, Randle K, Pope S. Young pigs can discriminate individual differences in odours from conspecific urine. Anim Behav 2002;64:97–101.
7. Meese GB, Ewbank R. The establishment and nature of the dominance hierarchy in the domesticated pig. Anim Behav 1973;21:326–34.
8. Meese GB, Baldwin BA. The effect of ablation of the olfactory bulbs on aggressive behaviour in pigs. Appl Anim Ethol 1975;1:251–62.
9. Kennedy JM, Baldwin BA. Taste preferences in pigs for nutritive and non-nutritive sweet solutions. Anim Behav 1972;20:706–18.
10. Houpt KA, Houpt TR. Comparative aspects of the ontogeny of taste. Chem Senses Flavor 1976;2:219–28.
11. Kare MR, Pond WC, Campbell J. Observations on the taste reactions in pigs. Anim Behav 1965;13:265–9.
12. Heffner RS, Heffner HH. Hearing in domestic pigs (*Sus scrofa*) and goats (*Capra hircus*). Hear Res 1990;48:231–40.
13. Weary DM, Braithwaite LA, Fraser D. Vocal response to pain in piglets. Appl Anim Behav Sci 1998;56:161–72.
14. Fraser D. The vocalizations and other behavior of growing pigs in an "open field" test. Appl Anim Ethol 1974;1:3–16.
15. Weary DM, Ross S, Fraser D. Vocalizations by isolated piglets: a reliable indicator of piglet need directed towards the sow. Appl Anim Behav Sci 1997;53:249–57.
16. Mills DS. Medical paradigms for the study of problem behaviour: a critical review. Appl Anim Behav Sci 2003;81:265–77.
17. Mauget R. Behavioural and reproductive strategies in wild forms of *Sus scrofa* (European Wild Boar and feral pigs). In: Sybesma W, editor. The welfare of pigs. Current Topics in Veterinary Medicine and Animal Science, vol 11. Dordrecht: Springer; 1981. p. 3–13.

18. Graves HB. Behavior and ecology of wild and feral swine (*Sus scrofa*). J Anim Sci 1984;58:482–92.
19. Giersing M, Andersson A. How does former acquaintance affect aggression in repeatedly mixed male and female pigs? Appl Anim Behav Sci 1998;59:297–306.
20. Stolba A, Wood-Gush DGM. The behavior of pigs in a semi-natural environment. Anim Prod 1989;48:419–25.
21. McBride G. The teat order and communication in young pigs. Anim Behav 1963; 11:53–6.
22. Hemsworth PH, Winfield CG, Mullaney PD. A study of the development of the teat order in piglets. Appl Anim Ethol 1976;2:225–33.
23. Scheel DE, Graves HB, Sherritt GW. Nursing order, social dominance and growth in swine. J Anim Sci 1977;45:219–29.
24. Ingram DL. Evaporative cooling in the pig. Nature 1965;207:415–6.
25. Blackshaw JK, Blackshaw AW. Shade seeking and lying behaviour in pigs of mixed sex and age, with access to outside pens. Appl Anim Behav Sci 1994; 39:249–57.
26. Heitman H, Hahn L, Bond TE, et al. The effect of modified summer environment on swine behavior. Anim Behav 1962;10:15–9.
27. Huynh TTT, Aarnink AJA, Gerrits WJJ, et al. Thermal behaviour of growing pigs in response to high temperature and humidity. Appl Anim Behav Sci 2005;91:1–16.
28. van Putten G. Comfort behavior in pigs: informative for their well-being. In: Folsch DW, editor. The ethology and ethic of farm animal production. Basel (Switzerland): Springer; 1978. p. 70–6.
29. Haugse CN, Dinusson WE, Erickson DO, et al. A day in the life of a pig. Feedstuffs North Dakota Farm Research 1965;23:18–23.
30. Andersen HM, Jorgensen E, Dybkjaer L, et al. The ear skin temperature as an indicator of the thermal comfort of pigs. Appl Anim Behav Sci 2008;113:43–56.
31. Fraser D. Selection of bedded and unbedded areas by pigs in relation to environmental temperatures and behaviour. Appl Anim Behav Sci 1985;14:117–26.
32. Whatson TS. The development of dunging preferences in piglets. Appl Anim Ethol 1978;4:293.
33. Hacker RR, Ogilvie JR, Morrison WD, et al. Factors affecting excretory behavior of pigs. J Anim Sci 1994;72:1455–60.
34. Buchenauer D, Luft C, Grauvogl A. Investigation of the eliminative behaviour of piglets. Appl Anim Ethol 1982/83;9:153–64.
35. Olsen AW, Dybkjaer L, Simonsen HB. The behavior of growing pigs kept in pens with outdoor runs II: Temperature regulatory behavior, comfort behavior and dunging preferences. Livest Prod Sci 2001;60:265–78.
36. Blasetti A, Boitani L, Riviello MC, et al. Activity budgets and use of enclosed space by wild boars (*Sus scrofa*) in captivity. Z Biol 1988;7:69–79.
37. Ingram DL, Stephens DB. The relative importance of thermal, osmotic and hypovolaemic factors in the control of drinking in the pig. J Physiol 1979;293:501–12.
38. Baldwin BA. The study of behaviour in pigs. Br Vet J 1969;125:281–8.
39. Yang TS, Howard B, MacFarlane WB. Effects of food on drinking behavior of growing pigs. Appl Anim Ethol 1981;7:259–70.
40. Studnitz M, Jensen MB, Pederson LJ. Why do pigs root and in what will they root? A review on the exploratory behavior of pigs in relation to environmental enrichment. Appl Anim Behav Sci 2007;107:183–97.
41. Beattie VE, O'Connell NE. Relationship between rooting behaviour and foraging in growing pigs. Anim Welf 2002;11:295–303.

42. Tynes VV, Hart BL, Bain MJ. Human directed aggression in miniature pet pigs. J Am Vet Med Assoc 2007;230:385–9.

43. Newberry RC, Wood-Gush DG. The suckling behaviour of domestic pigs in a semi-natural environment. Behaviour 1985;95:11–25.

44. Fraser D. Observations on the behavioural development of suckling and early-weaned piglets during the first six weeks after birth. Anim Behav 1978;26:22–30.

45. Worsaae H, Schmidt M. Plasma cortisol and behaviour in early weaned piglets. Acta Vet Scand 1980;21:640–57.

46. Donaldson TM, Newberry RC, Špinka M, et al. Effects of early play experience on play behaviour of piglets after weaning. Appl Anim Behav Sci 2002;79:221–31.

47. D'Eath RB. Socializing piglets before weaning improves social hierarchy formation when pigs are mixed post-weaning. Appl Anim Behav Sci 2005;93:199–211.

48. Parratt CA, Chapmen KJ, Turner C, et al. The fighting behaviour of piglets mixed before and after weaning in the presence or absence of a sow. Appl Anim Behav Sci 2006;101:54–67.

49. Melottis L, Oostindjer M, Bolhuis EJ, et al. Coping personality type and environmental enrichment affect aggression at weaning in pigs. Appl Anim Behav Sci 2011;133:144–53.

50. Clark CA, D'Eath RB. Age over experience: consistency of aggression and mounting behavior in male and female pigs. Appl Anim Behav Sci 2013;47:81–93.

51. Prunier A, Averos X, Dimitrov I. Review: early life predisposing factors for biting in pigs. Animal 2020;14(3):570–87.

52. D'Eath RB. Consistency of aggressive temperament in domestic pigs: the effects of social experience and social disruption. Aggress Behav 2004;30:435–48.

53. Erhard HW, Mendl M, Ashley DD. Individual aggressiveness of pigs can be measured and used to reduce aggression after mixing. Appl Anim Behav Sci 1997;54(2):137–51.

54. Turner SP, Roehe R, D'Eath RB, et al. Genetic validation of post-mixing skin injuries in pigs as an indicator of aggressiveness and the relationship with injuries under more stable social conditions. J Anim Sci 2009;87:3076–82.

55. Erhard HW, Mendl M. Measuring aggressiveness in growing pigs in a resident-intruder situation. Appl Anim Behav Sci 1997;54(2):123–36.

56. Camerlink I, Turner SP, Farish M, et al. Aggressiveness as a component of fighting ability in pigs (*Sus scrofa*) using a game-theoretical framework. Anim Behav 2015;108:183–91.

57. Dobao MT, Rodriganez J, Silio. Choice of companions in social play in piglets. Appl Anim Behav Sci 1984-1985;13:259–66.

Abnormal Repetitive Behaviors and Self-Mutilations in Small Mammals

Claire Vergneau-Grosset, Dr Med Vet, IPSAV, CES, DACZM[a],*,
Hélène Ruel, Dr Med Vet, MSc, DACVIM (Neurology), PhD Candidate[b]

KEYWORDS

- Stereotypies • Small mammals • Rat • Chinchilla

KEY POINTS

- Primary causes of self-mutilation may be medical and/or environmental.
- Cerebral mechanisms are involved in the development and persistence of these behaviors; thus, resolving the primary cause is not always sufficient to solve the problem.
- Treatment should include environmental changes and therapeutic drugs as needed, including analgesics.

Abnormal repetitive behaviors (ARBs) and self-mutilations are regularly observed in small mammals by owners, breeders, and veterinarians. These behaviors are primarily coping mechanisms associated with stress and anxiety, and may constitute clinical signs of pain. When physical damages are absent, ARBs may not be easily acknowledged by owners. Therefore, a detailed history and/or at-home videos are important to detect these behaviors.

DESCRIPTION OF ABNORMAL REPETITIVE BEHAVIORS AND SELF-MUTILATION
Definitions

- Self-mutilation is an intentional and impulsive self-inflicted destruction of tissue or alteration of the body (**Fig. 1**).[1]
- In humans, ARBs include stereotypies (voluntary repetitive seemingly purposeless behavioral pattern that cannot be interrupted by an external stimulus[1]) and obsessive-compulsive disorders (an anxiety disorder in which recurring, unwanted thoughts, ideas, or sensations make the subject feel driven to do something repetitively).[2]

[a] Service de Médecine Zoologique, Clinical Sciences Department, Université de Montréal, 3200 rue Sicotte, Saint-Hyacinthe, Montreal, Québec J2S 2M2, Canada; [b] Clinical Sciences Department, Université de Montréal, 3200 rue Sicotte, Saint-Hyacinthe, Québec J2S 2M2, Canada
* Corresponding author.
E-mail address: claire.grosset@umontreal.ca

Vet Clin Exot Anim 24 (2021) 87–102
https://doi.org/10.1016/j.cvex.2020.09.003
1094-9194/21/© 2020 Elsevier Inc. All rights reserved.

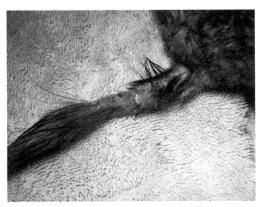

Fig. 1. Tail of a chinchilla (*Chinchilla lanigera*) presented for self-mutilation. (*Courtesy of* C. Vergneau-Grosset, med vet, IPSAV, CES, dipl ACZM, Saint-Hyacinthe, Canada.)

Most Frequently Observed Abnormal Repetitive Behaviors in Small Mammals

- Excessive grooming: excessive amount of time spent grooming the fur, associated or not with dermatopathy (**Fig. 2**).
- Barbering, also called hair plucking: action of pulling hair, including, but not limited to, whiskers (**Fig. 3**).[2]
- Fur chewing, mainly observed in chinchillas: action of breaking hair with the teeth, which makes the underfur visible (**Fig. 4**).
- Self-biting: action of repetitively biting a part of the body (**Fig. 5**). For more information regarding various dermatopathies secondary to behavioral problem in small mammals, the readers are referred to a previous comprehensive review.[2]
- Bar mouthing: repetitive biting of cage bars.
- Somersaulting: action of doing repetitive backflips.
- Corner digging, which is mainly reported in laboratory gerbils raised in absence of burrows: action of repetitively digging substrate in the corner of the cage.[3] Videos of these behaviors are available to online (see: http://animalbiosciences.uoguelph.ca/~gmason/StereotypicAnimalBehaviour/library.shtml).[4]

ETIOLOGIES OF ABNORMAL REPETITIVE BEHAVIORS AND SELF-MUTILATION

Maladaptive behaviors owing to an inadequate environment should be distinguished from malfunctioning behaviors resulting from brain dysfunctions.[5] The former is an

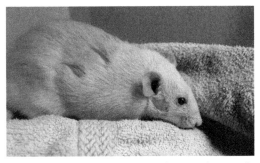

Fig. 2. Alopecia associated with excessive grooming in a rat (*Rattus domesticus*). (*Courtesy of* C. Vergneau-Grosset, med vet, IPSAV, CES, dipl ACZM, Saint-Hyacinthe, Canada.)

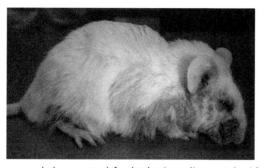

Fig. 3. Mouse (*Mus musculus*) presented for barbering, diagnosed with a cutaneous lymphoma. (*Courtesy of* C. Vergneau-Grosset, med vet, IPSAV, CES, dipl ACZM, Saint-Hyacinthe, Canada.)

expression of coping mechanism to stress or fear in "normal" individuals, whereas the latter is the consequence of neurologic or neuropsychological changes.

Pain

A study by Blumenkopf and Lipman[6] showed that the neurectomy of the sciatic nerve leads to self-mutilation of the ipsilateral foot, whereas chronic functional denervation secondary to local block (with lidocaine 2%) of the sciatic nerve was not associated with autotomy. This experiment proved that autotomy in rats is a behavior associated with pain.

In Bennett and Xie's[7] model of neuropathic pain induced by loose ligation of the sciatic nerve in rats, autotomy was described in 70% of cases, but was never seen on the sham-operated paw. In this case, dysesthesias (abnormal sensations) are believed to induce this behavior.

Stress

Some stressors of mild intensity (eg, novelty, handling, and transportation) causing excessive grooming, have been associated to the release of adrenocorticotropin hormone in the brain.[8] Of note, lesions involving the substantia nigra or the hippocampus reduce this behavior. It has been suggested that stressors that do not induce

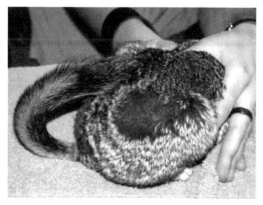

Fig. 4. Fur chewing in a chinchilla (*Chinchilla lanigera*). (*Courtesy of* Clinique des Animaux Exotiques, Saint-Hyacinthe, Canada.)

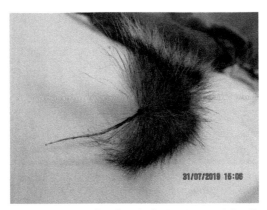

Fig. 5. Self-biting of the tail associated with a degloving injury of the distal tail in an Eastern gray squirrel (*Sciurus carolinensis*): self-biting resulted in exposure of the coccygeal vertebrae. (*Courtesy of* C. Vergneau-Grosset, med vet, IPSAV, CES, dipl ACZM, Saint-Hyacinthe, Canada.)

excessive grooming likely elicit antagonistic activity, in addition to the release of adrenocorticotropin hormone.[8] Although this reaction to stress is normal, persistent stress factors may lead to chronic excessive grooming and dermatologic complications.

Boredom

Boredom has been associated with stereotypies in zoo animals as it was found that increasing foraging opportunities could decrease stereotypic behaviors.[1] Similarly, highly enriched environments significantly decrease the occurrence of stereotypic behaviors in laboratory female mice.[9] Some stereotypies are considered as redirected behaviors associated with a lack of environmental elements essential to express a normal behavior.[1]

Stereotypic Movement Disorder

In humans, stereotypic movement disorder is due to a dysfunction of the prefronto-corticobasal ganglia circuits or cortico-striatal-thalamo-cortical pathways.[10] Similar central lesions could potentially cause stereotypies in small mammals as well, but it has not been documented to date.

Secondary Stereotypies (ie, a Consequence of a Primary Neuro[psycho]logical Dysfunction)

In humans with borderline personality disorders, self-mutilation in the form of self-cutting has been shown to decrease the activity in the amygdala, thus decreasing emotional activity.[11] In addition, it normalizes the functional connectivity with superior functional gyri, which also regulates emotional activity. This effect is particularly potent in certain cases of mental illness, which can explain why some individuals are more prone to developing stereotypic behaviors.

In humans, impulse control disorders have been linked to basal ganglia and prefrontal cortex malfunctions, leading to an inability to switch goals.[12] The dopaminergic system is one of the neurologic systems involved in impulse control.[13] This system has also been incriminated in self-mutilation behaviors after demonstrating that, in rats with damaged dopaminergic neurons, the administration of dopamine agonists induces self-mutilation.[14] Individual predispositions to develop self-mutilation and ARBs also include exposition to early stressors in life, such as early or abrupt weaning, and a lack of early tactile stimulations in rats.[15] However, because cerebral plasticity is now well-documented in rodents,[16] these cases can be successfully treated. Cerebral plasticity is a process by which cerebral connections established in early life can change based on the environment.

Genetic factors
Although no specific gene had been linked to stereotypies in humans, it was found that up to 40% of affected children have a family member with stereotypies.[10] Similarly, a genetic transmission of the fur-chewing behavior has been documented in chinchillas.[17]

Endocrine factors
Certain stereotypies have been associated with endocrine factors. For instance, female chinchillas are more prone to exhibit fur chewing than males.[18] In addition, all chinchillas displaying fur-chewing behavior had evidence of adrenal gland hyperplasia compared with controls in a study including 11 affected individuals and 3 controls.[19] It is unknown whether stress was the cause of the fur chewing and was associated to secondary adrenal gland hyperplasia, or whether an intrinsic endocrine problem was the reason behind this abnormal behavior.

Perpetuation of abnormal repetitive behaviors and self-mutilations
Regardless of the primary cause leading to ARBs and self-mutilations, these behaviors can be perpetuated either by generating pain (eg, nociceptive pain after a wound, neuropathic pain after autotomy) or by human intervention causing reinforcement of an abnormal behavior. Indeed, owners tend to pay more attention to their companion animal while the behavior is happening. Some owners may involuntarily encourage the behavior by talking to their pet or taking it out of the cage, or feed to offer a distraction.

MEDICAL APPROACH AND THERAPEUTIC MANAGEMENT

Small mammals may be presented to practitioners for traumatic wounds or dermatopathies caused by self-mutilation.[2] ARBs may not always be easily identified at home, particularly in nocturnal small mammals where ARBs occur more often at night, during their peak of activity.[20] Therefore, a detailed history and/or videos recorded at home are important to detect these behaviors. Owners also may not seek advice from veterinarians when noticing ARB in their pet, unless physical consequences are already present, as reported in avian medicine.[21]

Detailed Medical History

Self-mutilation may be noticed by the caretakers or suspected in case of chronic cutaneous lesions including alopecia, excoriation, wounds, or ulcerations. Care should be taken to rule out trauma from a conspecific or from the environment. If the behavior has not been observed directly, video recordings of the activity of the patient at home may be useful to confirm the suspicion.

When the animal history is collected, it is important to discriminate between normal and abnormal behaviors, for instance, normal grooming versus barbering associated with alopecia. It is also key to precisely quantify the frequency of each specific behavior, pattern, and duration. This information will allow one to monitor progression overtime. If the problem has been noted for years, seasonality may be important to record to rule out any association with reproductive status, photoperiod, or presence of allergens, such as pollens in particular. If the behavior occurs daily, identifying sensitive times of the day is also helpful. When pets are unattended (at night or while owners are not at home), video recording the animal's behavior may be useful to detect trigger factors, such as boredom.

Some small mammal species may target specific body parts during their episodes of self-mutilation. For instance, it is common for chinchillas to pluck and bite their tail (see **Fig. 1**), whereas rats will more often be presented with digital amputation or thoracic lesions.[22] Sugar gliders are particularly prone to injure themselves on the genital area (scrotum and penis).[23] Commonly reported patterns of ARB also vary depending on the species. Rats may repeatedly sit and chew litter, make repetitive movements of the forelimbs or lateral head movements.[22] Ferrets may sniff repeatedly and show rhythmic head movements.[24]

As for any other medical problems, a complete review of the environment should be performed. If wounds are associated with hemorrhages, the volume and frequency should be recorded to calculate blood loss and determine whether hematologic tests are required. Any potential toxin in the environment should be listed. For example, intoxications by coffee are reported to lead to self-injuries and should be ruled out.[25]

Management

Environmental improvements

Environmental changes should aim at decreasing the number of stressful factors while avoiding boredom. It is also important to maintain a high quality of substrates provided. Indeed, an increased frequency of substrate and dust bath change has been associated with a lower incidence of fur chewing in farm chinchillas.[26] Depending on the case, improving the environment may include changing the setting of the habitat, adapting the social structure of the group, or adding enrichment. For instance, if a rodent is troubled by the constant presence of a cat in the environment, the cage should be placed in an area that the predator cannot access. Nocturnal small mammals, such as hamsters, hedgehogs, and sugar gliders, should be placed in a quiet environment during the day.[23] Intact male rats subject to aggression by male congeners could be moved to an alternative group of neutered female rats to limit conflicts. Social animals such as rats or sugar gliders should be housed in groups because isolation has been proven in the latter species to contribute to the occurrence of self-mutilation.[23] Small mammals should be provided with a daily rotation of enrichment items, for instance, by hiding food in cardboard boxes or pipes in muridae, providing different food displays, such as burrows made of hay for rabbits or hanging hay in the cage. Of note, enrichment items do not decrease the prevalence of self-mutilation once this behavior is present, as shown in an experiment conducted in rats with pemoline-induced self-mutilation.[22] These 24 rats did not interact with the enrichment items and avoided tactile stimuli. Conversely, foraging is intended to avoid boredom and prevent the development of abnormal behaviors. A detailed description of adequate environments and possible enrichments for small mammals may be found elsewhere.[27]

Owners should also be instructed to stop any reinforcing behavior that could perpetuate self-mutilation or ARB. They should ignore the abnormal behavior once it has started ,but if the history revealed a specific window of time when ARBs or mutilation occur, owners should be told to offer enrichment before this time as an attempt to avoid boredom.

Finally, in case of genital self-mutilation in sugar gliders kept in groups, neutering has been recommended in an attempt to decrease sexual frustration.[23]

The presence of stereotypies and ARBs always warrants a thorough investigation of the animal's welfare. However, in some cases stereotypies in companion, research or farmed small mammals can substitute for normal behaviors[28] and reduce frustrations. Thus, stereotypies should be considered as red flags, but cannot be used to quantify welfare.

Drugs

Medical treatment of self-mutilation and ARB include specific treatments of the underlying cause when possible, antinociceptive drug administration and application of physical barriers to break the vicious circle of self-injuries if severe cutaneous lesions are present.

When patients are presented in emergency for acute self-mutilation, hospitalization and analgesia with injectable opioids are often required. Dosages for exotic small mammals can be found elsewhere.[29] Antinociceptive drugs may also be used long term in small mammals presented with self-mutilation. Suggested doses are summarized in **Table 1**. Readers may refer to previous reviews regarding recommended administration techniques for small mammal patients.[30]

Gabapentin is a structural analog of the gamma-aminobutyric acid commonly used for the treatment pain. Its oral bioavailability varies between 47% and 79% in mice and rats,[31,32] which is lower than the oral bioavailability described in dogs.[33] Although its effect on the central nervous system is well-studied, its analgesic effect is mediated by complex peripheral mechanisms of action.[34] Gabapentin administered at 100 mg/kg every 12 hours by mouth for 5 days decreased hyperalgesia in an experimental model of neuropathic pain in guinea pigs and rats.[35] Similarly in neuropathic mice, a dose of 100 mg/kg gabapentin by mouth decreased cold and mechanical allodynia.[36] In 7 clinical cases of cats presented with self-mutilation of the tail of undetermined origin (feline hyperesthesia), gabapentin treatment, alone or combined with other drugs, was also associated with clinical improvement in 6 cases.[37] In rats, no interaction between morphine and gabapentin pharmacokinetics has been found.[38]

In case of vasculitis, treatment with pentoxifylline may be attempted (**Fig. 6**). Pentoxyfylline is a xanthine derivative that increases erythrocyte flexibility.[39] A dosage of 10 mg/kg of pentoxifylline every 12 hours for 10 days has been published in an experimental study in chinchillas,[40] and this dose has been used by one of the authors in clinical cases without noticeable adverse effects.

Naloxone has been reported to decrease self-mutilation behaviors in some rodents.[41] The proposed mechanism is that it increases pain perception associated with self-mutilation by antagonizing enkephalinergic (endogenous opioid) systems. Thus, rodents may be less prone to self-mutilate.[42] However, it should be noted that naloxone compromises animal welfare rather than improves it, because the underlying cause of self-mutilation is not addressed, and the pain experienced may be potentiated by this drug. Therefore, the authors do not recommend the use of naloxone to treat self-mutilation.

Psychotropic drugs For general recommendations regarding psychopharmacology for the exotic practitioner, readers should refer to the article on this topic in this issue.

Treatment of self-mutilation with psychotropic drugs may include the use of selective serotonin reuptake inhibitor antidepressants, such as fluoxetine. These drugs block the serotonin reuptake at presynaptic membrane level.[43] Many selective serotonin reuptake inhibitors also act on other serotoninergic receptors, such as the $5HT_{2A}$ for fluoxetine, indirectly enhancing dopaminergic and noradrenergic pathways.[43] Finally, serotoninergic and enkephalinergic (endogenous opioid) systems are now known to be interrelated.[44] The use of selective serotonin reuptake inhibitors to treat ABR is therefore potentially using a multimodal approach working on reducing anxiety,

Table 1
Examples of suggested analgesic drugs dosages in exotic small mammals (species are in alphabetical order)

Agents	Dosage	Comments
African pygmy hedgehogs		
Buprenorphine	0.03 mg/kg SC q12 h in the mantle[55]	
Meloxicam	0.5 mg/kg PO q12 h or 0.5 mg/kg SC q24 h[56]	
Chinchillas		
Hydromorphone	2 mg/kg SC q4 h[57]	
Buprenorphine	0.2 mg/kg SC q4 h[58]	
Ferrets		
Meloxicam	0.2 mg/kg PO q24 h[59]	Shorter treatment interval may be needed in female
Tramadol	5 mg/kg PO q12–24 h[60]	Empirical use
Gabapentin	3–5 mg/kg PO q8–24 h[60]	Empirical use
Hydromorphone	0.1–0.2 mg/kg SC, IM, IV[60]	Empirical use
Guinea pigs		
Carbamazepine	0.3–30 mg/kg PO q 12 h[35]	Reduces hyperalgesia
Meloxicam	1.5 mg/kg PO q 12 h[76]	Hydration status must be restored before administration, empirical use
Gabapentin	100 mg/kg PO q 12 h[35]	
Buprenorphine	0.05–0.1 mg/kg PO, SC q6–12 h or 0.1 mg/kg TM q2–3 h[61]	
Hydromorphone	0.3 mg/kg IM q4h or 0.3 mg/kg IV q2 h[62]	
Mice		
Meloxicam	5 mg/kg PO, SC q24 h[63,64]	
Gabapentin	10–50 mg/kg PO q 12–24 h[31,65]	
Sustained-release buprenorphine[a]	1.5 mg/kg SC q48 h[66]	
Rabbits		
Gabapentin	30 mg/kg PO q12–24 h[65]	
Meloxicam	1 mg/kg PO q24 h[66] or 0.5 mg/kg PO q12 h	
Tramadol	12–15 mg/kg PO q12 h	Empirical use, an 11 mg/kg oral dose did not reach plasmatic concentration consistent with analgesia in humans[67]
Buprenorphine	0.03–0.05 mg/kg IM, SC, IV q6–8 h[60]	
Hydromorphone	0.1–0.2 mg/kg IM, SC, IV q6–8 h[60]	
Rats		
Gabapentin	60–120 mg/kg PO q12–24 h[35,68]	
Meloxicam	1 mg/kg PO/SC q12 h[69]	

(continued on next page)

Table 1
(continued)

Agents	Dosage	Comments
Tramadol	10–40 mg/kg PO[70] 10 mg/kg IP[71]	Significant thermal antinociception 1 h later. Unknown duration and toxicology. Hepatotoxicity and nephrotoxicity reported in rats after a single dose of 25 mg/kg IP.[71] Sedation has been anecdotally reported at a dose of 10 mg/kg
Sustained-release buprenorphine[a]	1.2 mg/kg SC q2–3 d[72]	No pica nor self-mutilation observed in an experimental study in rats
Sugar Gliders		
Meloxicam	0.3 mg/kg PO q24 h × 3 d[73]	Empirical used based on a case series
Syrian hamster		
Meloxicam	5 mg/kg PO q24 h[74]	
Gabapentin	50 mg/kg PO q24 h[75]	Empirical use based on a single case report

Abbreviations: IM, intramuscularly; IP, intraperitoneally; IV, intravenously; PO, by mouth; q, every; SC, subcutaneously.
[a] WildPharm, Windsor, CO, USA.
Data from Refs.[31,35,55–63,65–75]

regulating the dopamine system, while modulating pain pathways. Fluoxetine at 0.5 to 1.0 mg/kg by mouth every 24 hours has been reported anecdotally in sugar gliders presented with self-mutilation but pharmacokinetic is unknown in this species.[2] Higher doses, ranging from 10 to 20 mg/kg by mouth have been used experimentally in rats and pharmacokinetic has been studied.[45] At higher doses, oral bioavailability increased in rats and a prolonged half-life was observed.[45] Pharmacokinetic and

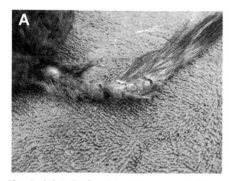
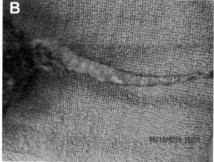

Fig. 6. (*A*) Tail of a chinchilla presented for self-mutilation. Histology of a skin biopsy was consistent with vasculitis. (*B*) Tail of the same individual after a 3-week treatment with pentoxifylline 10 mg/kg by mouth 2 times per day, chloramphenicol 30 mg/kg by mouth 2 times per day, meloxicam 0.5 mg/kg. (*Courtesy of* C. Vergneau-Grosset, med vet, IPSAV, CES, dipl ACZM, Saint-Hyacinthe, Canada.)

pharmacodynamic of fluoxetine administered at 10 to 20 mg/kg intravenously, intraperitoneally, and subcutaneously has also been studied in mice.[46] In rats, a pharmacodynamic study showed a significant reduction of intracerebral proinflammatory cytokines after administration of fluoxetine at 42 mg/kg by mouth once a day for 90 days. No adverse effects were detected clinically in these rats for the 120-day duration of this study.[47] At extremely high dosages, fluoxetine may cause anorexia in rodents: intraperitoneal doses causing anorexia in 50% of animals range from 8 g/kg in guinea pigs to 12 g/kg in mice.[48] Another serotonin reuptake inhibitor, sertraline, has been tested in rabbits. Sertraline administered orally at 4 mg/kg/d (approximately twice the recommended dose for humans) for 9 weeks was associated with hepatotoxicity in rabbits.[49] Whenever long-term studies toxicology studies are not available, patients administered these drugs should be monitored closely. Recheck examination should include biochemistry panels.

Reports of clinical use of antidepressant drugs in exotic small mammals remain scarce. However, use of these drugs should be considered when dosages have been established in laboratory animals. Of note, these drugs should be used in the early stage of patients' management, because they may significantly improve animal welfare when anxiety is the underlying cause. However, owners should be informed that the use of these drugs does not replace the need for environmental changes.[50]

Physical barriers

When there is a risk of fatal hemorrhage secondary to recurrent trauma to the same area, the placement of protective bandages or Elizabethan collar in parallel to medical treatments should be considered (**Fig. 7**) until recovery. For rodent species who use their forepaws to eat, such as rats and chinchillas, padded body bandages are preferred to an Elizabethan collar (**Fig. 8**). These bandages, placed with the animal under sedation, are made of multiple layers of padding covered by Vetrap and Telfa dressing material (Tyco Healthcare Group, Baie-D'Urfe, Quebec, Canada). This system prevents the animal to bend the cranial part of its body to reach its pelvic limb, rear part of the body, or thorax. Care should be taken to allow normal breathing movement. If the bandage tends to slip cranially, a cross over the thoracic inlet can be added (**Fig. 9**). Some patients require close monitoring and a low dose of midazolam to adjust to this type of bandage initially. In rabbits, an alternative to avoid using Elizabethan

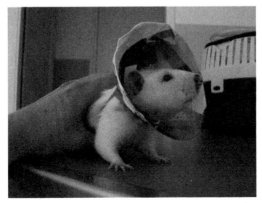

Fig. 7. Home-made Elizabethan collar placed on a rat with scrotal self-mutilation secondary to funiculitis. (*Courtesy of* C. Vergneau-Grosset, med vet, IPSAV, CES, dipl ACZM, Saint-Hyacinthe, Canada.)

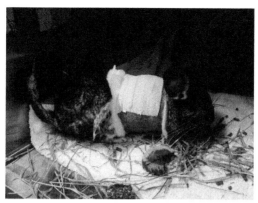

Fig. 8. Body wrap placed on a chinchilla presented for tail self-mutilation. This bandage should always be associated with analgesic and etiologic treatments. (*Courtesy of* C. Vergneau-Grosset, med vet, IPSAV, CES, dipl ACZM, Saint-Hyacinthe, Canada.)

collar has been described to prevent postoperative self-mutilation after laparotomy: some authors have successfully use infant pants as physical barriers against wound by self-mutilation.[51] Bandages on the cervical and thoracic area can be used to prevent rabbits from reaching their ears in case of self-injuries of the pinnae (**Fig. 10**).

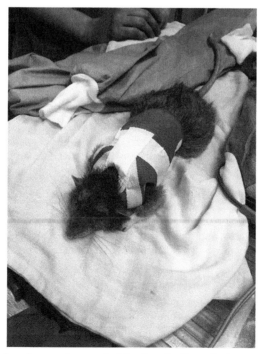

Fig. 9. Body wrap placed on a rat presented for dorsal self-mutilation associated with severe dermatitis. This bandage should always be associated with antinociceptive and etiologic treatments. (*Courtesy of* C. Vergneau-Grosset, med vet, IPSAV, CES, dipl ACZM, Saint-Hyacinthe, Canada.)

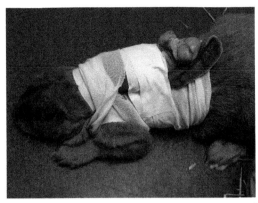

Fig. 10. Protective bandage to prevent ear self-mutilation in an English lop rabbit with chronic cellulitis of the right pinna secondary to a cat bite. (*Courtesy of* C. Vergneau-Grosset, med vet, IPSAV, CES, dipl ACZM, Saint-Hyacinthe, Canada.)

It is also important to remove water bowls from the environment and to train patients to drink from water bottles instead before using this type of bandage. In all case, pain monitoring is critical in this situation and antinociceptive medications should be adjusted on a case by case basis. Criteria used by clinician to assess patient comfort may include appetite, foraging activity while in hospitalization or grimace scales, especially in rats, mice, ferrets, and rabbits.[52–54]

SUMMARY

Although self-mutilation and ARBs are well-known issues in exotic small animals, the underlying causes remain poorly understood. Species and individual predisposition to develop these problems exist, however cerebral plasticity and learning abilities are 2 natural preventive mechanisms that clinicians and owners of small mammals should understand to provide the best care for these animals. Although diagnostic tests, treatment of the underlying cause (if any identified), and analgesia constitute the initial phase of medical management in cases brought to the clinic, environmental improvements and owners education about small mammals' welfare are the most effective ways in the long term to avoid the perpetuation of these abnormal behaviors.

CLINICS CARE POINTS

- Abnormal repetitive behaviors are multifactorial.
- In some cases, abnormal behaviors activate the dopaminergic system.
- Cerebral plasticity may allow predisposed animals to be successful treated.

DISCLOSURE

No conflict of interest to disclose.

REFERENCES

1. Fernandez EJ, Timberlake W. Foraging devices as enrichment in captive walruses (*Odobenus rosmarus*). Behav Processes 2019;168:103943.
2. Tynes VV. Behavioral dermatopathies. Vet Clin North Am Exot Anim Pract 2013; 16(3):801–20.

3. Wiedenmayer C. Stereotypies resulting from a deviation in the ontogenetic development of gerbils. Behav Processes 1997;39(3):215–21.
4. Colgoni A. Abnormal Repetitive Behaviour in captive animals. 2003. Available at: http://animalbiosciences.uoguelph.ca/~gmason/StereotypicAnimalBehaviour/library.shtml. Accessed March 2020.
5. Garner JP. Stereotypies and other abnormal repetitive behaviors: potential impact on validity, reliability, and replicability of scientific outcomes. ILAR J 2005;46(2):106–17.
6. Blumenkopf B, Lipman JJ. Studies in autotomy: its pathophysiology and usefulness as a model of chronic pain. Pain 1991;45(2):203–9.
7. Bennett GJ, Xie YK. A peripheral mononeuropathy in rat that produces disorders of pain sensation like those seen in man. Pain 1988;33(1):87–107.
8. Gispen WH, Isaacson RL. ACTH-induced excessive grooming in the rat. Pharmacol Ther 1981;12(1):209–46.
9. Bailoo JD, Murphy E, Boada-Sana M, et al. Effects of cage enrichment on behavior, welfare and outcome variability in female mice. Front Behav Neurosci 2018;12:232.
10. Mackenzie K. Stereotypic movement disorders. Semin Pediatr Neurol 2018;25:19–24.
11. Reitz S, Kluetsch R, Niedtfeld I, et al. Incision and stress regulation in borderline personality disorder: neurobiological mechanisms of self-injurious behaviour. Br J Psychiatry 2015;207:165–72.
12. Garner J. Perseveration and stereotypy - systems level insights from clinical psychology. In: Mason G, Rushen J, editors. Stereotypic animal behavior, fundamentals and applications to welfare. Oxfordshire (United Kingdom): CAB International; 2006. p. 121–53.
13. Weintraub D. Dopamine and impulse control disorders in Parkinson's disease. Ann Neurol 2008;64(Suppl 2):S93–100.
14. Breese GR, Criswell HE, Duncan GE, et al. Dopamine deficiency in self-injurious behavior. Psychopharmacol Bull 1989;25(3):353–7.
15. Aguirre-Benitez EL, Porras MG, Parra L, et al. Disruption of behavior and brain metabolism in artificially reared rats. Dev Neurobiol 2017;77:1413–29.
16. Papadakakis A, Sidiropoulou K, Panagis G. Music exposure attenuates anxiety- and depression-like behaviors and increases hippocampal spine density in male rats. Behav Brain Res 2019;372:112023.
17. Gonzalez C, Yanez JM, Tadich T. Determination of the genetic component of fur-chewing in chinchillas (Chinchilla lanigera) and its economic impact. Animals (Basel) 2018;8(9):144.
18. Ponzio MF, Monfort SL, Busso JM, et al. Adrenal activity and anxiety-like behavior in fur-chewing chinchillas (Chinchilla lanigera). Horm Behav 2012;61(5):758–62.
19. Tisljar M, Janic D, Grabarevic Z, et al. Stress-induced Cushing's syndrome in fur-chewing chinchillas. Acta Vet Hung 2002;50(2):133–42.
20. Franchi V, Aleuy OA, Tadich TA. Fur chewing and other abnormal repetitive behaviors in chinchillas (Chinchilla lanigera), under commercila fur-farming conditions. J Vet Behav 2016;11:60–4.
21. Gaskins LA, Bergman L. Surveys of avian practitioners and pet owners regarding common behavior problems in psittacine birds. J Avian Med Surg 2011;25(2):111–8.
22. Mueller K, Hsiao S. Pemoline-induced self-biting in rats and self-mutilation in the deLange syndrome. Pharmacol Biochem Behav 1980;13(5):627–31.

23. Ness RD, Johnson-Delaney CA. Chapter 29: Sugar gliders. In: Quesenberry KE, Carpenter JW, editors. Ferrets, rabbits and rodents clinical medicine and surgery. St Louis (MO): Elsevier; 2012. p. 393–410.

24. Harrer S, Schmidt WJ. Oestrogen modulates dopamine-controlled behaviours in the male ferret. Eur J Pharmacol 1986;128(1–2):129–32.

25. Mueller K, Saboda S, Palmour R, et al. Self-injurious behavior produced in rats by daily caffeine and continuous amphetamine. Pharmacol Biochem Behav 1982; 17(4):613–7.

26. Ponzio MF, Busso J, Ruiz RD, et al. A survey assessment of the incidence of fur-chewing in commercial chinchilla (*Chinchilla lanigera*) farms. Animal Welfare 2007;16(4):471–9.

27. Pilny A. Small exotic companion mammal wellness management and environmental enrichment. Vet Clin North Am Exot Anim Pract 2015;18(2):245–54.

28. Masson GJ, Latham NR. Can't stop, won't stop: is stereotypy a reliable animal welfare indicator? Animal Welfare 2004;13:57–69.

29. Hawkins MG. Advances in exotic mammals clinical therapeutics. Vet Clin North Am Exot Anim Pract 2015;18(2):323–37.

30. Coutant T, Vergneau-Grosset C, Langlois I. Overview of drug delivery methods in exotics, including their anatomic and physiologic considerations. Vet Clin North Am Exot Anim Pract 2018;21(2):215–59.

31. Radulovic LL, Turck D, von Hodenberg A, et al. Disposition of gabapentin (neurontin) in mice, rats, dogs, and monkeys. Drug Metab Dispos 1995;23(4):441–8.

32. Aryal B, Tae-Hyun K, Yoon-Gyoon K, et al. A comparative study of the pharmacokinetics of traditional and automated dosing/blood sampling systems using gabapentin. Indian J Pharmacol 2011;43(3):262–9.

33. Ruel HLM, Steagall PV. Adjuvant Analgesics in Acute Pain Management. Vet Clin North Am Small Anim Pract 2019;49(6):1127–41.

34. Camara CC, Ramos HF, da Silva AP, et al. Oral gabapentin treatment accentuates nerve and peripheral inflammatory responses following experimental nerve constriction in Wistar rats. Neurosci Lett 2013;556:93–8.

35. Fox A, Gentry C, Patel S, et al. Comparative activity of the anti-convulsants oxcarbazepine, carbamazepine, lamotrigine and gabapentin in a model of neuropathic pain in the rat and guinea-pig. Pain 2003;105(1–2):355–62.

36. Atwal N, Casey SL, Mitchell VA, et al. THC and gabapentin interactions in a mouse neuropathic pain model. Neuropharmacology 2019;144:115–21.

37. Amengual Batle P, Rusbridge C, Nuttall T, et al. Feline hyperaesthesia syndrome with self-trauma to the tail: retrospective study of seven cases and proposal for an integrated multidisciplinary diagnostic approach. J Feline Med Surg 2019;21(2): 178–85.

38. Papathanasiou T, Juul RV, Gabel-Jensen C, et al. Population pharmacokinetic modelling of morphine, gabapentin and their combination in the rat. Pharm Res 2016;33(11):2630–43.

39. Plumb DC. Pentoxyfylline. In: Plumb DC, editor. Plumb's veterinary drug handbook. 6th edition. Ames (IA): Wiley-Blackwell; 2015. p. 714–5.

40. Ramalho JR, Bento RF. Healing of subacute tympanic membrane perforations in chinchillas treated with epidermal growth factor and pentoxifylline. Otol Neurotol 2006;27(5):720–7.

41. Kenny DE. Use of naltrexone for treatment of psychogenically induced dermatoses in five zoo animals. J Am Vet Med Assoc 1994;205(7):1021–3.

42. Jain S, Sharma R. Analgesia in phasic and tonic pain tests in a pharmacological model of autotomy. Indian J Exp Biol 2002;40(11):1269–74.

43. Stahl SM. Stahl's essential psychopharmacology. New York: Cambridge University Press; 2013.
44. Diniz DA, Petrocchi JA, Navarro LC, et al. Serotonin induces peripheral antinociception via the opioidergic system. Biomed Pharmacother 2018;97:1434–7.
45. Caccia S, Cappi M, Fracasso C, et al. Influence of dose and route of administration on the kinetics of fluoxetine and its metabolite norfluoxetine in the rat. Psychopharmacology (Berl) 1990;100(4):509–14.
46. Holladay JW, Dewey MJ, Yoo SD. Pharmacokinetics and antidepressant activity of fluoxetine in transgenic mice with elevated serum alpha-1-acid glycoprotein levels. Drug Metab Dispos 1998;26(1):20–4.
47. Lu Y, Ho CS, Liu X, et al. Chronic administration of fluoxetine and pro-inflammatory cytokine change in a rat model of depression. PLoS One 2017;12(10):e0186700.
48. Anelli M, Bizzi A, Caccia S, et al. Anorectic activity of fluoxetine and norfluoxetine in mice, rats and guinea-pigs. J Pharm Pharmacol 1992;44(8):696–8.
49. Almansour MI, Jarrar YB, Jarrar BM. In vivo investigation on the chronic hepatotoxicity induced by sertraline. Environ Toxicol Pharmacol 2018;61:107–15.
50. Galeano MG, Ruiz RD, de Cuneo MF. Effectiveness of fluoxetine to control fur-chewing behaviour in the chinchilla (*Chinchilla lanigera*). Appl Anim Behav Sci 2013;146(1–4):112–7.
51. Bartley KA, Johnson CH. Human Infant pants for postoperative protection during social housing of New Zealand white Rabbits (*Oryctolagus cuniculus*). J Am Assoc Lab Anim Sci 2019;58(4):510–6.
52. Sotocinal SG, Sorge RE, Zaloum A, et al. The rat grimace scale: a partially automated method for quantifying pain in the laboratory rat via facial expressions. Mol Pain 2011;7:55.
53. Keating SC, Thomas AA, Flecknell PA, et al. Evaluation of EMLA cream for preventing pain during tattooing of rabbits: changes in physiological, behavioural and facial expression responses. PLoS One 2012;7(9):e44437.
54. Reijgwart ML, Schoemaker NJ, Pascuzzo R, et al. The composition and initial evaluation of a grimace scale in ferrets after surgical implantation of a telemetry probe. PLoS One 2017;12(11):e0187986.
55. Doss G, Mans C. Analgesic efficacy of buprenorphine in African pygmy hedgehogs (*Atelerix albiventris*). Paper presented at: ICARE; London, United Kingdom, April 28th - May 1st, 2019.
56. Abada C, Cuerela J, Gilabertb J, et al. Pharmacokinetics of oral and subcutaneous meloxicam (Metacam) in African pygmy hedgehogs (*Atelerix albiventris*). Paper presented at: ICARE2017; Venice, Italy.
57. Evenson EA, Mans C. Analgesic efficacy and safety of hydromorphone in chinchillas (*Chinchilla lanigera*). J Am Assoc Lab Anim Sci 2018;57(3):282–5.
58. Fox L, Mans C. Analgesic efficacy and safety of buprenorphine in chinchillas (*Chinchilla lanigera*). J Am Assoc Lab Anim Sci 2018;57(3):286–90.
59. Chinnadurai SK, Messenger KM, Papich MG, et al. Meloxicam pharmacokinetics using nonlinear mixed-effects modeling in ferrets after single subcutaneous administration. J Vet Pharmacol Ther 2014;37(4):382–7.
60. Carpenter JW, Marion CJ. Exotic animal formulary. St Louis (MO): Elsevier; 2018.
61. Sadar MJ, Knych H, Drazenovich T, et al. Pharmacokinetics of buprenorphine in the guinea pig (*Cavia porcellus*): intravenous and oral transmucal administration. Paper presented at: Association of Exotic Mammal Veterinarians 13th Conference Proceedings; Disney's Coronado Springs Resort, October 18-24th, 2014.

62. Ambros BB, Knych HK, Sadar MJ. Pharmacokinetics of hydromorphone hydrochloride after intravenous and intramuscular administration in guinea pigs (*Cavia porcellus*). Am J Vet Res 2020;81(4):361–6.

63. Roughan JV, Bertrand HG, Isles HM. Meloxicam prevents COX-2-mediated postsurgical inflammation but not pain following laparotomy in mice. Eur J Pain 2016; 20(2):231–40.

64. Ostadhadi S, Akbarian R, Norouzi-Javidan A, et al. Possible involvement of ATP-sensitive potassium channels in the antidepressant-like effects of gabapentin in mouse forced swimming test. Can J Physiol Pharmacol 2017;95(7):795–802.

65. Healy JR, Tonkin JL, Kamarec SR, et al. Evaluation of an improved sustained-release buprenorphine formulation for use in mice. Am J Vet Res 2014;75(7): 619–25.

66. Korkmaz M, Saritas TB, Sevimli A, et al. The effect of gabapentin and pregabalin on intestinal incision wound healing in rabbits. Vet World 2015;8(3):279–83.

67. Delk KW, Carpenter JW, KuKanich B, et al. Pharmacokinetics of meloxicam administered orally to rabbits (*Oryctolagus cuniculus*) for 29 days. Am J Vet Res 2014;75(2):195–9.

68. Souza MJ, Greenacre CB, Cox SK. Pharmacokinetics of orally administered tramadol in domestic rabbits (*Oryctolagus cuniculus*). Am J Vet Res 2008;69(8): 979–82.

69. Roughan JV, Flecknell PA. Evaluation of a short duration behaviour-based postoperative pain scoring system in rats. Eur J Pain 2003;7(5):397–406.

70. Taylor BF, Ramirez HE, Battles AH, et al. Analgesic activity of tramadol and buprenorphine after voluntary ingestion by rats (*Rattus norvegicus*). J Am Assoc Lab Anim Sci 2016;55(1):74–82.

71. Barbosa J, Faria J, Leal S, et al. Acute administration of tramadol and tapentadol at effective analgesic and maximum tolerated doses causes hepato- and nephrotoxic effects in Wistar rats. Toxicology 2017;389:118–29.

72. Foley PL, Liang H, Crichlow AR. Evaluation of a sustained-release formulation of buprenorphine for analgesia in rats. J Am Assoc Lab Anim Sci 2011;50(2): 198–204.

73. Morges MA, Grant KR, MacPhail CM, et al. A novel technique for orchiectomy and scrotal ablation in the sugar glider (*Petaurus breviceps*). J Zoo Wildl Med 2009;40(1):204–6.

74. Tsuchida A, Itoi T, Kasuya K, et al. Inhibitory effect of meloxicam, a cyclooxygenase-2 inhibitor, on N-nitrosobis (2-oxopropyl) amine induced biliary carcinogenesis in Syrian hamsters. Carcinogenesis 2005;26(11):1922–8.

75. Granson H. Gabapentin for tail trauma in a Syrian hamster (*Mesocricetus auratus*). Paper presented at: Proceedings of the Annual Conference of the AAV and the AEMV, August 1, 2010; San Diego, CA.

76. Moeremans I, Devreese M, De Baere S, et al. Pharmacokinetics and absolute oral bioavailability of meloxicam in guinea pigs (Cavia porcellus). Vet Anaesth Analg 2019;46(4):548–55.

Avian Behavior Consultation for Exotic Pet Practitioners

Elizabeth Stelow, DVM

KEYWORDS

- Psittacine behavior • Feather damaging • Vocalizations

KEY POINTS

- The most commonly reported behavior problems in psittacine birds include feather damaging, aggression toward people, excessive vocalization, and chronic egg laying (reproductive behaviors). In addition, fear/phobias and stereotypic behaviors indicate a welfare problem for the bird.
- Reduced-stress veterinary appointments are better for the bird's welfare and the veterinary staff's safety, but they require good planning and staff training.
- The veterinary team should be prepared to make general recommendations about psittacine husbandry and enrichment, regardless of the problem behavior being addressed.
- Physical and social enrichment play a key role in the behavioral health and overall welfare of pet psittacines.

 Video content accompanies this article at http://www.vetexotic.theclinics.com.

INTRODUCTION

The behavior of a pet affects its relationship with its owner and is a measure of overall psychological well-being. Psittacine birds are no exception to this. It stands to reason, then, that identifying and treating problem behaviors in these pets is an effective way of enhancing their relationships with their owners and increasing the chances of their retention in their homes. There is also a benefit to the veterinary team in understanding and treating problem behaviors in psittacines: safer and more efficient veterinary examinations and necessary medical treatments.

With all of the benefit to be gained from identifying and treating behavioral disorders in pet psittacines, it is important that the veterinary team is prepared to conduct a well-planned and thorough behavior appointment. Planning for such an appointment requires team training, preparing the examination space to be comfortable for the patient, stocking it with all necessary equipment, learning and

University of California, Davis, 1 Shields Avenue, Davis, CA 95616, USA
E-mail address: eastelow@ucdavis.edu

Vet Clin Exot Anim 24 (2021) 103–117
https://doi.org/10.1016/j.cvex.2020.09.006

practicing the principles of reduced-stress handling techniques, sending a detailed form to the owner to collect relevant history germane to the perceived behavior issues, requesting video evidence of behaviors not likely to be seen on examination, and having the knowledge necessary to diagnose and treat whatever the history form uncovers. Although this is a daunting list, some of these necessities (preparing a comfortable examination room, learning and practicing reduced-stress handling techniques, and gathering working knowledge about behavior diagnoses and treatments) need be done only once.

Another aspect of behavior in psittacines (perhaps in veterinary visits by all species) requiring greater attention is the failure of medical records to gather information about behavior, either during the appointment or as reported by the caregiver.[1] Recording this information is an aid during subsequent appointments and can track successes and weaknesses in the treatment plan sent home with the caregivers.

WHY PROBLEM BEHAVIORS ARISE

Most psittacines are not domestic; they retain the need for many of the daily maintenance behaviors of their wild parents or grandparents.[1,2] However, the environment in which they live, both the husbandry and the human relationships, is usually not sufficient or appropriate for engaging in those species-typical behaviors.[3,4] Birds that lack opportunities for foraging, lack a routine, lack sufficient sleep, were raised in an isolated setting (hand reared with little contact with parent birds), or crave attention are more likely to develop behavior problems.[5,6] These shortcomings can allow the development of fears and phobias, aggression, abnormal repetitive behaviors, self-mutilation, and screaming.[3] Inappropriate relationships with caregivers can exacerbate aggression and lead to reproductive behavior issues; many caregivers do not realize that petting or cuddling with or sharing food with their birds can be perceived by the bird as courting behaviors.[7]

Globally, the solution is to acknowledge and meet the needs of these gregarious, intelligent, nondomesticated pets; for people who raise young birds, this burden also requires provision of an environment supportive of normal psittacine brain development. However, little is known about the elements of enrichment necessary to improve a captive psittacine's welfare, although studies have confirmed that increased foraging, environmental complexity, and social contact can play a role.[3]

In addition to examining behavior problem diagnoses and treatment, this article also considers how to prepare for avian behavior examinations, how to minimize stress during the appointment, and how to counsel caregivers on the needs of their birds.

PREPARING FOR THE APPOINTMENT

In advance of the bird being presented, it is important for the caregivers to complete a behavior history form (**Box 1**). Along with observations in person or via video, this form is the primary tool for diagnosis during the appointment, as well as formulation of the treatment plan.[8,9]

The role of the history form is 2-fold. It helps the caregivers to organize pertinent information into a single document; this process helps to trigger memories, allow disagreements among household members to emerge for discussion, and prod caregivers into gathering medical records or other documentation that may be useful during the appointment. It also gives the clinician a good deal of information from which to begin to narrow differentials to be further explored during the appointment. The work the caregivers put into the document is time saved randomly probing for useful information during the appointment.

Box 1
The history form

A comprehensive behavior history form should include, at a minimum:

- Signalment
- Disease history
- Diet, environment, daily regimen
- Rearing history
- Relationships with each caregiver and other animals in the house
- History of reproductive activity, wing clips, and molting
- History of the current problem and other current patterns of behavior
- Whether caregiver must be present for the undesirable behavior (to determine whether there is an attention-seeking component); conversely, whether certain behaviors are worse when 1 or more owners leave.

Ideally, this form is made available to the clinician and team in advance of the appointment, so that special arrangements may be made if veterinary visits are of concern.

Data from Refs.[15,16,35]

Asking for a video of the behavior is another important step toward having the whole story. Often, birds do not perform a behavior of concern during the appointment, so the only way for a clinician to see it is to watch a video of it. Observation is important to make certain that the caregiver is not interpreting the behavior differently than the clinician would. Mistakes in diagnosis lead to inappropriate treatment plans.[8]

In addition, it is important that the examination room is prepared for an avian visit. The examination area should be arranged with all the necessary tools close at hand. If a table is to be used, it should have a nonslip cover. Similarly, the scale should be placed nearby with an appropriate perch on it. All laboratory sample and venipuncture supplies should be together. Any staff should have already been trained in reduced-stress handling techniques, as discussed later.

DURING THE APPOINTMENT

Early in the appointment, the medical team should be assessing the patient and looking for signs of fear, anxiety, and stress. These signs may include:

- Freezing: tense muscles, crouched posture, vigilant watching of the threat
- Escape or avoidance behaviors: leaning or flying away from the source of stress, attempting to hide, flapping wings, falling off the perch, or screaming
- Aggression: eye pinning, kicking with feet while lying on back, lunging forward while thrusting beak, biting, or screaming
- Abnormal repetitive behaviors: some birds engage is patterned behaviors caused by the stress of the appointment (Video 1)

At any of these signs, the clinician must change both tactics and expectations.[10]

To perform an examination that helps to rule out medical differentials, restraint and handling are necessary. There is ample evidence that low-stress techniques are better for the patient, the caregivers, and the medical team, but may not represent the standard of care in some clinics.[1,4,10] Even 20 years ago, many psittacines were wild caught and challenging to restrain for examination. Many pet psittacines are now captive-bred family members that can be examined and treated with far less restraint.[11]

It is, therefore, incumbent on veterinarians to maintain a less-is-more approach to the examination and avoid all painful or threatening handling.[11] During the examination, the client can be made aware of handling techniques that can be practiced in the comfort of home that can make the next veterinary visit even less stressful (beak, feet, eye/ear/nares, and wings).[11] In addition, the client can be instructed on how to give medications using food items or how to use desensitization and counter-conditioning to help the bird view medication administration or other medical treatment in a more positive light.[10]

Client counseling about psittacines as pets often includes some basic information in addition to specifics of a treatment plan for particular problem behaviors. These general points of information are included in **Box 2**.

One element of the treatment plan to be fully explored before the client leaves is the family's understanding of and commitment to the particulars of the plan being prescribed. Outcome depends on the willingness of the family members to embrace and implement the plan as written.[7,8]

MAKING THE DIAGNOSIS AND PLANNING THE TREATMENT

As with all behavior diagnoses, medical problems that could account for the behaviors should be explored, and ruled out wherever possible. If all that is left on the differentials list is "behavior problem," it is time to explore for an underlying motivation.

Box 2
Important general information for psittacine caregivers

The veterinary team should be prepared to discuss the following with each caregiver of a pet psittacine:

- Predisposing factors for behavior issues (lack of foraging opportunities, unstimulating physical environment, lack of a routine, insufficient sleep, inappropriate relationships with caregivers, hand rearing, and so forth)
- That not all households are a good fit for a psittacine bird[8]
- What birds need to learn before they make good pets:[1]
  ○ Normal social behaviors for flock interactions
  ○ Appropriate means to resolve conflicts
  ○ Understanding of what behaviors are acceptable and what behaviors are unacceptable
  ○ Other maintenance/social behaviors, as needed
- What to train the bird to do and how to train it with positive reinforcement[20]
- That food sharing and mutual grooming between the caregiver and the bird indicates to the bird that they are mates (ie, sexual partners),[28] and that much undesirable behavior can be caused by this inappropriate bond[8]
- That caregivers may have inadvertently reinforced bad behaviors when the bird was young
- That neonates should be socialized[28]
- That, because of the lack of generations to be domesticated, psittacines see humans as flock members rather than humans; they never develop the human-animal bonds that people enjoy with cats and dogs[28]

Ideally, medical teams practice these elements of client counseling before presenting them during an appointment. Some of these messages may be uncomfortable for the clients.[28]

Data from Refs.[1,8,20,28]

It is best to start behavior work-ups with a functional assessment based on the history form, caregiver interrogation, and observation. In this, look for the ABCs of the behavior in question: what are the antecedents (what happens before this behavior?), the behavior itself (in great detail, including body postures and accompanying vocalizations), and the consequences (outcome for the bird) for this behavior? Knowing these can give insight into the cause of the behavior.[12] An example might be that, when the caregiver leaves the living room to cook dinner (antecedent), the bird starts screaming while pacing and flapping its wings (behavior), so the caregiver comes back to the living room to scold the bird to be quiet (consequence). The suggestion here would be that the motivation for the bird is to get the caregiver back into the room. If the caregiver had fed the bird when he returned to the living room, the motivation might have been about the caregiver returning or about the food; more questions would be useful.[12]

The second step is to design an intervention for this behavior, based on the ABCs of it. The goal is to change the physical and social context. It is important that the bird be taught new skills to perform as an alternate rather than trying to quash the behavior. The plan should be scientifically sound and within the ability of the caregiver to implement. Ideally, it will have a way to evaluate its success[12] (for details of behavior modification, see "Animal Behavior and Learning: Support from Applied Behavior Analysis," by Friedman colleagues in this issue).

Studies have shown that the behavior problems most often noted by practitioners are different from those that concern the birds' caregivers. Practitioners surveyed reported feather damaging behavior (FDB) as the most common behavioral problem presented, followed by chronic egg laying, aggression toward humans, and screaming. By contrast, bird caregivers reported aggression toward humans most often, followed by screaming, then FDB.[13] However they are ranked by frequency of presentation, these represent the 4 most common behavioral problems in psittacines birds seen in medical practices. In addition to these 4, this article also discusses abnormal repetitive behaviors and fears and phobias.[1]

Presented in this article are diagnostic and treatment plans for:

- FDB and self-mutilation
- Aggression toward humans
- Reproductive behavior problems
- Excessive vocalization
- Abnormal repetitive behaviors
- Fears and phobias

With this information, clinicians are better able to address problems that create tension between caregivers and their birds.

Feather Damaging and Self-mutilation

Kenneth Martin[14] calls FDB a disorder of captivity. In that 1 phrase, he sums up the behavioral motivations for this behavior issue. It is estimated that approximately 15% of the captive parrot population shows FDB.[15] Self-mutilation is considered an extension of FDB in which the bird damages its skin, often to the point of bleeding; it is a life-threatening problem that must be addressed acutely and monitored carefully.

Further history exploration

Depending on how much time caregivers spend with their birds, and how observant they are, they may not be able to say whether observed feather loss is caused by the bird actively pulling out feathers. These cases force clinicians to rely more on diagnostics to rule out medical causes before determining that the cause is behavioral.[7]

If it is not on the behavior history form, be certain to ask the caregivers whether the bird has shown regurgitation or mating postures toward any of the caregivers.[16]

Predisposing factors

Although FDB is often attributed to boredom, the constellations of factors influencing this behavior makes the disorder far more complex. There is some debate about what predisposing factors are relevant to the development of FDB[15]; however, it seems that sleep deprivation, lack of foraging opportunities, lack of environmental complexity, and inadequate or inappropriate social relationships can lay the groundwork for FDB or self-mutilative behaviors.[5,6] In addition, age, breed, and socialization with other birds as a juvenile can influence the likelihood of FDB. The prevalence of this problem increases with age, with it being higher in adolescents than in juveniles, and higher still in adults.[15] Breed matters: FDB is more prevalent in macaw, African gray, eclectus, cockatoo, and conure species.[6,9,15] Socialization in the form of preening knowledge acquired from adults is more likely to be lacking in feather damaging birds; this puts hand-reared individuals at risk.[6] Interestingly, Kinkaid and colleagues[15] found that hatch origin (wild caught, parent reared, hand reared) and sex of the bird did not seem to contribute to the development of FDB.

Differential diagnoses

Medical differentials are discussed elsewhere in this issue in relation to medical causes of feather picking behavior for.

Anxiety/phobia, including separation anxiety There are many signs of anxiety in birds; (discussed later), and some birds engage in FDB when they are afraid or anxious. This behavior is to be contrasted with displacement behaviors, which occur from the stress of captivity, rather than other concerns, such as fear of the household dog, garbage trucks, strangers, or caregivers leaving.[5,6,9]

Attention-seeking behavior It is important to ask how the caregiver responds to the behavior and whether the caregiver must be present for the behavior to occur. Video can help to determine when the behavior is happening, but evidence of feather loss when the caregiver is gone is sufficient to rule out attention seeking as a sole cause.[5,6]

Displacement behavior This indicates a motivationally ambivalent response to the stress of a confinement situation that provides insufficient opportunity for species-typical behaviors, such as foraging, locomotion, and reproduction.[9,17]

Impulse control disorder This is a human psychiatric construct characterized by impulses that cannot be controlled.[18] Such a diagnosis equates FDB to hair pulling (trichotillomania) in humans.[5,17]

Prolonged reproductive behavior Especially in cockatoos, macaws, conures, and grey-cheeked parakeets, prolonged reproductive behavior can be the root cause of FDB. This behavior can occur with unnatural (artificially lengthened) photoperiods, high-fat diets, frustrated mating impulses caused by loss of a mate or inappropriate mate selection (including a caregiver), or the presence of mating pairs in the environment.[9]

Treatment

Certain predisposing factors, such as genetics and rearing history, cannot be undone. However, the history form and client interview are likely to uncover elements of the bird's living situation suspected of contributing to the FDB; these elements are the targets of an effective treatment plan. In general, the clinician should ensure that the bird is given a sufficiently stimulating environment and equally stimulating tasks to do.[5,7]

When planning for the environment, attention should be paid to the location and furnishings of the bird's home cage.[7] There should be a variety of opportunities for engaging in feeding behaviors,[7] because psittacines should be foraging most of day.[19] Species-typical foraging behaviors can be enhanced by providing a variety of foods from which to choose[5,19]; naturally, every food selected should be healthy for the specific species of bird. There should also be opportunities for self-play in the form of interactive toys that are rotated to keep them interesting.[5,19]

Appropriate tasks can involve provision of things to be chewed or destroyed, locomotory opportunities with ladders/perches, or the interactive training of specific behaviors.[7,20,21] The added benefit of training is that it allows for interactions between the bird and its caregivers that are unlikely to be misconstrued as courtship behaviors.

One type of enrichment caregivers can consider is pair housing, which has been shown to reduce many of the stressors that lead to problem behaviors.[22] The challenge is finding 1 or more additional birds that the patient would enjoying having as a companion. This author has a few clients with multiple single psittacines in their households because of pairings that never gelled.

If the patient presenting for FDB is also self-mutilating, the clinician must consider whether a protective Elizabethan-like collar is advisable.[5] Many types of commercial and home-made collars are available. The benefit is that a collar reduces the likelihood of serious blood loss. The challenge is that birds can become aggressive to caregivers because of the caregiver's need to check for good fit and pressure sores.

Clinicians can consider psychopharmacology as an intervention. Although they can be life changing for many patients, behavior medications should be used with some caution because of the lack of controlled trials of human psychotropic medication on psittacine patients.[23]

Aggression

There are several reasons a bird might become aggressive toward a human or another bird. The most common reasons are fear and conditioned/learned, territorial, mate-related, and redirected behaviors. Each of these is discussed in detail later; of these, fear is by far the most common (as in most species).

Predisposing factors for aggression include poor socialization with people or other birds, overattachment (inappropriate pair bonding) to a caregiver, and previous mishandling (including painful procedures or inappropriate wing trims).[24,25]

Aggressive behaviors include lunging, growling, and biting. Depending on the cause, the bird may chase down the victim; however, most aggression occurs when the bird is being approached (or even handled) by the person.[24,25]

Further history exploration

The clinician should ask the caregiver for a video showing the settings of the aggression, if not an example of the aggression itself. Such a video is helpful because, unless the aggression is triggered by vet visits, the clinician is not likely to see it manifested during the appointment. The caregiver should avoid intentionally triggering the aggression to get a video, particularly if someone might be injured by so doing.

The history form should ask for any known triggers, as well as the ABCs of notable incidents. However, the clinician may wish to explore some of these points if there is any doubt about the motivation for the aggression.

Behavioral differentials/possible causes

Fear Caregivers may note that the aggression happens most when the bird is unable to retreat from a situation. Examples include being reached for, medical treatments being administered, or being scared by things such as new toys being placed in the housing with the bird. The caregivers may also note overt signs of fear (eg, body tensing, hunched posture, staring at the threat, leaning away, looking for an opportunity to escape, and/or screaming).[10]

Conditioned/learned Biting is a very effective way to get people to stop doing things the bird does not like. The first bite is a response that can be based in fear, frustration, redirection, or any other motivation. However, the bird sees that the human stops the undesirable interaction when bit. Now, the bird can use biting (or the threat thereof) to keep the undesirable thing from happening again. The caregiver may or may not have noted signs of fear before the first bite. There may be no particular behavior change or warning before this type of aggression. Also, this type of aggression may target only 1, or all, members of the human family. There has been some speculation that this type of aggression is more commonly seen toward people with less bird experience and those who may appear meeker around birds.[24]

This type of aggression has mistakenly been called dominance aggression by some investigators. That term is not currently in favor because it implies a social hierarchical relationship between birds can humans that does not exist.

Territorial It is normal for most wild psittacines to establish and protect certain areas of their habitats.[25] Aggression that is directed toward people, birds, or other animals entering the bird's territory (cage, play area, and so forth) may have at least a component of territoriality. These birds are often relaxed and affiliative when away from the territory they guard.[25] This type of aggression may be more prevalent in breeding stock or during breeding season.[24]

Mate related (sexual) Single psittacines in a home lack suitable mate choices and may engage in pair-bonding behavior directed at one of their caregivers.[24,25] Any resulting aggression, therefore, may be directed at "rival" humans or, occasionally, the human "mate." It is often triggered when the bird's favorite person is approached by another person. This type of aggression can be exacerbated if the mate human is the sole caregiver, as well as during breeding season for the given species, particularly with increasing daylight.[24]

Redirected This type of aggression occurs when the cause/target of the aggression is unreachable (because of barriers or distance) or too scary to approach. The bird then becomes aggressive to the human (or bird) that is within range and not overly intimidating. It is important for the caregivers to identify the actual motivation for the aggression and address it; in cases of redirection, it is often mate-related or fear aggression being expressed.[24]

Treatment

The treatment depends on the motivation for the aggression:

Fear aggression Desensitization and counterconditioning to the scary objects, sounds, situations, and so forth are the primary treatments of fears that lead to aggression. While working on behavior modification, the caregivers should refrain from forcing the bird to face its fears by exposure to whatever is causing fear. Such exposure can deepen the fear, which is counterproductive.[25]

Conditioned/learned aggression It is important for caregivers to note the specific triggers for the aggression. Those triggers that can be avoided should be, because the bird has clearly expressed its preference to avoid these things.[25] For the unavoidable, such as medical treatments, behavior modification, including desensitization and counterconditioning, as well as positive-reinforcement training, can help these things to be less concerning to the bird.[10]

Territorial aggression Behavior modification and counterconditioning to people/birds/ and so forth in the home territory constitutes most of the treatment plan. In the meantime, the bird should be asked to step onto a perch to be removed from its territory before being invited to interact with people or other birds. This way, the territoriality is not engaged while behavior modification is changing the bird's emotional perception of its territory.[25]

Mate-related aggression Possibilities for treatment include having nonpreferred family members take over daily care for the bird, having the preferred human develop a more arms-length relationship through less cuddling and more training interactions, and, if necessary, hormone therapy.[24]

Redirected aggression Treatment of redirected aggression is treatment of the underlying cause, whether fear, mate related, or another motivation. Therefore, it is crucial that the diagnostic plan uncover the actual target and motivation for the aggression. Then, a plan can be developed based on that motivation.[24]

Reproductive Behavior Problems

This category of behavior problem is an amalgam of several previously discussed problem behaviors induced by hormonal, environmental, and social cues.[25] Behavior changes that comes with puberty (6 months to 6 years, depending on species) can include screaming, irritability, favoring 1 caregiver more than all others, territorial aggression, and overt sexual behaviors (regurgitation, masturbation). These behaviors can be reinforced or escalated by affection from the caregiver in the form of petting, cuddling, and food sharing. Coupled with the environmental cues of long daylight and plentiful food, the sexual behavior can persist for extended periods of time.[25]

Although it involves behaviors that are undesirable for the caregiver, this condition can also cause medical problems. In females, persistent sexual behaviors can lead to dystocia, cloacal prolapse, pathologic fractures, and coelomitis. In males, they can lead to cloacal prolapse and orchitis.[26]

Further history exploration
The caregiver may be presenting the bird for overt sexual behaviors or for the medical problems that can result. It is important to find out as much as possible about the bird's relationship with each caregiver in the household, in addition to the duration and progression of the problem.

Treatment
There is a 2-pronged approach to treating prolonged reproductive behaviors:

1. The caregivers should alter their relationships with the bird to provide more platonic interactions, including positive-reinforcement training, less petting or cuddling, and sharing of resources.
2. The environment should be altered to include an improved diet, shorter daylight, and removal of any actual or potential nesting sites.

If these elements are ineffective, direct modulation of reproductive hormones can be done via leuprolide acetate or similar intervention.[25]

Excessive Vocalization/Screaming

Psittacines, in general, are loud. They vocalize most at dawn, when the flock is waking up, and dusk, when the flock settles down together after a day of foraging; they are typically quiet overnight.[27] They engage in several different types of vocalizations, including contact calls, flight calls, alarm calls, food begging calls, and agonistic screams; they learn these from their parents and other nearby adults.[25,27]

Excessive vocalization is a common complaint by caregivers and is purported to be a leading cause of rehoming pet parrots.[4] However, because vocalization is a normal psittacine behavior, how is it determined to be excessive?[28] This decision depends on what the caregivers can tolerate as much as determining whether poor welfare is leading to the vocalizations. If it is the latter, here are some things to look for:

Some caregivers note that their birds make contact calls every time they leave the room; if they do not respond, some of these birds change from contact calling to alarm or distress calling, as their attempts to maintain contact fail. Other caregivers find that the escalating contact calls occur only when they leave the house. Either way, the frequency and intensity of these behaviors can help clinicians decide when to intervene.[27]

Some caregivers note alarm calls when certain people or other pets are present. Similarly, birds may alarm in new settings or when new objects are presented. These calls suggest anxiety about or fear of the person, pet, setting, object, and so forth that should be addressed for the welfare of the bird.[27]

One additional issue can be undesirable words or phrases that the bird has learned from its current or past caregivers, or noises that it has heard in its environment. These things can be inappropriate or simply annoying when spoken repeatedly.[27]

Further history exploration

It is important to find out what the vocalizations are and when they are happening. Video or audio recording is helpful, because some caregivers are not good at attributing the correct meaning to a specific vocalization. It is crucial to know what each person in the family does in response to the vocalizations, to focus on any attention-seeking aspects of the behavior.[27]

Behavioral differentials/possible causes

Anxiety/phobia, including separation anxiety There are many signs of anxiety in birds (discussed later), but some birds scream or otherwise vocalize when they are afraid or anxious. Separation anxiety occurs when key caregivers (or all caregivers) are separated from the bird. Some birds tolerate separation as long as it is clear the caregiver is still at home. Others seem to panic when the caregiver leaves the room.[25,27]

Inappropriate pair bonds with people Birds that form bonds with caregivers that mimic pair bonds seem to be more likely to vocalize when caregivers leave the room or leave the house. In the wild, contact calls keep the pair in communication with each other, so these vocalizations may take the form of excessive contact calling or may (if the bird is very concerned about the mate's absence) be distress calls.[3,25,27]

Attention-seeking behavior This motivation for vocalizations may result in vocalizations when the caregiver is in the same room or in an attempt to get the caregiver to return.[4] The attention they receive does not need to be positive to be rewarding; yelling, squirting with a water bottle, or other attempts to make the bird stop are all in the category of attention.[4] Therefore, it is important to ask how the caregiver responds to the behavior and whether the caregiver must be present for the behavior to occur. Video can help to determine whether the vocalization ever occurs when the bird is alone in the house (thus indicating a motivation other than attention seeking).[4,25]

Lack of appropriate enrichment or stimulation In short, the bird might not have anything better to do than call out.[25]

Treatment

Before developing a treatment plan, it is important to determine whether the vocalization is indeed excessive. It is equally important to counsel the caregiver that, even with appropriate treatment, the bird is likely to be vocal at dusk and dawn, simply by virtue of it being a psittacine.

Next, it is crucial to find the motivation for the vocalizations. Distress calls should never be ignored, whereas ignoring nuisance calls is a key part of the treatment plan for attention-seeking behaviors.[25]

For anxieties, including separation anxiety, see the treatment plan outlined earlier in relation to feather damaging.

For persistent contact calls, it may be helpful for the caregiver to speak occasionally to the bird from whatever other location they go to. This method allows the bird to limit its contact calls and engage in other, quieter behaviors.[27]

If the motivation is determined to be lack of stimulation or enrichment, a change in husbandry that allows more variety in activities is necessary. Enrichment can take many forms, including a more complex cage and play area[29] or pair/group housing.[22]

Stereotypic Behaviors

Stereotypic behavior is a type of abnormal repetitive behavior typically shown by captive wild animals or livestock kept in small quarters (horse stalls, farrowing crates, and so forth). Although the specific neural pathways have not been completely identified, it has long been suggested that the tight housing of these animals prevents species-typical behaviors in the realm of locomotion, foraging, or social engagement with others of their kind.[30]

The hallmark of stereotypic behaviors, and what sets them apart from other abnormal repetitive behaviors such as compulsive behaviors, is their patterned nature. What is meant by this is that the pattern that the behavior takes on is repeated nearly precisely the same way each and every time. This finding explains the very specific paths worn by pacing polar bears in their zoo enclosures and the particular damage done to stall doors by cribbing horses.[3]

Once a stereotypic behavior takes hold, it may be possible to reduce the frequency of the behavior but may not be possible to extinguish it completely.[31] With current research, it is hoped that better treatments will be available in the future.

Further history exploration

In addition to the history form exploring the circumstances under which the behavior started and continues, the clinician should request video of the specific behavior thought to be problematic. In this way, the clinician can judge the patterned nature of the behavior to make an accurate diagnosis. It is also important to have a clear understanding of the physical and social environment of the bird to best understand whether inadequacies exist.

Behavioral differentials/possible causes

Stereotypical behavior in psittacines has been divided into 3 main categories:

- Oral stereotypic behaviors include cage biting or tongue rolling. These behaviors are most likely caused by frustrations about foraging opportunities.
- Locomotory stereotypies include pacing, bobbing, spinning, and route tracing (Video 1). These behaviors are often secondary to limited space for movement/flight or lack of social interactions.[3,32]
- Object-directed stereotypies include repeated, patterned manipulation of a toy, feeder, or other item in the bird's cage or play space. These behaviors may indicate a lack of both environmental complexity and foraging opportunities.[3]

If the clinician determines that the pattern is not sufficient to consider the behavior stereotypic, consider displacement or attention seeking as alternative causes.

Treatment

There is little written about how to treat stereotypies in psittacines, save the findings of the aforementioned studies by combinations of Meehan and Mench.[2,3,22,29] However, if a clinician is to deduce treatment from those findings, the first step in treating stereotypies is to correct the identified shortcomings of the patient's environment, including its foraging and exercise regimen.

Fears/Phobias

Psittacine birds are prey species, so the individuals with the most reproductive success are the ones that were most suspicious of new things. This suspicion still persists in many pet psittacines. Fear in these birds can be caused by any of several possible factors: sharing a home with predatory species (humans, cats, dogs, and so forth), being invited out of the safety of their cage, being carried by people (sometimes strangers), facing people who are as anxious about the bird as the bird is about them, and so forth. Specific triggers can be as seemingly innocuous as new artwork in the room or a new toy in the bird's cage. This fear can be exacerbated when the caregivers do not take it seriously enough to keep the bird out of troubling situations until a treatment plan can be developed and implemented.[33]

Note that a fear response is considered normal (even if undesirable) if it is shown toward a stimulus that could actually be harmful, such as a dog or cat, vacuum cleaner, or a person running through the house with a stick. If the fear response is extreme, and seen as a response to an innocuous stimulus (a new toy, the caregiver's new hat, a telephone ringing, and so forth), it is considered a phobia.[33]

Phobic birds have been documented as having many similar personality characteristics and common elements in their behavioral histories. These characteristics include excitability, reactivity to eye contact, overreaction to noises and movement, and consistent attempts to escape rather than face (or fight) the stimulus.[33]

Fear responses to novelty have been shown to be more extreme in parrots living in less enriched environments, including birds who lack physical complexity in their housing and those who lack social stimulation.[3] This fact plays a role in the treatment plan for birds presented for fear.

Further history exploration

The behavior history form ascertains how the problem started, how it is progressing, and what response there has been to attempts to correct it. However, there may be confusion about the underlying cause of the behaviors. Psittacines have many possible fear responses, including a variety of postures associated with either fight or flight; and it is possible for caregivers to miss or misinterpret these.[33] The caregiver may not fully understand why the bird is frightened, or even that the behaviors of concern are a result of fear that manifests in aggression or escape behaviors; this is particularly true if the bird is afraid of items or situations that the caregiver believes the bird should find innocuous. The clinician is therefore best served by a video of the bird's response to a possible source of concern; this provides information beyond what the caregiver's interpretation allows.

Behavioral differentials/possible causes

Behavioral differentials are mainly about the extent of the fear, as well as its triggers. For instance, is the bird mildly concerned about the family's pet Yorkie, or is its response far out of scale for that type of trigger? Was the bird previously comfortable walking around the house on the hand of the teenage daughter, but is now panicking in her presence? Is the bird afraid of the lawnmower (understandable) or the purple octopus toy now hanging in its cage (perhaps a phobia)?

The diagnosis should therefore include the intensity (mild, moderate, severe), the scale (fear, phobia), and the triggering stimuli (dogs, noises, hands, and so forth).

Treatment

In the case of psittacine birds, the first order of business is to address the need for enrichment, both environmental and social. As discussed earlier, many psittacines live environmentally and socially deprived lives, compared with those of their wild counterparts. Studies have shown that individuals who live in enriched environments are, overall, less fearful.[22,29] One study found that individuals living in cages with ample foraging opportunities and sufficient complexity to the cage furnishings showed far more interest in (and therefore less fear of) new objects presented to them.[29] A second study showed that pair housing these individuals also leads to lessened signs of fear over a novel object if the pair was together when the object was presented. This finding is supported by similar research on other types of animals (rats, chickens, and monkeys), in which having a social partner decreased signs of fear in response to environmental novelty.[3]

Once any husbandry or enrichment problems have been addressed, the most effective treatment of fears and phobias is a combination of avoidance and behavior modification in the form of desensitization and counterconditioning (see "Animal Behavior and Learning: Support from Applied Behavior Analysis," by Friedman colleagues in this issue).

Some clinicians have had success using psychopharmacologic agents, such as benzodiazepines, selective serotonin reuptake inhibitors, and tricyclic antidepressants, to treat fears and phobias[14]; there are few clinical trials to support any specific claims about safety or effectiveness of these medications.[34] All psychotropic medications must be compounded, leading to more opportunity for error or variability of effect. However, there is some instructive literature describing the use of these medications in psittacines.

SUMMARY

The behavior of an individual bird is, essentially, a reflection of the quality of its life. Those who show problem behaviors may be experiencing poor husbandry, may lack the ability to engage in 1 or more species-typical behaviors, or may have experienced traumatic events in the past. The exotic animal veterinary team is in a position to explore these behavior issues, identify the underlying causes, and assemble a series of treatment options to help the bird (and its caregivers) experience a better quality of life.

DISCLOSURE

The author has nothing to disclose.

SUPPLEMENTARY DATA

Supplementary data related to this article can be found online at https://doi.org/10.1016/j.cvex.2020.09.006.

REFERENCES

1. Speer B. Normal and abnormal parrot behavior. J Exot Pet Med 2014;23(3): 230–3.
2. Meehan CL, Millam JR, Mench JA. Foraging opportunity and increased physical complexity both prevent and reduce psychogenic heather picking by young Amazon parrots. Appl Anim Behav Sci 2003;80(1):71–85.
3. Meehan C, Mench J. Captive parrot welfare. In: Leuscher AU, editor. Manual of parrot behavior. Ames (IA): Blackwell Publishing Professional; 2006. p. 301–18.
4. Welle KR. Behaviour and behavioural disorders. In: Harcourt-Brown N, Chitty J, editors. BSAVA Manual of psittacine birds. 2nd edition. Gloucester (England): British Small Animal Veterinary Association; 2005. p. 205–21.
5. Seibert LM. Psittacine feather picking. Presented at the Western Veterinary Conference, Las Vegas, NV, February 17-20, 2003.
6. Chitty J. Feather plucking in psittacine birds: 2. Social, environmental and behavioural considerations. Pract 2003;25(9):550–5.
7. Rubenstein J, Lightfoot T. Feather loss and feather destructive behavior in pet birds. J Exot Pet Med 2012;21(3):219–34.
8. Welle KR, Wilson L. Clinical evaluation of psittacine behavioral disorders. In: Leuscher AU, editor. Manual of parrot behavior. Ames (IA): Blackwell Publishing Professional; 2006. p. 175–85.
9. Seibert LM. Feather-picking disorder in pet birds. In: Leuscher AU, editor. Manual of parrot behavior. Ames (IA): Blackwell Publishing Professional; 2006. p. 255–65.
10. Speer BL, Hennigh M, Muntz B, et al. Low-stress medication techniques in birds and small mammals. Vet Clin N Am Exot Anim Pract 2018;21(2):261–85.
11. Davis C. New handling techniques for the avian patient. Semin Avian Exot Pet Med 1999;8(4):178–82.
12. Friedman SG, Hess L. A clinic-based protocol for solving behavior problem. Proc Annu Conf Assoc Avian Vet March 10-13, 2009. Milwaukee (WI). p 251–62.
13. Gaskins LA, Bergman L. Surveys of avian practitioners and pet owners regarding common behavior problems in psittacine birds. J Avian Med Surg 2011;25(2): 111–8.
14. Martin KM. Psittacine behavioral pharmacotherapy. In: Leuscher AU, editor. Manual of parrot behavior. Ames (IA): Blackwell Publishing Professional; 2006. p. 267–79.
15. Kinkaid HYMD, Mills DS, Nichols SG, et al. Feather-damaging behavior in companion parrots: an initial analysis of potential demographic risk factors. Avian Biol Res 2013;6(4):289–96.
16. Eatwell K. How to…investigate and treat a feather plucking parrot. J Small Anim Pract 2009;50(12):p12–6.
17. van Zeeland YRA, Spruit BM, Rodenburg TB, et al. Feather damaging behavior in parrots: A review with consideration of comparative aspects. Appl Anim Behav Sci 2009;121(2):75–95.

18. American Psychiatric Association. Diagnostic and statistical manual of mental disorders, 4th edition, text-revised (DSM-IV-TR). Washington, DC: American Psychiatric Publishing, Inc; 2000.
19. Bauck L. Psittacine diets and behavioral enrichment. Semin Avian Exot Pet Med 1998;7(3):135–40.
20. Heidenreich B. An introduction to positive reinforcement training and its benefits. J Exot Pet Med 2007;16(1):19–23.
21. Heidenreich B. Solving companion parrot behavior problems. Proc Annu Conf Assoc Avian Vet August 9-11, 2005; Monterey, CA. pp. 219-227.
22. Meehan CL, Garner JP, Mench JA. Isosexual pair housing improves the welfare of young Amazon parrots. Appl Anim Behav Sci 2003;81(1):73–88.
23. Seibert LM. Pharmacotherapy for behavioral disorders in pet birds. J Exot Pet Med 2007;16(1):30–7.
24. Welle KR, Leuscher AU. Aggression in pet birds. In: Leuscher AU, editor. Manual of parrot behavior. Ames (IA): Blackwell Publishing Professional; 2006. p. 211–7.
25. Seibert LM, Sung W. Psittacines. In: Tynes VV, editor. Behavior of exotic pets. Ames (IA): Wiley-Blackwell; 2010. p. 1–11.
26. Speer B. Sex and the single bird. Presented at the North American Veterinary Conference, Orlando, FL, January 14-18, 2012.
27. Bergman L, Reinisch US. Parrot vocalization. In: Leuscher AU, editor. Manual of parrot behavior. Ames (IA): Blackwell Publishing Professional; 2006. p. 219–23.
28. Welle KR. Behavior classes in the veterinary hospital: preventing problems before they start. In: Leuscher AU, editor. Manual of parrot behavior. Ames (IA): Blackwell Publishing Professional; 2006. p. 165–74.
29. Meehan CL, Mench JA. Environmental enrichment affects the fear and exploratory responses to novelty of young Amazon parrots. Appl Anim Behav Sci 2002;79(1):75–88.
30. Mason GJ. Stereotypies: a critical review. Anim Behav 1991;41(6):1015–37.
31. Cooper JJ, Odberg F, Nicol C. Limitations on the effectiveness of environmental improvement in reducing stereotypic behavior in bank voles (*Clethrionomys glareolus*). Appl Anim Behav Sci 1996;48(3–4):237–48.
32. Cussen VA, Mench JA. The relationship between personality dimensions and resiliency to environmental stress in Orange-Winged Amazon parrots (*Amazona amazonica*), as indicated by the development of abnormal behaviors. PLOS one 2015;10(6):e0126170.
33. Wilson L, Leuscher AU. Parrots and fear. In: Leuscher AU, editor. Manual of parrot behavior. Ames (IA): Blackwell Publishing Professional; 2006. p. 225–31.
34. Seibert LM. Behavioral pharmacology in exotic pets. In: Tynes VV, editor. Behavior of exotic pets. Ames (IA): Wiley Blackwell; 2010. p. 200–14.
35. Chitty J. Feather plucking in psittacine birds: 1. Presentation and medical investigation. In Pract 2003;25(8):484–93.

Medical Causes of Feather Damaging Behavior

Isabelle Langlois, DMV, DABVP (Avian)*

KEYWORDS

- Feather damaging behavior • Feather destructive behavior • Feather picking
- Medical causes • Diseases

KEY POINTS

- Any localized or systemic medical condition that affects brain function or causes pain, irritation, discomfort, and/or pruritus may result in the bird damaging its feathers.
- Thorough physical examination of the integumentary system as well as all other systems is crucial to identify medical causes of feather damaging behavior.
- Medical causes of feather damaging behavior are excluded or are identified by performing a series of diagnostic tests adapted to each patient's clinical presentation.
- As a portion of the sound medical evaluation, the initial aspects of behavioral assessment should be evaluated.
- Treatment plan of the medical causes of feather damaging behavior should be multifaceted and not directed strictly toward the diagnosed medical condition.

INTRODUCTION

Feather damaging behavior (FDB), also referred to as feather picking, feather plucking, or pterotillomania, is one of the most common and frustrating clinical presentations in captive psittacines. The prevalence in companion parrots from private homes varies from 10% to 17.5%.[1–5] By definition, FDB is a condition in which the parrot damages its feathers with the beak. The feathers of the head are typically unchanged because these are inaccessible to the bird's beak, although, in rare cases, parrots have been seen pulling the head feathers with their feet.[6–11]

The diagnosis of medical causes of FDB requires a meaningful logical process including a thorough history, complete physical examination with emphasis on the evaluation of the integument, and additional diagnostic tests.[8,12] Initial behavioral assessment including, but not limited to, the way the behavior is manifested, the time of the day or year the behavior is most intense, social interactions among the

Centre Hospitalier Universitaire Vétérinaire (CHUV), Université de Montréal, Saint-Hyacinthe, Quebec, Canada
* 3200 rue Sicotte, Saint-Hyacinthe, Quebec J2S 2M2 Canada.
E-mail address: Isabelle.langlois@umontreal.ca

Vet Clin Exot Anim 24 (2021) 119–152
https://doi.org/10.1016/j.cvex.2020.09.005
1094-9194/21/© 2020 Elsevier Inc. All rights reserved.

vetexotic.theclinics.com

bird's household, and early life experiences should be an integral part of the FDB consultation as well (see "Avian Behavior Consultation for the Exotic Pet Practitioner," by Elizabeth Stelow in this issue).

CLINICAL APPROACH

The history taking is important in determining a list of differential diagnosis and the possible implication of a medical cause to the FDB.[10,13] The onset, duration, progression, and distribution may provide some valuable clues as to the cause.[14] The gathering of pertinent information requires more time than the usual anamnesis. Therefore, the use of a questionnaire that can be sent to the client before the veterinary visit is helpful.[12,14,15] Several examples are available.[9,14,15]

The first crucial step is to confirm that the feather damage is self-inflicted as opposed to other conditions that causes loss or damage to the bird's feathers irrespective of the bird's behavior (**Box 1**). If the veterinarian is able to confirm that the feather abnormalities or loss is self-inflicted, the next challenge is to identify whether the plumage deterioration (1) results from husbandry management, (2) primarily originates from a medical condition, (3) consists of a primary behavioral problem, or (4) is caused by a combination of 2 or more of these options.[9]

Environmental inadequacies identified may act as a contributing factor for FDB. A small cage or poor cage design may cause damage to the feathers. As a result, the bird may remove the damaged feathers, which should be regarded as normal behavior.[8] Low humidity levels, lack of bathing opportunities, and abnormal photoperiods may also contribute to FDB.[16] For example, Amazon parrots need to be bathed, showered, or misted at least once a week to allow the expression of natural bathing behavior.[17] Any changes in the bird's routine that coincide with the onset of feather picking should be investigated as a possible trigger for initiating FDB.

Box 1
Clinical approach to determine whether feather damage is self-inflicted

- Question the owner regarding the typical amount of time the bird spends preening.
  - Normal grooming and normal removal of feather sheaths from growing feathers must be differentiated from FDB. Owners may not be familiar with the typical amount of time birds spend preening and may confuse FDB with normal preening and molt-related feather loss. To complicate this further, birds with plumage problems may spend more time on comfort activities such as preening.[119]

- Determine whether the owner might confuse the apterylae with zones of feather plucking.
  - Birds naturally have areas of skin with no feathers between feather tracts. These featherless areas might be visible only during molt because the loss of feathers makes them visible to the owner.

- Ensure the feathers covering the head are clinically normal.
  - Only the feathers accessible to the bird's beak are typically damaged.
  - In rare instances, some birds damage head feathers with their feet.

- Confirm feather anomalies are compatible with self-inflicted damage.
  - Evidence of chewed, cut, plucked, and/or frayed feathers must be distinguished from normal plumage or feather loss

- Verify whether the owner witnesses the bird damaging its plumage.
  - Video recordings of the bird at home, in its own environment, in the presence and absence of the owner, are helpful in some instances to allow objective evaluation.

Avian physical examination consists of 2 parts: observation and the hands-on examination. The observation phase is best performed at the beginning of the visit with the bird at rest in a nonthreatening situation in the consultation room, whereas the history data are discussed with the owner. The bird should be evaluated for the presence of pruritus/discomfort. The bird's mentation, posture, and stance are important indicators of disease.[12]

During the hands-on physical examination, all systems should be evaluated in a systematic manner to determine whether anomalies compatible with a medical cause leading to FDB are present. Notation of dermatologic abnormalities involving the skin and feathers should be detailed to facilitate monitoring of the patient's progress. Pictures of the lesions may be included in the patient's medical record for objective monitoring. Feather scoring systems offer a reliable and practical alternative.[18,19] **Box 2** presents a list of physical examination findings that may suggest a medical cause to the FDB.

The diagnostic testing should be tailored to the individual patient. The diagnostic tests potentially indicated to identify medical causes of FDB and their indications are listed in **Table 1**. Test selection is based on the differential diagnosis established for the patient according to the species, age, sex, history, and clinical presentation. Multiple laboratory samples may be collected during the initial visit, but submission for laboratory testing may be staggered. Ultimately, this decreases the owner's financial burden and adapts the diagnostic investigation to each patient as pending results are received.

While performing the physical examination, various skin and feather samples may be collected. Skin scrapings and impression smears may be evaluated microscopically. Several blood feathers of an affected area can be gently pulled for pulp cytology and/or culture.[12,20] If folliculitis is suspected, aspiration of the follicle by sterile needle and syringe is necessary.[13] Remembering that feather pulp cytology does not replace culture or histological examination is crucial. Fine-needle aspiration of any cutaneous or subcutaneous mass lesion is indicated.

If a complete blood count or plasma biochemical analysis needs to be included in the work-up of the patient, it is best to collect the blood sample before a significant amount of handling time.[12,21] Avian species with heterophils as dominant granulocytes are reported to show increase in both white blood cell count and heterophil count after handling and transport.[22,23] Of note, the presence of an inflammatory

---

Box 2
Physical examination findings suggesting a medical cause of feather damaging behavior

Hands-off Physical Examination	Hands-on Physical Examination
Lethargy, depression	Skin erythema, exudation, crusting
Lameness, drooping wing	Swollen/dystrophic feather follicles
Obvious cutaneous/subcutaneous mass or displaced feathers	Skin wound
Abnormal breathing pattern	Cutaneous/subcutaneous mass or mass of other origin
Coelomic distension	Heart murmur
Abnormal feces (diarrhea, biliverdinuria, yellow-discolored urates)	Coelomic distention/mass effect/hepatomegaly
Abnormal feathering of the head	Joint crepitus, decreased range of motion
Discolored feathers	Abnormal respiratory auscultation, prolonged respiratory recovery time

Table 1
Diagnostic tests that may be used for identification of medical causes of feather damaging behavior

With Specific Focus on the Integumentary System	
Diagnostic Tests	Objectives
Skin scrapings	Evaluate for ectoparasites such as *Knemidocoptes, Metamichrolichus nudus*
Feather digestion	Evaluate for ectoparasites such as quill mites
Skin cytology (swab, tape, impression smear)	Evaluate for bacterial or fungal dermatitis, ectoparasites, pox virus
Feather pulp cytology	Evaluate for bacterial or fungal folliculitis, ectoparasites such as quill mites
Culture (skin swab, feather pulp, biopsy)	Evaluate for bacterial or fungal dermatitis/folliculitis
Fine-needle aspiration	Evaluate for a cyst, abscess, neoplasia
Biopsies for histologic evaluation (skin + follicle)	Consider submission of paired samples from unaffected (back of the head or neck) and affected area of the tegument Evaluate for infectious, inflammatory, and/or neoplastic skin disorder
With Specific Focus on a Systemic Evaluation	
Diagnostic Tests	Objectives
Complete blood count	Evaluate for generalized infection or inflammatory process
Biochemistry profiles General profile Lipid profile	Evaluate for hepatopathy, nephropathy, pancreatic disease Establish baseline when atherosclerosis is suspected
Fecal analysis (wet mount and flotation)	To evaluate for the presence of endoparasites and *Macrorhabdus ornithogaster*
Medical Imaging	
Radiology	To evaluate the gastrointestinal tract, reproductive disorder, organomegaly, airway disease, musculoskeletal disease
Ultrasonography	To evaluate the appearance of the liver, reproductive tract, kidneys, heart and major vessels, any coelomic mass effect, coelomic effusion
Computed tomography	To consider in the assessment of airway/cardiovascular disease, musculoskeletal anomaly, or any other coelomic anomalies
Endoscopy	To determine the cause of air sacculitis and disorders of the liver, kidneys, pancreas, spleen, and reproductive tract

(continued on next page)

Table 1
(continued)

With Specific Focus on a Systemic Evaluation	
Diagnostic Tests	**Objectives**
Lead and zinc levels	To rule out heavy metal intoxication only if exposure is documented with consistent medical imaging findings because no clear association has been demonstrated
Specific detection tests	• Psittacine beak and feather disease): PCR (blood, growing feather) • Polyomavirus: PCR (blood, cloacal swab, tissue) • Avian bornavirus: RT-PCR (crop and cloacal swab), serology • *Chlamydia psittaci*: PCR (conjunctival, choanal, cloacal swab; blood), serology

Abbreviation: PCR, polymerase chain reaction; RT-PCR; reverse transcription polymerase chain reaction.

leukogram is expected, especially when extensive lesions are present.[14] Increased levels of muscular enzymes (aspartate transaminase, lactate dehydrogenase, creatine kinase) may occur with handling and may be observed with FDB. Plasma butyrylcholinesterase, a glycoprotein enzyme, has been investigated in companion psittacine species with and without FDB.[24] No significant association between serum concentrations and FDB could be established except in lovebirds. Therefore, the use of this parameter is currently limited.

Skin biopsy provides useful diagnostic information for birds presenting FDB. A paired biopsy protocol is recommended with full-thickness biopsies of skin and feather from affected and unaffected sites (**Box 3**).[20,25,26] This technique allows discrimination between inflammatory changes secondary to FDB, in which an inflammatory component would be limited to the affected area, and generalized skin inflammation suggests hypersensitivity or cutaneous manifestation of systemic

---

Box 3
Paired biopsy protocol recommended to investigate feather damaging behavior

• Both affected and unaffected sites should be biopsied.
  ○ Affected sites are areas easily reached by the bird's beak and clinically abnormal.
  ○ Unaffected sites are areas clinically normal and unable to be reached by the bird's beak, such as the back of the neck and head.
• Use punch biopsy technique using tape to prevent the skin from rolling or balling up.[27]
  ○ Apply nontranslucent self-adhesive tape on the skin of the chosen sites before performing the biopsy.
  ○ Perform biopsy through the tape by applying gentle force to the biopsy punch as it is twisted clockwise and counterclockwise.
  ○ Once the tape is passed through, only minimal pressure is required to go through the skin.
  ○ Place each skin biopsy flat in small cassettes clearly identified (affected vs unaffected).
• Evaluate the need to collect additional skin biopsies for other tests (culture, polymerase chain reaction, and so forth).

inflammation.[20,25] This technique allows trimming at right angles and through the longitudinal diameter of the feather follicles for accurate histopathologic evaluation.[27]

Intradermal allergy testing has been investigated in psittacines but with ambiguous results.[28,29] The response to histamine was highly inconsistent in birds.[30] Endogenous cortisone production during the testing procedure may account for the weak wheal formation observed during skin testing.[31] For all these reasons, this diagnostic test is not performed routinely in avian patients.

Medical imaging may be indicated if the bird is picking intensely at 1 area on the body, if the picking began at 1 distinct area, or if no abnormalities have been found on the physical examination as part of an in-depth examination of the patient. Depending on the clinical presentation and species involved, tests for specific diseases should be considered.[14] If less invasive diagnostic tests have led to inconclusive results, endoscopy to evaluate the air sacs and other internal organs may be performed.

The information obtained during the clinical approach is useful to identify the body system or systems affected. The data collected enable determination of whether the integumentary system is most likely involved primarily or secondarily and sheds light on the involvement of other body systems.

MEDICAL CAUSES OF FEATHER DAMAGING BEHAVIOR

The causes of FDB have been classified in various way in the literature over the years: infectious versus noninfectious,[7,10] inflammatory versus noninflammatory,[12,21] medical causes versus behavioral (psychogenic).[24,32,33] This last classification may falsely give the impression that this artificial grouping makes these categories mutually exclusive. However, they are interrelated. This article presents the medical causes of FDB using the VITAMIN D algorithm (**Table 2**).

Vascular Causes

Atherosclerosis has been suggested as a cause of FDB. One author reports numerous cases of recurrent or nonresolving dermatologic conditions (eg, axillary or propatagial dermatitis, feather loss or abnormal growth, or self-inflicted feather damage or mutilation of the skin), wherein advanced atherosclerotic lesions were ultimately identified in vessels supplying the affected areas.[34] These conditions may potentially reflect tissue hypoperfusion or associated pain or unusual sensations such as tingling and numbness. Further, it is possible that myocardial ischemia could produce angina pectoris as in humans, which results in a disproportion between oxygen offered to and oxygen needed by the heart muscle.[34,35] Atherosclerosis should be investigated, especially if the patient is older, of female gender, and belongs to a species known to be atherosclerosis prone (African grey and Amazon parrots, cockatiels).[36]

Inflammatory Causes

In a retrospective study of birds presenting FDB, inflammatory skin disease was diagnosed histologically in 51% of cases.[25] The cause for inflammatory skin disease in the study was not determined, but it is likely that more than 1 cause exists. Current knowledge regarding inflammatory causes of FDB is discussed next.

Infectious causes
Parasites Reports of external parasites in captive pet birds are few and are presented in **Table 3**.[37,38] The burrowing mite *Knemidocoptes pilae* is the most common external parasite in the author's practice (**Fig. 1**). Mites are usually superficial and may be diagnosed by skin scrapings. However, mite infestation should not be ruled out just based on skin scrapings. Some species of mites may require deep scrapings or biopsy for

Table 2
Medical causes of feather damaging behavior using the VITAMIN D algorithm

	Algorithm		Medical Causes of FDB
V	Vascular		Atherosclerosis[a]
I	Infectious	Parasites	Ectoparasites (*Knemidocoptes* spp, *Sarcoptes* sp, quill mites, lice), endoparasites (*Giardia* spp)[a]
		Bacteria	*Staphylococcus* sp, *Mycobacterium* spp, *C psittaci*,[a] and so forth
		Fungi	*Trichophyton* spp, *Microsporum gypseum*, *Aspergillus* spp, *Mucor* spp, *Rhizopus* spp, *Penicillium* spp, *Cryptococcus neoformans*, *Malassezia* spp, and *Candida* spp
		Viruses	Avipoxvirus, polyomavirus, circovirus, bornavirus[a]
	Immune		Hypersensitivity, contact dermatitis
	Inherited		Feather cyst (some species of canaries), genetic predisposition (Amazon parrots)[a]
T	Traumatic		Fall/collision leading to skin wound, feather cyst; chronic fracture, luxation, soft tissue trauma
	Toxic		Inhalants, topicals, heavy metals[a]
A	Anomalous		Hamartoma
M	Metabolic		Liver disease,[a] reproductive activity/disease, kidney disease, pancreatic disorder, acute or chronic stress
I	Iatrogenic		Inappropriate trim of remiges, intramuscular microchip[a]
	Idiopathic		CUD, Amazon foot necrosis, polyfolliculitis
N	Neoplastic		Xanthoma, lipoma, basal cell tumor (associated with feather cyst), squamous cell carcinoma, fibrosarcoma, and so forth
	Nutritional		Various deficiencies may be contributing factors[a]
D	Degenerative		Osteoarthritis

Abbreviation: CUD, chronic ulcerative dermatitis.
[a] Circumstantial evidence, pathogenesis not shown.

diagnosis. Therefore, in order to exclude mite infestation, the clinical approach used in small animal dermatology, consisting of excluding mite infestation in the presence of negative skin scrapings by treating as such, is advisable in some cases.

Giardia psittaci has been linked to FDB and intense pruritus in cockatiel.[39,40] Some investigators report the axillary areas are most often affected.[39] The relationship between giardia infection and FDB in this species has not been proved scientifically and this syndrome is not observed in all cockatiels with giardiasis.[41] The proposed mechanism of pruritus is related to gastrointestinal malabsorption of fat-soluble vitamins.[42,43] Diagnosis is by direct examination (20–40×) of fresh fecal sample (<10 minutes) using warm saline to identify the motile trophozoites or zinc sulfate flotation test to detect infective cysts. The trophozoites are destroyed in salt or sugar flotation solutions.[40] Note that the trophozoites and cysts are shed intermittently. An enzyme-linked immunosorbent assay test for *Giardia* spp antigen in feces may be used, but false-negative results are possible so it should not be relied on as a sole mean of diagnosis.[44] Nested polymerase chain reaction (PCR) may also be performed.[45] Empiric treatment to eliminate this pathogen may be considered in some clinical situations if direct smear and flotation yielded negative results. Metronidazole is most commonly used, but resistance does occur.[46]

Table 3
External parasites that may be associated with feather damaging behavior

External Parasites	Species Affected	Clinical Presentation	Comments
Knemidocoptes pilae	Most commonly seen in budgerigars (*Melopsittacus undulatus*) and canaries (*Serinus canarius*)[12]	• Raised yellowish, honeycombed encrustations on unfeathered skin around the beak, cere, gular region, vent, legs and feet[7] • In severe infestations, feather follicles of the wing, tail, and body may all be affected[10,41] • FDB can occur with severe infestations	Concomitant infection (circovirus, *Mycobacterium* sp) is a predisposing factor to severe infestation[39,47]
Sarcoptes sp	Reported in a green-winged macaw[38]	Multifocal severe pyogranulomatous dermatitis along the leading edge of the wings and lower legs	The bird had a 1-y history of partially antibiotic-responsive feather picking
Quill mites (Laminosioptidae, Fainocoptinae, and so forth)	Passeriformes and Psittaciformes[12,39,40]	• Opaque quill appearance instead of transparent[7] • Thickened, easily split calamus[39] • May cause damage to developing feathers, most commonly the primaries	• Diagnosis may be obtained through microscopic examination of powdery quill material or a broken feather shaft[39] • Mites can also be seen in pulp material within a developing feather[121]
Lice	Uncommon in well-cared-for companion birds, but common in domestic gallinaceous birds, pigeons, and wild birds[47]	• Lice eggs may be observed on the remiges and feathers around the vent typically[12,39] • Mild to moderate pruritus and hyperkeratosis, which can lead to FDB depending on the degree of infestation[12,16]	Their significance as a cause of FDB in pet birds is vastly exaggerated

Data from Refs.[7,10,12,16,38–41,47,121]

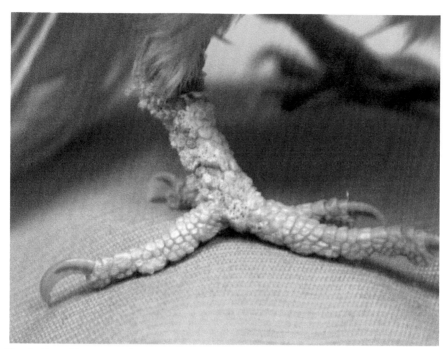

Fig. 1. *Knemidocoptes pilae* in a budgerigar (*Melopsittacus undulatus*). Raised yellowish, honeycombed encrustations are present with associated FDB proximal to the intertarsal joint.

Bacteria Bacterial skin disease in pet birds may be primary or secondary, and either can be confined to the feather follicle or be generalized.[12,47] In cases of folliculitis, swelling of the perifollicular skin with a variable amount of reddening is seen grossly.[47] Severe feather dystrophy and feather pulp inflammation,[48] as well as follicular abscessation, may also occur. Generalized bacterial dermatitis is associated with soft tissue swelling, reddening, induration, and crust formation (**Fig. 2**). These lesions are often pruritic, resulting in FDB or self-trauma.[12]

Skin infection may spread systemically. Vegetative valvular endocarditis and myocarditis developed in a macaw with chronic ulcerative dermatitis and FDB, presumably secondary to repeated trauma and low-rate bacteremia because translocation of *Staphylococcus aureus* skin infection may lead to subacute endocarditis in humans.[49] In a retrospective study of *S aureus* infections in psittacine birds, 2 out of 13 birds also developed septicemia in the presence of feather abnormalities.[50] Prompt optimal management of skin infection is therefore advisable.

Staphylococcus spp are the most common bacteria associated with folliculitis.[47] In a retrospective study of superficial chronic ulcerative dermatitis in psittacine birds, *Enterobacter cloacae* was most commonly isolated, followed by *Escherichia coli* and *S aureus*.[51] Mycobacterial infections of the skin and subcutis are described.[14,52] Infection may be primarily caused by localized invasion but also may indicate systemic bacterial disease.[47] Nonpainful and nonpruritic nodules may be seen.[53] Other clinical presentations include erythema, multiple pustules, and localized thickening and induration of the skin.[47,52] Feather loss and feathers that easily fall out are also described.[52]

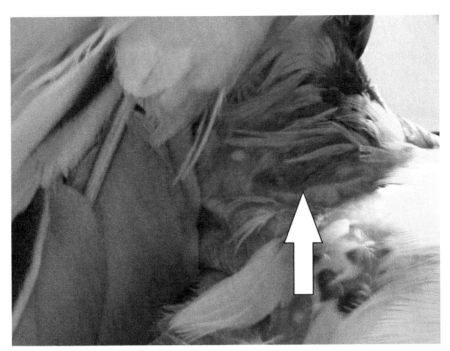

Fig. 2. Bacterial dermatitis involving the ventral propatagium in a blue and gold macaw (*Ara ararauna*). A crust (*arrow*) is covering the affected area. Heavy growth of *Klebsiella* sp was isolated from the lesion. (*Courtesy of* Service de médecine Zoologique, Université de Montréal, Saint-Hyacinthe, Canada.)

Diagnosis of most bacterial disease requires a culture using a swab of the lesion or a biopsy specimen. If mycobacterial infection is suspected, a biopsy specimen in preferred. PCR and Ziehl-Neelsen stain may assist in the diagnosis. An acid-fast stain on the feather pulp material may be considered.[54] Culture results must be interpreted judiciously, and key elements are summarized in **Box 4**.

Complete species identification and sensitivity testing in order to select the appropriate antibiotic is crucial when managing a primary or secondary bacterial infection. There have been reports of methicillin-resistant *S aureus* (MRSA) isolation from parrots.[55–57] Recently, MRSA was isolated from the tail base of an African grey parrot with ulcerative dermatitis and showing FDB toward this region.[58] MRSA is major problem in human medicine.[59,60] A study showed that a shared population of MRSA can infect both humans and companion animals (cats, dogs, horses) without undergoing host adaptation,[59,60] which raises zoonotic concerns. MRSA resistance patterns are influenced by different antibiotic usage patterns between human and veterinary medicine, which can shape the population of bacterial pathogens.[59,61] In the context of a One Health view of infectious diseases, it highlights how implementing appropriate use of antimicrobials is paramount.

Initial treatment plan may include wound debridement, systemic antibiotic therapy, topical therapy, analgesic, and bandages. Use of compounded poloxamer 407 antibiotic topical therapy shows promise for severe, infected, ulcerated skin lesions in birds when other therapies fail to achieve a cure.[57]

Box 4
Key elements to remember when interpreting bacterial culture from avian tegument

- Identification of microbial agents does not necessarily implicate these organisms as the precipitating cause of FDB because they may be secondary invaders.

- Bacterial organisms that reside on the integument of companion psittacine birds in a normal physiologic state may also be opportunistic pathogens.[126,127] Therefore, isolation of a commensal organism does not rule out infection.

- Bacteria isolated may represent local bacterial population in the bird's environment. In a study to characterize *Staphylococcus* spp isolated from commensal cutaneous microflora of privately owned birds and birds in a sanctuary, companion birds were twice as likely to have positive results for staphylococci as were sanctuary birds (71% vs 35%), and the species of *Staphylococcus* isolated from a captive parrot were more commonly isolated from people.[127] Researchers hypothesize that this was likely secondary colonization of birds by bacteria from their owners.[127]

Data from Lamb S, Sobczynski A, Starks D, et al. Bacteria isolated from the skin of Congo African grey parrots (*Psittacus erithacus*), budgerigars (*Melopsittacus undulatus*), and cockatiels (*Nymphicus hollandicus*). J Avian Med Surg. 2014;28(4):275-279 and Briscoe JA, Morris DO, Rosenthal KL, et al. Evaluation of mucosal and seborrheic sites for staphylococci in two populations of captive psittacines. J Am Vet Med Assoc. 2009;234(7):901-905.

In addition to bacterial infection involving the skin, systemic bacterial agents affecting various body systems, such as *Chlamydia psittaci*, have been associated with internal discomfort from airsacculitis and hepatitis leading to FDB.[6,8,16,62]

Fungi Fungal diseases affecting the integumentary system are uncommon in companion birds.[12,39,47,63] Yeasts were identified infrequently via acetate tape strips from the skin surface of psittacine birds with chronic FDB.[64] Fungal organisms associated with skin or feather disease in the companion bird are listed in **Table 2**.[12,39] According to one author, *Candida albicans* often affects the commissures of the beak, and occasionally feather follicles on the head, back, and ventrum.[65] *Microsporum gypseum* was reported in a budgerigar with feather loss on the head, neck, and breast.[39] The same microorganism was isolated from a lesion on the owner's hand.[39] *Malassezia* has been associated with a pruritic condition in galahs and responded well to miconazole washes.[41]

The diagnosis is complicated by many fungi being found on the feathers and skin of healthy birds. Furthermore, heavy fungal growth may be seen on old and soiled feathers without causing disease. Repeated isolation of the fungus and histopathologic changes supporting lesions are required for a definitive diagnosis.

Viruses Poxviruses affect most of the avian families and each virus has the ability to infect a limited number of species.[47] Since importation of wild-caught parrots has ceased, this disease in rarely seen. *Agapornis* (lovebird) pox produces lesions in the oral and nasal cavities, and on the palpebrae, axillae, shoulders, and/or abdomen.[66] These lesions are dark, discolored areas of skin, and, when secondary infections exist, are very pruritic.[39] Therefore, FDB may be present. Diagnosis is based on the gross proliferative appearance of the lesions and histopathology showing characteristic intracytoplasmic eosinophilic inclusion bodies.[12,47]

It is common to find Old World psittacines infected with polyomavirus or circovirus with FDB.[67] Polyomavirus can infect all psittacine birds. Abnormal feathering occurs in budgerigars infected between 7 and 15 days of age and is referred to as French molt, or runners, with underdevelopment or absence of remiges and rectrices (**Fig. 3**). Feather abnormalities are uncommon in other psittacine species. However, polyomavirus can produce feather dystrophy, which may be confused with psittacine beak and feather disease (PBFD) in chronic cases. Affected birds may lack down feathers on the back and the abdomen.[41] Contour feathers grow slowly, lack barbs, and are shorter than normal.[41]

Circoviruses are hardy, nonenveloped DNA viruses causing PBFD.[68] Old World species are most commonly affected.[12] The disease usually affects young birds and the chronic form is characterized by progressive replacement of normal feathers by dystrophic feathers. Eventually, the feathers of the head become abnormal in appearance, which helps to indicate that there is a medical cause for the FDB. Abnormal feathering includes dystrophic feathers with hyperkeratotic retained sheaths, blood in the umbilicus of the feather shaft, clubbing of the feathers, annular constrictions at the calamus, and curled and abnormally pigmented feathers (**Fig. 4**).

In North America, lovebirds and budgerigars are frequently affected and diagnosed with this disease.[33] One laboratory reported an incidence of positive DNA probe test exceeding 30% in lovebirds.[69] Feather abnormalities in these species are more subtle, and may be limited to an unthrifty appearance, delayed molt, and loss of feathers.[33] In the early stages, feather abnormalities may be limited to the legs.[65] Affected lovebirds are usually older juvenile to young adult birds.[32]

Because mutilated feathers may mimic the appearance of dystrophic feathers found on birds infected with polyomavirus or PBFD, it is indicated to perform viral assay to rule out these diseases. Key elements to remember are listed in **Box 5**.

Early observation showed some birds with proventricular dilatation disease may be pruritic and show FDB.[70] Recently, several studies detected parrot bornaviruses

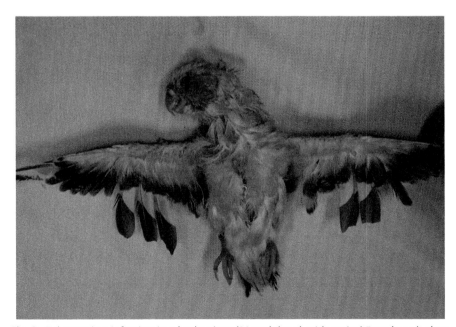

Fig. 3. Polyomavirus infection in a budgerigar (*M undulatus*) with typical French molt characterized by the underdevelopment or absence of remiges and rectrices. (*Courtesy of* Service de médecine Zoologique, Université de Montréal, Saint-Hyacinthe, Canada.)

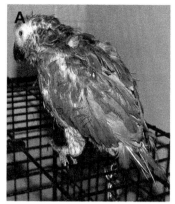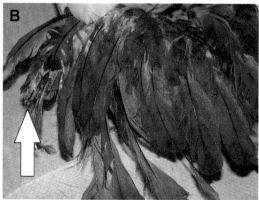

Fig. 4. Circovirus infection in a Congo African gray parrot (*Psittacus erithacus*). Abnormal feathering and replacement of grey feathers by red feathers also involve the head (*A*). Curled growing primary feathers with constriction of the calamus (*arrow*) are visible (*B*). (*Courtesy of* Service de médecine Zoologique, Université de Montréal, Saint-Hyacinthe, Canada.)

(PaBVs) in parrots showing FDB.[71–74] More recently, PaBV-2 was identified in a cockatoo with peripheral neuropathy showing autophagia.[75] Consequently, this circumstantial evidence leads to the speculation that PaBV infection may be a cause of FDB, but this remains to be proved scientifically.[32,33,71,76] Fluck and colleagues[78] showed a correlation between PaBV-specific antibody titer and the severity of clinical signs in birds showing feather picking of unknown cause, but this does not necessarily imply a causal link. It has been postulated that PaBV could lead to FDB through peripheral neuritis, but this hypothesis has not been investigated.[77] Nevertheless, testing for the presence of PaBV is possibly indicated for birds showing FDB with no identified cause.[76,78]

Immune-mediated causes

A seasonal recurrence of FDB may be related to the influence of factors that are limited to a specific season. For example, mosquitoes, biting flies, and ants may cause mild to severe hypersensitivity reaction. In a study evaluating feather-picking psittacines,

---

Box 5
Key elements to remember when performing viral assay for polyomavirus and circovirus

- For polyomavirus, PCR analysis of both whole blood and a combined choanal/cloacal swab are recommended.[128]

- For circovirus, feather sample, cloacal swab, along with a blood sample should all be submitted together.[68] In budgerigars, feather and cloacal samples were preferred.[129]

- Biopsy with histopathologic examination is another available diagnostic method. This method should be considered when PCR analysis yields negative results in the presence of feather dystrophy.

- Although the results from most laboratories are highly accurate, both false-positive and false-negative results are occasionally reported by some laboratories.[130,131] Therefore, veterinarians should contact their diagnostic laboratories to discuss their internal quality control measures.

Data from Refs.[68,128–131]

histologic pattern and the cellular constituents of inflammation were most suggestive of cutaneous delayed-type hypersensitivity.[25,79] These birds showed perivascular inflammation in the superficial or deep dermis of clinically affected and unaffected sites. Results of this study are in contrast with those of a previously published report that did not associate inflammatory skin disease with feather-picking birds.[80] However, in the later study, a paired sampling technique with multilevel histologic examination was not used. Whether the inflammation in the former study is a primary or a secondary lesion and how it might be related to allergens remain to be clarified.

In birds, hypersensitivity reactions can be elicited to a variety of antigens and occur at least 24 hours after antigen contact with sensitized T cells.[25,79] These reactions might be a source of discomfort or pruritus for birds and potentially play a role in FDB. Preliminary data suggest that there is a greater incidence in macaws (*Ara* spp) and Amazon parrots (*Amazona* spp).[25] Some investigators report that approximately 20% to 25% of the feather-picking birds in which a behavioral origin was originally suspected turned out to have a histologic diagnosis of hypersensitivity dermatitis.[81]

Initial treatment is preferably designed to decrease or eliminate exposure to the suspected allergens. In addition, the use of antihistamines and corticosteroids may be considered, the latter with caution considering the immunosuppressive side effects.[82] One author reported a combination of hydroxyzine hydrochloride and Derm Caps (eicosapentaenoic acid supplement) to be effective in controlling FDB of presumed hypersensitivity origin.[82]

Inherited causes

Feather cysts in soft-feathered canary breed (Norwich, Gloucester) result from inherited predisposition that is associated with color.[13] Feather cysts develop as a result of the inability of a feather to break through the skin surface.[83] While the feather continues to grow, it curls up within the follicle leading to the accumulation of yellow-white material. Eventually, it may rupture, revealing the contents (**Fig. 5**). Secondary infection and hemorrhage may occur. Differential diagnosis includes neoplasia (basal

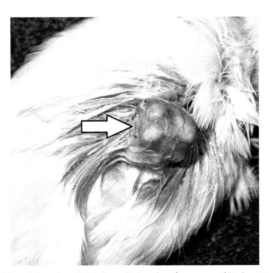

Fig. 5. Feather cyst involving the right dorsal pteryla of a canary (*Serinus canaria domestica*). The cyst has ruptured, revealing its contents (*arrow*). (*Courtesy of* Service de médecine Zoologique, Université de Montréal, Saint-Hyacinthe, Canada.)

cell tumor) and follicular infection. The cystic lesion may cause discomfort/pain, thereby resulting in FDB.[83] Surgical resection is the treatment of choice. Recurrence is common when a genetic component exists.[41,84]

A study in a colony of Amazon parrots showed a high heritability for feather picking, suggesting that a genetic basis exists.[6,85] However, the potential effects of parental behavior on feather picking of offspring were not evaluated in this study. In poultry, feather pecking has been shown to be heritable and the genetic regions involved in feather pecking have been identified.[86,87] Selection process proved to be successful in decreasing individual predisposition to this behavior.[88]

Traumatic Causes

Tearing and avulsion of the skin and muscles from their attachments on the ventral tail base, caudal to the vent, is most commonly seen in cockatiels (*Nymphicus hollandicus*) (**Fig. 6**). It may also occur in conures (*Aratinga* spp), cockatoos (*Cacatua* spp), and African grey parrots (*Psittacus erithacus*).[39] Laceration of the skin over the cranial portion of the keel occurs most commonly in heavy-bodied birds such as African grey and Amazon parrots. Both clinical presentations typically occur following an uncontrolled landing caused by inappropriate wing feather trim or obesity. Birds often show FDB in the affected area leading to, or caused by, secondary infection.[39]

Repeated damage to feather and feather follicle may lead to abnormal feather regrowth and feather cyst formation.[39] The remiges and rectrices are most susceptible

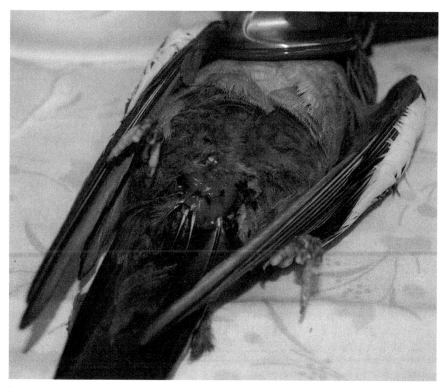

Fig. 6. Laceration of the ventral tail base caudal to the vent in a cockatiel (*N hollandicus*) following surgical debridement and closure. The bird had fallen on the ground following drastic trimming of the primary feathers. (*Courtesy of* Service de médecine Zoologique, Université de Montréal, Saint-Hyacinthe, Canada.)

to trauma when bumped or damaged,[39] and associated discomfort may lead to FDB.[83] Treatment of choice consists of surgical excision of the affected feather follicle, taking care not to damage any adjacent follicles.

Chronic fracture, luxation, and soft tissue trauma may be associated with FDB, particularly if proper reduction has not been achieved and mechanical/nervous impediment persists.

Toxic Causes

Toxins, both airborne (eg, cigarette smoke, scented candles, perfume, air fresheners, hairspray) and topical (eg, hand lotion, hand creams), have been implicated in FDB, although the association remains anecdotal.[32,33] Zinc toxicity has been proposed as a cause of FDB, but this has not been confirmed.[16,67] In a study presenting clinical histories and postmortem findings associated with zinc toxicosis, only 4 out of 28 birds with confirmed zinc toxicosis were reportedly feather pickers.[89] Gill[41] reports that some patients showing FDB have responded to chelation therapy, but a direct cause-and-effect relationship has not been described. Other than anecdotal reports, there is no known association between these heavy metals and FDB.[90]

Anomalous Causes

A dermal vascular hamartoma is reported in a 19-month-old sun conure (*Aratinga solstitialis*).[91] The lesion was located on the dorsal aspect of the right shoulder and the bird presented with feather picking of the ventral thoracic region. FDB resolved following surgical excision.

Metabolic Causes

Hepatic disease may either engender feather damage that is limited to the ventrum (**Fig. 7**) or follow a more diffuse, generalized pattern.[8,92] Pruritus is a prominent symptom in humans with chronic cholestatic liver disorders.[93] The potent neuronal activator lysophosphatidic acid and its forming enzyme, autotaxin (ATX), have been evaluated in the serum of humans with cholestatic pruritus,[94] and ATX activity correlated with itch severity.[93] Whether pruritus is caused by similar mechanism in birds with liver disease remains to be investigated.

Renal diseases have been associated with localized FDB in the region of the synsacrum.[8,95] Feather picking over the back and dorsal wings in a 5-year-old male greater sulphur-crested cockatoo (*Cacatua galerita galerita*) with pancreatitis was reported.[96] The bird stopped feather picking following appropriate antimicrobial therapy and dietary modification.

FDB involving the breast, abdomen, and legs has been observed during the breeding season.[14,42,97] Self-plucking for nesting can occur if there is no other nesting material or may be related to increases in reproductive hormone levels.[98] The pathophysiology remains unknown. In some cases, this may be associated with ventral abdominal hernia (**Fig. 8**). In contrast with their wild counterparts, birds in captivity are not subjected to many of the factors limiting reproduction that are typically present in their natural habitat; they may even be exposed to many stimuli promoting reproductive behavior, such as (1) nutrient-rich diet, (2) nesting material/site, (3) perceived mate mimicking pair bond behavior. The history may reveal the presence of stimuli that are known to promote reproductive behavior. Medical imaging techniques and endoscopy may be considered to investigate for the presence of an underlying reproductive disorder. Therapy including altering the photoperiod, diet offered, and nest/nesting material access,[97] in addition to modification of social interactions with the bird and

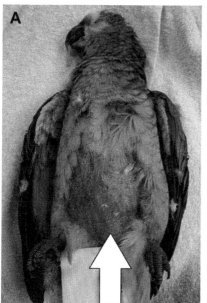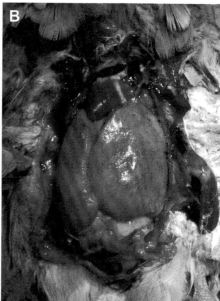

Fig. 7. FDB in a blue-fronted Amazon parrot (*Amazona aestiva*) with hepatic disease. The ventrum is apteric (*arrow*) with severe coelomic distension (*A*). Severe hepatomegaly with rounded liver margins caused by hepatic lipidosis was present (*B*). (*Courtesy of* Service de médecine Zoologique, Université de Montréal, Saint-Hyacinthe, Canada.)

the use of gonadotropin-releasing hormone agonist to reduce reproductive drive, is successful in some avian patients.[97,98]

Studies found that African grey parrots showing FDB have higher baseline corticosterone levels.[99,100] The link between FDB and corticosterone levels has also been observed in cockatoos.[101] Other studies showed that birds presenting FDB may have a higher stress response to handling than birds with normal plumage.[102] FDB was associated with stress, as reflected by an increased heterophil/lymphocyte ratio in a group of golden conures (*Guaruba guarouba*) and decreased significantly following social restructuring, which consisted in reduction of the male/female ratio.[103] Higher chronic stress levels in birds with abnormal feathering may play a role in the development and maintenance of this syndrome, which must be taken into account in the therapeutic approach of any bird with FDB. The bird may be unable to perform appropriate behavior to eliminate or avoid stress. The results of 1 survey support this assumption, with up to two-thirds of owners reporting a changing or tumultuous environment at the time their birds began FDB.[104]

Endocrine disorders, such as hypothyroidism and hyperadrenocorticism, are associated with feather loss or lack of feather growth as opposed to FDB.[105,106] Functional hypothyroidism in companion birds is rare,[107] with only 1 well-documented, confirmed case in the avian literature.[106] Clinical findings in this patient, an adult male Scarlet macaw, were obesity, thickening of the skin over the legs and ventral portion of the abdomen, and progressive nonpruritic feather loss, although there had been a history of some feather pulling. In an experimental model of hypothyroidism developed in cockatiels, poor feathering was either absent or mild 48 days after radiothyroidectomy, and no FDB was observed.[108] Lesions of the thyroid have been associated

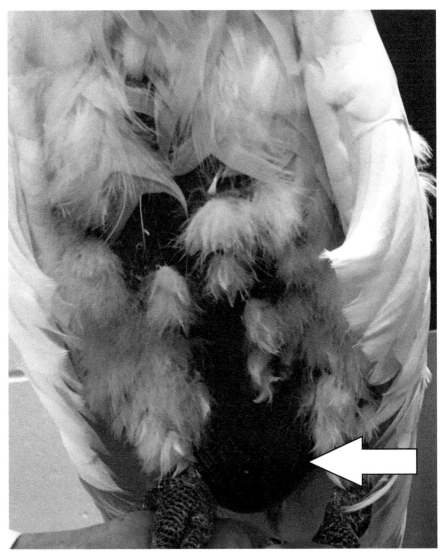

Fig. 8. FDB involving the breast, abdomen, and legs in a female umbrella cockatoo (*Cacatua alba*) presumably caused by sexual hyperstimulation with associated ventral abdominal hernia (*arrow*). (*Courtesy of* Service de médecine Zoologique, Université de Montréal, Saint-Hyacinthe, Canada.)

with atherosclerosis in older, obese Amazon parrots, but hypothyroidism was not confirmed.[109]

Idiopathic Causes

Idiopathic causes of FDB, including chronic ulcerative dermatitis (CUD), Amazon foot necrosis, and polyfolliculitis are summarized in **Table 4**. Visual examples of CUD (**Fig. 9**) and polyfolliculitis (**Fig. 10**) are provided.

Table 4
Idiopathic conditions associated with feather damaging behavior

Conditions	Species Involved	Affected Areas	Clinical Presentation	Suggested Causes	Proposed Treatment	Comments
CUD	• Most commonly lovebirds and cockatiels[7,13] • Less commonly grey-cheeked parakeet (*Brotogeris pyrrhoptera*), Amazon parrots, and cockatoos[7]	• Metapatagium, propatagium, and interscapular area[7,13]	• Intensely pruritic • Repeatedly damaging affected areas with beak • Hemorrhage and secondary infections associated with altered feathers, skin, and underlying musculature	• Malnutrition, hypovitaminosis E, herpes virus, poxvirus, giardiasis[42] • A recent study on a population of 32 lovebirds indicated that polyomavirus, circovirus, or both may be involved in this syndrome. More than 50% of the birds with CUD were positive for polyomavirus and approximately 20% were positive for circovirus[122]	• Various topical treatments (wound dressing, topical antimicrobial) may be implemented	• Even when the primary lesion is healed, scar tissue often restricts movement and recurrence of FDB or mutilation is common Photodynamic therapy may be considered for these patients

(continued on next page)

Table 4
(continued)

Conditions	Species Involved	Affected Areas	Clinical Presentation	Suggested Causes	Proposed Treatment	Comments
Amazon foot necrosis	• Most commonly yellow-naped Amazons (*Amazona auropalliata*) and double yellow-headed Amazons (*Amazona oratrix*)[123] • Conures • Quakers (*Myiopsitta monachus*)	• Feet and lower legs	• Affected birds suddenly begin chewing at their feet and lower legs • Associated FDB is restricted to the legs	• Delayed hypersensitivity reaction following staphylococcal dermatitis[47] • Circumstantial evidence suggests this might be a contact dermatitis with nicotine or tobacco smoke because lesions are restricted to the feet or legs and many owners of affected parrots were smokers[13,47] • Crack cocaine exposure[124] • Nutritional deficiencies, toxicities, hormonal influences[13]	• Environmental assessment to prevent exposure to contact irritants • Various topical along with systemic antimicrobials, antiinflammatories, and analgesics[7,13] • Topical therapy with a spray containing antibiotic and antiinflammatory has been shown to be helpful in some cases[123]	• Recurrence and seasonality commonly reported[13]
Polyfolliculitis	• Lovebirds • Budgerigars • Parrotlets • Cockatiels	• Rump, flank, and neck[16,125]	• Multiple quills projecting from a single feather follicle • Appears pruritic because affected patients preen with intensity, damage feathers and/or soft tissue in the affected area[7,125]	• Viral association in lovebirds[16,39,125]	• A combination of various systemic/topical treatment to alleviate skin irritation and pruritus	• Polyfolliculitis is a diagnosis of exclusion based on the clinical presentation along with histopathologic examination of a skin biopsy including a feather follicle

Data from Refs.[7,13,16,39,42,47,122–125]

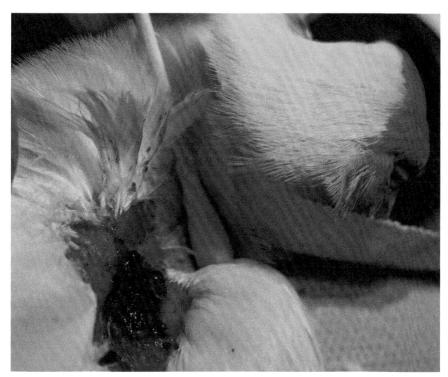

Fig. 9. CUD in a rosy-faced lovebird (*Agapornis roseicollis*) involving the dorsal propatagium. (*Courtesy of* Service de médecine Zoologique, Université de Montréal, Saint-Hyacinthe, Canada.)

Iatrogenic Causes

Trimming of wing feathers may have several detrimental effects on the behavior of the bird, including an increased risk of developing FDB.[9] As discussed previously, inappropriate trimming of wing feathers may lead to skin laceration of the tail ventrally or the keel region. In addition, because emerging feathers have little protection, a bumped feather may trigger a pain response resulting in FDB directed toward the traumatized feather and/or other feathers around it.[84]

In anseriformes, short trimming of remiges, exposing the hollow calamus, may allow water and algae to collect within the calamus and cause irritation of the follicle.[110] Excessive preening may be observed.

The author has also seen iatrogenic feather picking over the pectoral area following microchip placement in an African grey parrot (**Fig. 11**). The FDB resumed following surgical removal of the microchip under fluoroscopic guidance. It was hypothesized that the microchip was causing nerve or muscular irritation.

Neoplastic Causes

Various primary skin neoplasms may be associated with FDB (**Fig. 12**) and are not limited to the neoplasms discussed here or listed in **Table 2**. Once excised, if the FDB was related to the lesion, regrowth of feathers typically occurs. Practitioners should keep in mind that cutaneous masses may be the tip of the iceberg and a

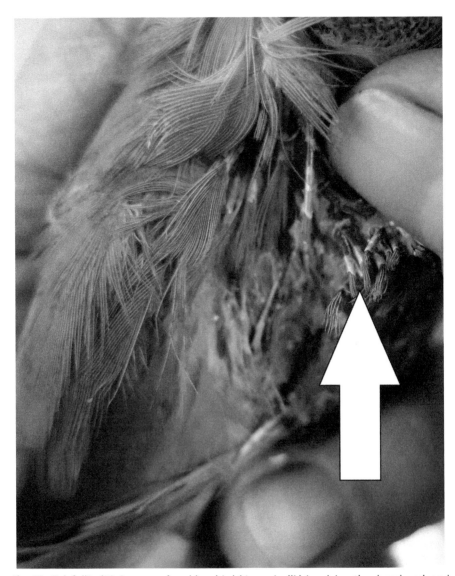

Fig. 10. Polyfolliculitis in a rosy-faced lovebird (*A roseicollis*) involving the dorsal neck and propatagium. Multiple quills projecting from a single feather follicle are seen (*arrow*). (*Courtesy of* Service de médecine Zoologique, Université de Montréal, Saint-Hyacinthe, Canada.)

systemic work-up is often warranted. Musculoskeletal neoplasia as well as internal neoplasia may also be associated with FDB.

As previously mentioned, basal cell tumors often develop in feather cysts. Although expansile, they are usually benign.[13] Multiple lesions or those causing irritation or discomfort should be excised surgically.[16,41]

Areas of chronic irritation and inflammation may promote squamous cell carcinomas, such as sites of chronic feather picking. Two integumentary squamous cell

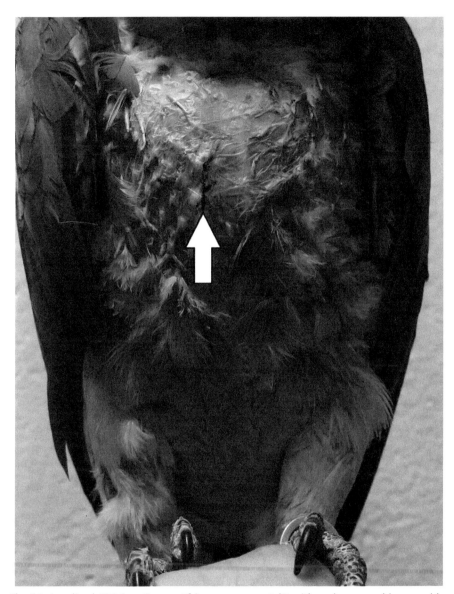

Fig. 11. Localized FDB in a Congo African grey parrot (*P erithacus*) presumably caused by intramuscular microchip. The surgical incision to retrieve the device is visible (*arrow*). (*Courtesy of* Service de médecine Zoologique, Université de Montréal, Saint-Hyacinthe, Canada.)

carcinomas were described in an African gray parrot with known episodes of feather picking and self-mutilation of 10-year duration.[111] Often, skin carcinomas are confused with delayed or nonhealing cutaneous infection. Practitioners should consider biopsy for any skin lesion not responding to treatment as expected to avoid delayed diagnosis.

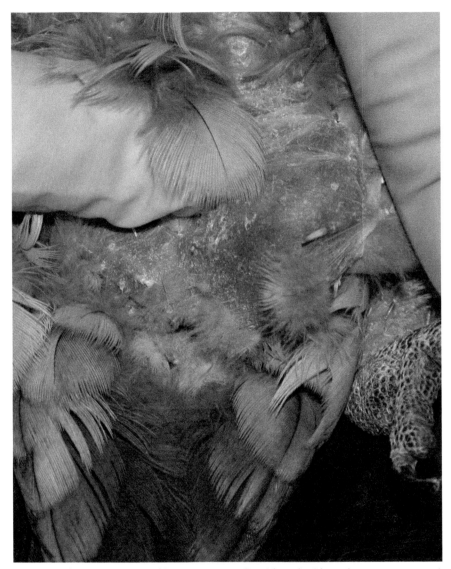

Fig. 12. Focal FDB in a Congo African grey parrot (*P erithacus*) with a subcutaneous tumor in the right inguinal area. (*Courtesy of* Service de médecine Zoologique, Université de Montréal, Saint-Hyacinthe, Canada.)

Nutritional Causes

Malnutrition is seen in captive psittacine birds both with and without FDB. Therefore, other factors are involved in the development of FDB. Scientific research into the potential mechanisms as to how deficiencies may lead to FDB are lacking.[33] Vitamin A deficiency, which causes squamous metaplasia, has been linked to subsequent behavioral disorders such as feather picking.[112] In a study, Hispaniolan Amazon parrots (*Amazona ventralis*) housed outdoors had significantly higher calcifediol levels compared with birds kept indoors. Self-inflicted feather damage was less present in the outdoor groups, although the difference was not statistically significant and numerous alternative potential variables may have accounted for the discrepancy.[113] Deficiencies in certain sulfur-containing amino acids can lead to abnormalities of the rachis, retained sheath, and misshapen vanes.[114] However, experiments in which specific amino acid deficiencies have been induced have not resulted in increased feather picking.[115] Overall, a poor plane of nutrition may act as a stressor and/or restrict the ability of the bird to regrow feathers.[15]

Degenerative Causes

Osteoarthritis may be associated with FDB.[116] One author described an Amazon parrot with severe osteoarthritis of the right hip.[12] This patient bore most of its weight on the left leg on presentation. The right side of the bird was mostly plucked over the back, hip, chest, and medial and right thigh.[12]

GENERAL THERAPEUTIC PRINCIPLES

The clinical management of FDB, whether a medical origin is identified or not, is multifaceted and is based on the findings gathered from the history, physical examination, initial behavioral assessment, and diagnostic tests. **Table 5** summarizes the various facets to consider when managing FDB of medical origin.

Treatment of FDB is challenging and most likely to respond if therapy is initiated promptly after the behavior develops (**Fig. 13**). In some cases, the behavior persists after the medical condition is cured. Owners often inadvertently reward the FDB by giving the bird attention when it damages its plumage. What owners might perceive as punishers (eg, screaming at the bird) can act as reinforcing conditions that contribute to maintaining the problem behavior.[9] In this situation, behavior analysis to identify antecedents and reinforcing consequences that may contribute to

Table 5 Multifaceted approach to medical causes of feather damaging behavior	
Treat/manage medical conditions	• According to diagnosis
Assess/improve environment	• Design, furnishing, location, and surroundings of the cage • Presence/absence of visual/auditory stimuli that may be perceived as stimulating/threatening
Decrease physical stress	• Correct/improve nutrition • Ensure sufficient sleep • Provide exercise opportunities
Promote occupational therapy	• Provide various types of toys to promote physical exercise and foraging: chewing (destructible) toys, climbing toys, manipulating (foot) toys, and cognition (puzzle) toys
Improve social environment and interactions with owners and other animals	• Optimize the type and quality of interactions with owners and other animals • Encourage daily routine with established activities • Promote activities such as training, verbal games and exercise
Behavior modification	• Operant learning using positive reinforcement • Teaching and reinforcing an alternative behavior that requires less effort and provides equivalent or superior reinforcement

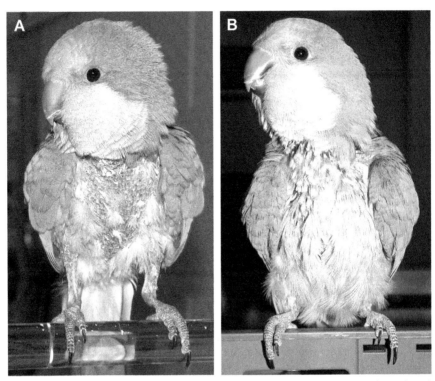

Fig. 13. FDB in a Quaker parrot (*Myiopsitta monachus*). The bird presented 7 days after the onset (*A*). Various topical irritants along with undesirable stressful social interactions were addressed through implementation of a multifaceted therapeutic approach. Plumage appearance 6 weeks following initial presentation (*B*). (*Courtesy of* Service de médecine Zoologique, Université de Montréal, Saint-Hyacinthe, Canada.)

maintenance of the undesired behavior can provided the basis for an adapted behavior modification plan.

When a medical origin is identified, appropriate clinical management must be implemented to address the bird's disorder. The mechanical prevention of feather damaging with the use of collars must be used judiciously. The pros and cons must be weighed because collars are a source of stress for avian patients.[98] Their short-term use may be indicated if the bird's behavior is assessed as possibly delaying recovery. All birds should be hospitalized to ensure proper placement/adjustment of the collar, and it should be confirmed that the bird is able to eat, drink, and ambulate in a satisfactory manner.

In addition, environmental enrichment should be part of the general management plan for these patients. Reduction of behavioral disorders such as feather picking using physical and foraging enrichments is possible.[18,117,118] Foraging enrichment is preferred to physical enrichment. In crimson-bellied conures (*Pyrrhura perlata perlata*), the severity of feather damage was correlated with the time spent preening, and environmental enrichment contributed to stabilization of the picking behavior.[119] Adding fruit baskets and willow branches of various sizes increased exploration and manipulation with feet and beak, which competed with other activities such as preening and vocalizing.

Behavior modification techniques should be used to replace the FDB with more desirable behaviors. Short training sessions may be initiated on a regular schedule to provide the bird with stimulating tasks to accomplish. It was found to be the most successful treatment in sulphur-crested cockatoos (*C galerita*).[101] These techniques, through providing the patient with alternative behavior, may be beneficial in reducing FDB.[9]

Pharmacologic intervention, with the use of psychotropic drugs, is indicated only when a behavioral diagnosis has been correctly established and if used concurrently with appropriate treatment of medical illnesses, environmental and social adjustments, and a sound behavior modification plan.[120] In that sense, early collaborative work between the avian veterinarian and the avian behaviorist is beneficial for some patients with FDB because the identification of a medical cause to the behavior does not rule out a behavioral anomaly. These patients may require concurrent use of psychotropic drugs to maximize the chances of a positive outcome.

SUMMARY/PROGNOSIS

Primary feather or skin diseases as well as systemic diseases, either localized or involving more than 1 system, may lead to FDB by causing pain, irritation, discomfort, or pruritus. The diagnostic approach must be adapted to each patient's clinical presentation.

The therapeutic plan depends mainly on the presumptive or definitive diagnosis. In all cases, additional contributing factors, such as suboptimal diet, environment, social interactions, and management should be addressed as well.

Prognosis varies considerably and depends on the medical condition involved, as well as all potential contributing factors. FDB may result in permanent damage to the feather follicle, thereby preventing feather regrowth. Overall, the prognosis may vary from fair to poor according to the bird's response the first few weeks after implementing the multifaceted therapeutic management plan.

DISCLOSURE

The author has nothing to disclose.

REFERENCES

1. Gaskins LA, Bergman L. Surveys of Avian Practitioners and Pet Owners Regarding Common Behavior Problems in Psittacine Birds. J Avian Med Surg 2011;25(2):111–8.

2. Grindlinger HM. Compulsive Feather Picking in Birds. Arch Gen Psychiatry 1991;48(9):857.

3. Kinkaid HMY, Mills DS, Nichols SG, et al. Feather-damaging behaviour in companion parrots: an initial analysis of potential demographic risk factors. Avian Biol Res 2013;6(4):289–96.

4. Costa P, Macchi E, Tomassone L, et al. Feather picking in pet parrots: sensitive species, risk factor and ethological evidence. Ital J Anim Sci 2016;15(3):473–80.

5. MacWhirter P, Muelle R, Gill J. Ongoing research report: Allergen testing as part of diagnostic protocol in self-mutilating Psittaciformes. Proceedings of the Annual Conference of the Association of Avian Veterinarians. New Orleans, LA, August 25-29, 1999. p. 125–8.

6. van Zeeland YRA, Schoemaker N. Feather damaging behavior and self-injurious behavior. In: Graham JE, editor. Blackwell's five-minute veterinary consult: avian. Ames (IO): John Wiley & Sons; 2016. p. 113–6.

7. Burgmann PM. Common psittacine dermatologic diseases. J Exot Pet Med 1995;4(4):169–83.

8. van Zeeland YRA, Schoemaker NJ. Plumage disorders in psittacine birds - Part 2: Feather damaging behaviour. European Journal of Companion Animal Practice 2014;24(2):24–36.

9. van Zeeland YRA, Friedman SG, Bergman L. Behavior. In: Speer BL, editor. Current therapy in avian medicine and surgery. St Louis (MI): Elsevier; 2016. p. 177–251.

10. Nett CS, Tully TN. Anatomy, clinical presentation, and diagnostic approach to feather-picking pet birds. Compend Contin Educ Pract Vet 2003;25(3):206–18.

11. Rosenthal K. Differential diagnosis of feather-picking in pet birds. Proceedings of the Annual Conference of the Association of Avian Veterinarians. Nashville, TN, August 31 - September 4, 1993. p. 108–12.

12. Orosz SE. Diagnostic workup of suspected behavioral problems. In: Luescher AU, editor. Manual of parrot behavior. Ames (IO): Blackwell publishing; 2006. p. 195–210.

13. Schmidt RE, Lightfoot TL. Integument. In: Harrison GJ, Lightfoot TL, editors. Clinical avian medicine, vol. 1. Palm Beach (FL): Spix Publishing; 2006. p. 395–410.

14. Lamberski N. A diagnostic approach to feather picking. Sem Avian Exotic Pet Med 1995;4(4):161–8.

15. Chitty J. Feather plucking in psittacine birds 1. Presentation and medical investigation. In Pract 2003;25(8):484–93.

16. Koski MA. Dermatologic diseases in psittacine birds: An investigational approach. Sem Avian Exotic Pet Med 2002;11(3):105–24.

17. Murphy SM, Braun JV, Millam JR. Bathing behavior of captive Orange-winged Amazon parrots (Amazona amazonica). Appl Anim Behav Sci 2011;132(3–4): 200–10.

18. Meehan C, Millam J, Mench J. Foraging opportunity and increased physical complexity both prevent and reduce psychogenic feather picking by young Amazon parrots. Appl Anim Behav Sci 2003;80(1):71–85.

19. van Zeeland YRA, Bergers MJ, van der Valk L, et al. Evaluation of a novel feather scoring system for monitoring feather damaging behaviour in parrots. Vet J 2013;196(2):247–52.

20. Garner MM. Inflammatory skin disease in feather picking birds: Histopathology and species predispositions. Proceedings of the Annual Conference of the Association of Avian Veterinarians. San Antonio, TX, August 27 - September 1, 2006. p. 17-20.

21. Orosz SE. Not another feather picker! The North American Veterinary Conference 2006. p. 1568. Gainesville (FL).

22. Speer BL, Kass PH. The influence of travel on hematologic parameters in hyacinth macaws. Proceedings of the Annual Conference of the Association of Avian Veterinarians, Nashville, Tennessee, August 31 - September 4, 1995. p. 43–9.

23. Woerpel RW, Rosskopf WJ Jr. Clinical experience with avian laboratory diagnostics. Vet Clin North Am Small Anim Pract 1984;14(2):249–86.

24. Grosset C, Bougerol C, Kass PH, et al. Plasma Butyrylcholinesterase Concentrations in Psittacine Birds: Reference Values, Factors of Variation, and Association With Feather-damaging Behavior. J Avian Med Surg 2014;28(1):6–15.
25. Garner MM, Clubb SL, Mitchell MA, et al. Feather-picking Psittacines: Histopathology and Species Trends. Vet Pathol 2008;45(3):401–8.
26. Clubb SL, Garner MM, Cray C. Detection of inflammatory skin disease in psittacine birds using paired skin biopsies. Proceedings of the Annual Conference of the Association of Avian Veterinarians. Monterey, CA, August 26-30, 2002. p. 193–9.
27. Nett CS, Hodgin EC, Foil CS, et al. A modified biopsy technique to improve histopathological evaluation of avian skin. Vet Dermatol 2003;14(3):147–51.
28. Nett CS, Hosgood G, Heatley JJ, et al. Evaluation of intravenous fluorescein in intradermal allergy testing in psittacines. Vet Dermatol 2003;14(6):323–32.
29. Colombini S, Foil CS, Hosgood G, et al. Intradermal skin testing in Hispaniolan parrots (*Amazona ventralis*). Vet Dermatol 2000;11(4):271–6.
30. Nett CS, Tully T. Hypersensitivity and intradermal allergy testing in Psittacines. Compend Contin Educ Pract Vet 2003;25(5):348–57.
31. Heatley JJ, Oliver JW, Hosgood G, et al. Serum corticosterone concentrations in response to restraint, anesthesia, and skin testing in Hispaniolan Amazon parrots (*Amazona ventralis*). J Avian Med Surg 2000;14(3):172–6.
32. Rubinstein J, Lightfoot T. Feather loss and feather destructive behavior in pet birds. Vet Clin North Am Exot Anim Pract 2014;17(1):77–101.
33. Rubinstein J, Lightfoot T. Feather loss and feather destructive behavior in pet birds. J Exot Pet Med 2012;21(3):219–34.
34. Fitzgerald BA, Beaufrere H. Cardiology. In: Speer BL, editor. Current therapy in avian medicine and surgery. St Louis (MI): Elsevier; 2015. p. 252–327.
35. Fricke C, Schmidt V, Cramer K, et al. Characterization of atherosclerosis by histochemical and immunohistochemical methods in African Grey parrots (*Psittacus erithacus*) and Amazon parrots (*Amazona* spp.). Avian Dis 2009;53(3): 466–72.
36. Beaufrère H. Avian atherosclerosis: parrots and beyond. J Exot Pet Med 2013; 22(4):336–47.
37. Barnes HJ. Parasites. In: Harrison GJ, Harrison LR, editors. Clinical avian medicine and surgery. Philadelphia: WB Saunders Co; 1986. p. 472–85.
38. Reavill DR, Schmidt RE, Fudge AM. Avian skin and feather disorders: A retrospective study. Proceedings of the Annual Conference of the Association of Avian Veterinarians. Phoenix, AR, September 10-15, 1990. p. 248–55.
39. Reavill D. Inflammatory skin diseases. Proceedings of the Annual Conference of the Association of Avian Veterinarians, Pittsburg, PA, August 26-28, 2003. p. 13-24.
40. Doneley RJ. Bacterial and parasitic diseases of parrots. Vet Clin North Am Exot Anim Pract 2009;12(3):417–32.
41. Gill JH. Avian skin diseases. Vet Clin North Am Exot Anim Pract 2001;4(2): 463–92.
42. Cooper JE, Harrison GJ. Dermatology. In: Ritchie BW, Harrison GJ, Harrison LR, editors. Avian medicine: principles and application. Lake Worth (FL): Wingers Publishing; 1994. p. 607–39.
43. Lumeij JT. Gastroenterology. In: Ritchie BW, Harrison GJ, Harrison LR, editors. Avian medicine: principles and application. Lake Worth (FL): Wingers Publishing; 1994. p. 482–521.

44. Clipsham R. Avian pathogenic flagellated enteric protozoa. Sem Avian Exotic Pet Med 1995;4(3):112–25.

45. Ichikawa RS, Santana BN, Ferrari ED, et al. Detection and molecular characterization of *Giardia* spp. in captive Psittaciformes in Brazil. Prev Vet Med 2019; 164:10–2.

46. Clyde VL, Patton S. Diagnosis, treatment, and control of common parasites in companion and aviary birds. Sem Avian Exotic Pet Med 1996;5(2):75–84.

47. Schmidt RE, Reavill DR, Phalen DN. Pathology of pet and aviary birds. Ames, Iowa: John Wiley & Sons; 2015.

48. Oglesbee BL, Oglesbee MJ. Feather dystrophy in a cockatiel (*Nymphicus hollandicus*). J Assoc Avian Vet 1994;8(1):16–20.

49. Huynh M, Carnaccini S, Driggers T, et al. Ulcerative dermatitis and valvular endocarditis associated with *Staphylococcus aureus* in a Hyacinth macaw (*Anadorhynchus hyacinthinus*). Avian Dis 2014;58(2):223–7, 225.

50. Hermans K, Devriese L, De Herdt P, et al. *Staphylococcus aureus* infections in psittacine birds. Avian Pathol 2000;29(5):411–5.

51. Abou-Zahr T, Carrasco DC, DVM NS, et al. Superficial chronic ulcerative dermatitis (SCUD) in psittacine birds: Review of 11 cases (2008-2016). J Avian Med Surg 2018;32(1):25–33.

52. Drew ML, Ramsay EC. Dermatitis associated with Mycobacterium spp. in a blue-fronted Amazon parrot. Proceedings of the Annual Conference of the Association of Avian Veterinarians. Chicago, IL, September 23-28, 1991. p. 252–4.

53. Ferrer L, Ramis A, Fernandez J, et al. Granulomatous dermatitis caused by *Mycobacterium genavense* in two psittacine birds. Vet Dermatol 1997;8(3): 213–9.

54. Johnson-Delaney C. Feather Picking: Diagnosis and Treatment. J Assoc Avian Vet 1992;6(2):82–3.

55. Walther B, Wieler LH, Friedrich AW, et al. Methicillin-resistant *Staphylococcus aureus* (MRSA) isolated from small and exotic animals at a university hospital during routine microbiological examinations. Vet Microbiol 2008;127(1–2): 171–8.

56. Loncaric I, Lepuschitz S, Ruppitsch W, et al. Increased genetic diversity of methicillin-resistant *Staphylococcus aureus* (MRSA) isolated from companion animals. Vet Microbiol 2019;235:118–26.

57. Pilny AA. Use of a Compounded Poloxamer 407 Antibiotic Topical Therapy as Part of the Successful Management of Chronic Ulcerative Dermatitis in a Congo African Grey Parrot (Psittacus erithacus). J Avian Med Surg 2018;32(1):45–50.

58. Briscoe JA, Morris DO, Rankin SC, et al. Methicillin-resistant *Staphylococcus aureus*-associated dermatitis in a Congo African grey parrot (*Psittacus erithacus erithacus*). J Avian Med Surg 2008;22(4):336–43.

59. Harrison EM, Weinert LA, Holden MTG, et al. A shared population of epidemic methicillin-resistant *Staphylococcus aureus* 15 circulates in humans and companion animals. MBio 2014;5(3):e00985-13.

60. Walther B, Tedin K, Lübke-Becker A. Multidrug-resistant opportunistic pathogens challenging veterinary infection control. Vet Microbiol 2017;200:71–8.

61. Rahman MM, Amin KB, Rahman SMM, et al. Investigation of methicillin-resistant *Staphylococcus aureus* among clinical isolates from humans and animals by culture methods and multiplex PCR. Vet Res 2018;14(1):300.

62. Kubiak M. Feather plucking in parrots. In Pract 2015;37(2):87–95.

63. Wade LL. Yeast dermatitis/conjunctivitis in a canary (Serinus canaria). Proceedings of the Annual Conference of the Association of Avian Veterinarians. Portland, OR, August 29 - September 2, 2000. p. 475–8.

64. Preziosi DE, Morris DO, Johnston MS, et al. Distribution of Malassezia organisms on the skin of unaffected psittacine birds and psittacine birds with feather-destructive behavior. J Am Vet Med Assoc 2006;228(2):216–21.

65. Perry RA, Gill J, Cross GM. Disorders of the avian integument. Vet Clin North Am Small Anim Pract 1991;21(6):1307–27.

66. Tsai SS, Chang TC, Yang SF, et al. Unusual lesions associated with avian poxvirus infection in rosy-faced lovebirds (*Agapornis roseicollis*). Avian Pathol 1997;26(1):75–82.

67. Jenkins JR. Feather picking and self-mutilation in psittacine birds. Vet Clin North Am Exot Anim Pract 2001;4(3):651–67.

68. Ritchie BW. Circoviridae. In: Ritchie BW, editor. Avian viruses: function and control. Lake Worth (FL): Wingers Publishing; 1995. p. 223–52.

69. Dalhausen R, Radabaugh S. Update on psittacine beak and feather disease and avian polyomavirus testing. Proceedings of the Annual Conference of the Association of Avian Veterinarians. Nashville, TN, August 31 - September 4, 1993. p. 5–7.

70. Rosenthal KL. Diagnostics: Please let there be an answer. Proceedings of the Annual Conference of the Association of Avian Veterinarians: Avian Specialty Advanced Program - Another feather picker: That sinking feeling. Pittsburg, PA, August 26-28, 2003. p. 25-30.

71. Horie M, Ueda K, Ueda A, et al. Detection of Avian bornavirus 5 RNA in *Eclectus roratus* with feather picking disorder. Microbiol Immunol 2012;56(5):346–9.

72. Philadelpho NA, Rubbenstroth D, Guimarães MB, et al. Survey of bornaviruses in pet psittacines in Brazil reveals a novel parrot bornavirus. Vet Microbiol 2014; 174(3):584–90.

73. Gancz AY, Kistler AL, Greninger AL, et al. Experimental induction of proventricular dilatation disease in cockatiels (*Nymphicus hollandicus*) inoculated with brain homogenates containing avian bornavirus 4. Virol J 2009;6:100.

74. Melillo A. An Interesting Neurologic Case in a Lovebird (*Agapornis fisheri*). Vet Clin North Am Exot Anim Pract 2006;9(3):539–44.

75. Sassa Y, Horie M, Fujino K, et al. Molecular epidemiology of avian bornavirus from pet birds in Japan. Virus Genes 2013;47(1):173–7.

76. Horie M. Parrot bornavirus infection: correlation with neurological signs and feather picking? Vet Rec 2019;184(15):473–5.

77. Rossi G, Dalhausen RD, Galosi L, et al. Avian Ganglioneuritis in Clinical Practice. Vet Clin North Am Exot Anim Pract 2018;21(1):33–67.

78. Fluck A, Enderlein D, Piepenbring A, et al. Correlation of avian bornavirus-specific antibodies and viral ribonucleic acid shedding with neurological signs and feather-damaging behaviour in psittacine birds. Vet Rec 2019;184(15):476.

79. Parmentier HK, Reilingh GD, Nieuwland MGB. Kinetic and immunohistochemical characteristics of mitogen-induced cutaneous hypersensitivity in chickens selected for antibody responsiveness. Vet Immunol Immunopathol 1998; 66(3–4):367–76.

80. Rosenthal KL, Morris DO, Mauldin EA, et al. Cytologic, histologic, and microbiologic characterization of the feather pulp and follicles of feather-picking psittacine birds: a preliminary study. J Avian Med Surg 2004;18(3):137–44.

81. Bennett T. Herbal treatment of feather picking. Exotic DVM 2002;4(3):29–30.

82. Krinsley M. Use of Dermcaps liquid and hydroxyzine hcl for the treatment of feather picking. J Assoc Avian Vet 1993;7(4):221.

83. van Zeeland YRA, Schoemaker N. Feather cyst. Blackwell's five-minute veterinary consult: avian. Ames (IO): John Wiley & Sons; 2016. p. 111–2.

84. Bauck L. Avian dermatology. In: Altman RB, Clubb SL, Dorrestein GM, et al, editors. Avian medicine and surgery. Philadelphia: W.B. Saunders Company; 1997. p. 548–62.

85. Garner JP, Meehan CL, Famula TR, et al. Genetic, environmental, and neighbor effects on the severity of stereotypies and feather picking in Orange-winged Amazon parrots (*Amazona amazonica*): An epidemiological study. Appl Anim Behav Sci 2006;96(1–2):153–68.

86. Rodenburg T, Van Hierden Y, Buitenhuis A, et al. Feather pecking in laying hens: new insights and directions for research? Appl Anim Behav Sci 2004;86(3–4): 291–8.

87. Jensen P, Keeling L, Schütz K, et al. Feather pecking in chickens is genetically related to behavioural and developmental traits. Physiol Behav 2005;86(1–2): 52–60.

88. Rodenburg TB, Komen H, Ellen ED, et al. Selection method and early-life history affect behavioural development, feather pecking and cannibalism in laying hens: A review. Appl Anim Behav Sci 2008;110(3–4):217–28.

89. Puschner B, St. Judy L, Galey FD. Normal and toxic zinc concentrations in serum/plasma and liver of psittacines with respect to genus differences. J Vet Diagn Invest 1999;11(6):522–7.

90. Rosenthal KL. Medical aspects of feather picking. Proceedings of the North American Veterinary Conference. Orlando, FL, January 8-12, 2005. p. 1211–2.

91. Steinberg H, Paré JA, Paul-Murphy J. A Dermal Vascular Hamartoma in a Sun Conure (*Aratinga solstitialis*). J Avian Med Surg 2006;20(3):161–6.

92. Grunkemeyer VL. Advanced diagnostic approaches and current management of avian hepatic disorders. Vet Clin North Am Exot Anim Pract 2010;13(3): 413–27.

93. Kremer AE, Namer B, Bolier R, et al. Pathogenesis and Management of Pruritus in PBC and PSC. Dig Dis 2015;33(suppl 2):164–75.

94. Mittal A. Cholestatic Itch Management. Curr Probl Dermatol 2016;50:142–8.

95. Burgos-Rodriguez AG. Avian renal system: clinical implications. Vet Clin North Am Exot Anim Pract 2010;13(3):393–411.

96. Doneley R. Acute pancreatitis in parrots. Aust Vet J 2001;79(6):409–11.

97. Bowles HL. Reproductive hormone related feather picking in a Monk parakeet. Proceedings of the North American Veterinary Conference. Orlando, FL, January 18-22, 2003. p. 1177.

98. Chitty J. Feather plucking in psittacine birds 2. Social, environmental and behavioural considerations. Practice 2003;25(9):550–5.

99. Owen D, Lane J. High levels of corticosterone in feather-plucking parrots (*Psittacus erithacus*). Vet Rec 2006;158(23):804.

100. Costa P, Macchi E, Valle E, et al. An association between feather damaging behavior and corticosterone metabolite excretion in captive African grey parrots (*Psittacus erithacus*). Peer J 2016;4:e2462.

101. Peng J, Hessey J, Tsay T, et al. Assessment and treatment of feather plucking in sulphur-crested cockatoos (*Cacatua galerita*). J Anim Vet Adv 2014;13(1): 51–61.

102. Clubb SL, Cray C, Arheart KL, et al. Comparison of selected diagnostic parameters in African grey parrots (*Psittacus erithacus*) with normal plumage and

those exhibiting feather damaging behavior. J Avian Med Surg 2007;21(4): 259–64.

103. Dislich M, Neumann U, Crosta L. Successful reduction of feather-damaging behavior by social restructuring in a group of golden conures (*Guaruba guarouba*). J Zoo Wildl Med 2017;48(3):859–67.

104. Jayson SL, Williams DL, Wood JLN. Prevalence and risk factors of feather plucking in African Grey parrots (*Psittacus Erithacus* and *Psittacus Erithacus Timneh*) and Cockatoos (*Cacatua* spp.). J Exot Pet Med 2014;23(3):250–7.

105. van Zeeland YRA, Bastiaansen P, Schoemaker NJ. Diagnosis and treatment of Cushing's syndrome in a Senegal parrot. 1st International Conference on Avian, Herpetological, and Exotic Mammal Medicine (ICARE). Wiesbaden, Germany, April 20-26, 2013. p. 303–4.

106. Oglesbee BL. Hypothyroidism in a scarlet macaw. J Am Vet Med Assoc 1992; 201(10):1599–601.

107. Schmidt RE, Reavill DR. The avian thyroid gland. Vet Clin North Am Exot Anim Pract 2008;11(1):15–23, v.

108. Harms CA, Hoskinson JJ, Bruyette DS, et al. Development of an experimental model of hypothyroidism in cockatiels (*Nymphicus hollandicus*). Am J Vet Res 1994;55(3):399–404.

109. Rae M. Endocrine disease in pet birds. Sem Avian Exotic Pet Med 1995; 4(1):32–8.

110. Suedmeyer WK. Trimming Wings in Waterfowl. J Assoc Avian Vet 1992;6(4):205.

111. Klaphake E, Beazley-Keane SL, Jones M, et al. Multisite integumentary squamous cell carcinoma in an African grey parrot (*Psittacus erithacus erithacus*). Vet Rec 2006;158(17):593–6.

112. Péron F, Grosset C. The diet of adult psittacids: veterinarian and ethological approaches. J Anim Physiol Anim Nutr 2014;98(3):403–16.

113. West JA, Tully TN, Nevarez JG, et al. Effects of fluorescent lighting versus sunlight exposure on calcium, magnesium, vitamin D, and feather destructive behavior in Hispaniolan Amazon parrots (*Amazona ventralis*). J Avian Med Surg 2019;33(3):235–44.

114. Koutsos EA, Matson KD, Klasing KC. Nutrition of birds in the order Psittaciformes: a review. J Avian Med Surg 2001;15(4):257–76.

115. Klasing KC. Comparative avian nutrition. Wallingford (United Kingdom): CAB International; 1998.

116. Hoppes S. Geriatric Avian Medicine. Proceedings of the Annual Conference of the Association of Avian Veterinarians. Washington, DC, July 29 - August 2, 2017. p. 23–32.

117. Lumeij JT, Hommers CJ. Foraging 'enrichment' as treatment for pterotillomania. Appl Anim Behav Sci 2008;111(1–2):85–94.

118. Coulton L, Waran N, Young R. Effects of foraging enrichment on the behaviour of parrots. Anim Welf 1997;6:357–64.

119. van Hoek CS, King CE. Causation and influence of environmental enrichment on feather picking of the crimson-bellied conure (*Pyrrhura perlata perlata*). Zoo Biol 1997;16(2):161–72.

120. Seibert LM. Pharmacotherapy for behavioral disorders in pet birds. J Exot Pet Med 2007;16(1):30–7.

121. Greiner EC, Ritchie BW. Parasites. In: Ritchie BW, Harrison GJ, Harrison LR, editors. Avian medicine: principles and application. Lake Worth (FL): Wingers Publishing; 1994. p. 1007–29.

122. Cornelissen JMM, Gerlach H, Miller H, et al. An investigation into the possible role of circo and avian polyoma virus infections in the etiology of three distinct skin and feather problems (CUD, FLS, PF) in the rose-faced lovebird (Agapornis roseicollis). Proc Euro Col Avian Med Surg. Munich, Germany, March 7-10, 2001. p. 3-5.

123. Worell AB. Dermatological Conditions Affecting the Beak, Claws, and Feet of Captive Avian Species. Vet Clin North Am Exot Anim Pract 2013;16(3):777–99.

124. Hasiri MA, Ahmadabadi HN, Tabrizi AS. Can Chronic Crack-Cocaine Exposure Cause Parrot Foot Necrosis? A Possible Hypothesis. Acta Sci Vet 2013; 41(1):1–4.

125. Perry RA. Pruritic polyfolliculosis and dermatitis in budgerigars (Melopsittacus undulatus) and african lovebirds (Agapornis spp.). Proceedings of the Annual Conference of the Association of Avian Veterinarians. Chicago, IL, September 23-28, 1991. p. 32–7.

126. Lamb S, Sobczynski A, Starks D, et al. Bacteria isolated from the skin of Congo African Grey parrots (*Psittacus erithacus*), budgerigars (*Melopsittacus undulatus*), and cockatiels (*Nymphicus hollandicus*). J Avian Med Surg 2014;28(4): 275–9.

127. Briscoe JA, Morris DO, Rosenthal KL, et al. Evaluation of mucosal and seborrheic sites for staphylococci in two populations of captive psittacines. J Am Vet Med Assoc 2009;234(7):901–5.

128. Phalen D. Implications of viruses in clinical disorders. In: Harrison GJ, Lightfoot TL, editors. Clinical avian medicine, vol. 2. Palm Beach (FL): Spix Publishing; 2006. p. 573–86.

129. Hess M, Scope A, Heincz U. Comparative sensitivity of polymerase chain reaction diagnosis of psittacine beak and feather disease on feather samples, cloacal swabs and blood from budgerigars (*Melopsittacus undulatus*). Avian Pathol 2004;33(5):477–81.

130. Olsen G, Speer B. Laboratory reporting accuracy of polymerase chain reaction testing for psittacine beak and feather disease virus. J Avian Med Surg 2009; 23(3):194–8.

131. Fitzgerald B, Olsen G, Speer B. Laboratory reporting accuracy of polymerase chain reaction testing for avian polyomavirus. J Avian Med Surg 2013; 27(1):32–7.

Behavior of Birds of Prey in Managed Care

Michael P. Jones, DVM, DABVP (Avian)[a],*, Barbara Heidenreich, BSc (Zoology)[b]

KEYWORDS

- Raptors • Behavior • Modal action patterns • Imprint • Learned behavior
- Resource guarding • Aggression • Territory

KEY POINTS

- Birds of prey are highly complex and intelligent species with many of their activities deeply rooted in modal action patterns such as foraging, courtship and nest building, migration, bathing, preening, and even prey selection.
- Behavioral imprinting is the long-term memory of stimuli encountered during early development and affects social preferences and behaviors in all species.
- Training birds of prey requires an understanding of how motivating operations work and how to use principles of behavior analysis to influence behavioral responses.
- Traditional approaches to behavior management can lead to adjunctive behaviors, feather damaging behavior, aggression, excessive vocalizations, and persistent juvenile behaviors.
- Understanding the components of behavior decreases the reliance on intrusive methods that are less conducive to positive animal welfare.

INTRODUCTION

Birds of prey are highly complex and intelligent species with many of their activities deeply rooted in modal action patterns, such as the foraging, courtship, nest building, migration, bathing, preening, and prey selection. Like other avian species, raptors in managed care are susceptible to presenting undesired behavior when the environment provides antecedents for these behaviors and consequences to maintain them. These behaviors can then be expressed on a regular basis due to a long and strong reinforcement history that may bring harm to the raptor or those who provide care for them. Behavioral problems often do not arise overnight, and it is important

This article is an update of Jones MP. Behavioral aspects of captive birds of prey. *Vet Clin Am Exot Anim Pract.* 2001;4(3):613–32.

[a] Department of Small Animal Clinical Sciences, Avian and Zoological Medicine, The University of Tennessee, College of Veterinary Medicine, 2407 River Drive, Room C247, Knoxville, TN 37996, USA; [b] Barbara's Force Free Animal Training, Austin, TX, USA
* Corresponding author.
E-mail address: mpjones@utk.edu

for avian veterinarians that care for birds of prey to understand how undesired behavior is influenced and maintained in birds of prey in managed care. This article discusses concepts of behavior in birds of prey in managed care, with inferences from the behavior of their wild conspecifics that will assist the veterinarian in understanding the etiologies and methods of managing these abnormal or undesired behaviors.[1]

MODAL ACTION PATTERNS

Modal action patterns are behaviors that do not require previous learning to be expressed for the first time.[1] These include behaviors such as predatory responses, play behaviors, sexual and courtship behavior, and nest building behaviors. However, they are called modal because they are modular and can be influenced by learning. Nest building becomes more refined with each season. Hunting skills improve with practice. Falconers play a significant role in improving the hunting skills of their birds by providing young or inexperienced raptors frequent opportunities to "develop" their hunting skills without some of the consequences that free-ranging raptors experience if they are unsuccessful. There are species-specific modal action patterns that show more rigidity than others. For example, the foraging methods of falcon will differ greatly from a large buteo, compared with goshawk or a great horned owl.

SPECIES-SPECIFIC BEHAVIORAL TRAITS

Behavioral tendencies, or traits, have been studied in dogs, nonhuman primates, and a number of other species.[2–6] It often involves adding labels for a class of behaviors and using that label to describe a personality type (sometimes used interchangeably with the word temperament).[7] Although some information is available to compare "personality" or behavioral traits in free-ranging avian species versus those in managed care,[8] very little information is available concerning birds of prey. Here, we provide an informal description linking hunting techniques of free-ranging raptors with behavioral traits or tendencies in managed care. Certainly, there must be some understanding that individuality exists even within species.[9] Buteos such as red-tailed hawks (*Buteo jamaicensis*) are opportunistic predators and from a conspicuous perch, will sit and wait for extended periods for prey to appear beneath them. In some instances, they may soar while searching for prey. Once prey is spotted they may attempt to capture it with short dive or a longer gliding flight. Red-tailed hawks, with the exception of species such as the Ferruginous hawk (*Buteo regalis*), broad-winged hawk (*Buteo platypterus*), and red-shouldered hawk (*Buteo lineatus*) seem to calm down quickly, are more mellow and easy-going than other raptors,[9] and exhibit more predictable behaviors while in managed care. Accipiters, such as the Northern goshawk (*Accipiter gentilis* spp), Cooper's hawk (*Accipiter cooperi*), and the sharp shinned hawk (*Accipiter striatus*) tend to be very secretive in the wild and hunt prey in a very dynamic manner, requiring quick reactions, swift maneuverability, and a high degree of alertness, all while chasing equally swift avian prey through dense foliage or wide-open spaces. Accipiters in managed care are often considered nervous, high-strung,[9] less-predictable, more fearful, and less forgiving of mistakes in handling than buteos. Accipiters more commonly exhibit aggressive behavior toward humans in managed care. This is especially true in the Cooper's hawk; they are notorious for exhibiting aggression toward their human caretaker.

Small falcons such as the American kestrel (*Falco sparverius*) and merlin (*Falco columbarius* spp) often hunt from conspicuous perches and are commonly found near human habitation, yet they are difficult to approach in the wild. American kestrels hunt a variety of prey including insects, small mammals, and even small birds. They are easily found near agricultural activity, and can be seen hovering above grassland or surveying an open area from a perch or telephone lines. Merlins are swift falcons, and although they will take larger prey such as pigeons, most of their diet consists of small birds and insects, including grasshoppers and dragonflies, taken in the air. Despite their aloof nature, both merlins and American kestrels become extremely tame in managed care and are enjoyable to fly as falconry birds.

The hunting style of large falcons, such as the peregrine falcons (*Falco peregrinus ssp*), gyrfalcons (*Falco rusticolus*), or prairie falcons(*Falco mexicanus*) can vary from direct pursuit and catching prey in the air, or soaring then stooping down on prey at great speed with intent to bind to, incapacitate, or kill prey in the strike. However, between hunts large falcons are often reported to calmly and patiently sit and watch for prey from the ground or conspicuous perches (eg, fence posts, trees, rocks, and cliffs). Most large falcons, such as peregrine falcons, are easier to handle in managed care, although the prairie falcon has developed the reputation of being more anxious, fearful, and unpredictable than other large falcons, especially during early stages of training. Gyrfalcons can also be more fearful and reactive compared with other falcons. Hybrids of large falcons, of which one of the most common is the gyrfalcon × peregrine, also seem to be relatively calm like purebred falcons, although, there are exceptions. These hybrids are bred to take advantage of behaviors exhibited by both parent birds. For example, the reactivity, power, climbing ability, and speed in pursuit of the gyrfalcon is balanced by the calm temperament and stooping ability of the peregrine. Although hybrids demonstrate physical characteristics of both parents, the male parent has a greater effect on the morphology than the female. In the case of gyrfalcon × peregrine falcon hybrids, both male and female hybrids will have a morphology closer to that of the gyrfalcons than of peregrines.[10]

Free-ranging owls lead a very solitary and sedentary life, but they are formidable and aggressive predators. Larger species such as great horned owls (*Bubo virginianus*) are capable of taking large prey such as rabbits, other raptors, and even skunks. Smaller species such as screech owls (*Megascops asio*) are equally, if not more, secretive and aggressive hunters. Given their behaviors exhibited in the wild, great horned owls can also be rather aggressive and unpredictable in managed care. Even imprinted owls, while many become very "tame" may exhibit aggressive/territorial behavior under certain conditions. For example, during breeding season or in defense of their territory, they may fly at the caregiver when the person enters the owl's enclosure. Wild snowy owls (*Bubo scandiacus*) and Northern hawk owls often show overt signs of stress in captivity (eg, anorexia, vocalizations, repeated escape attempts in their aviaries) and remain highly sensitive to environmental changes while under managed care. Other owl species such as boreal owls (*Aegolius funereus*) and barred owls (*Strix varia*) often display what is considered a calmer demeanor in captivity. However, immobility should not be interpreted, as tolerance to handling as it can be a natural way to escape predator in the wild and could be displayed by fearful individuals (Marion Desmarchelier, personal communication, 2020).

IMPRINTING PROCESS AND BEHAVIOR

Behavioral imprinting is the long-term memory of stimuli encountered during early development that affects social preferences and behaviors in all species.[11] Young raptors, on hatching, rapidly imprint on various sights and sounds (especially parent birds and their vocalizations) within their environment. As their visual acuity improves, social interactions with parents, siblings, conspecifics, and even predators are critical and necessary during this learning phase of development.[12] These cues will ultimately direct their filial behavior as well as future interactions with conspecifics (eg, territorial behavior, food preferences, mate selection, courtship, breeding behavior, nest site locations).[13] The length of the imprinting process may vary between species but is considered finite and often irreversible.[14] The process is generally thought to be longer in larger species such as eagles. Once the imprinting process has begun, young raptors may demonstrate varying degrees of fear toward objects that are not a parent, sibling, or conspecific.[12] As the raptor matures, recognition of breeding partners is influenced by imprinting and early-life experience. Courtship and nesting behaviors also play a significant role in pair bonding. Even raptors that were reared by species other than their own can often recognize conspecifics when they reach sexual maturity and begin to form pair bonds.[12] The time that the young raptor spends in the nest site also leads to environmental imprinting. The nest site, immediate surroundings, and environmental stimuli are firmly imprinted in the fledgling raptor's brain and affect future nest site choice and location.[12]

Imprinting Raptors to Humans

Raptors in managed care that are imprinted to humans or other unnatural objects should be classified as malimprints, and it is important to make that distinction. Imprinting raptors is a common practice in the sport of falconry. Falconers desire a young hawk or falcon that shows little to no fear of animate and inanimate objects (eg, humans or hunting companions, dogs, planes, trains, and automobiles), loud noises, or other disturbances, which might frighten a nonimprinted raptor, potentially resulting in the loss of the bird. In falconry, the imprinting process may occur over several months and requires frequent exposure (**Fig. 1**).

Filial imprinting is a process, readily observed in precocial birds, whereby a social attachment is established between a young animal and an object that is typically (although not necessarily) a parent.[11] These species hatch with their eyes open and can quickly imprint on and follow any animant object within the first few hours after hatching. In altricial birds (eg, raptors), the imprinting process is more variable and longer than precocial species.[11] The process naturally occurs at an early age, presumably during their second week after hatching, and varies between species.[15,16] Several investigators have provided guidelines regarding the imprinting process in raptors. For small falcons like the American kestrels, the imprinting process is believed to occur at approximately 10 to 14 days of age,[17] while larger falcon species, such as the peregrine falcons, become firmly imprinted at approximately 14 days of age, and before this time, they may react impartially to their human caregiver.[16] One falcon breeder suggests taking peregrine chicks at 12 to 15 days as ideal for imprinting for future breeding (Bill Meeker, personal communication, 2020). Sparrow hawks (*Accipiter nisus*) reportedly imprint to humans between days 1 and 8 and will most likely accept the human as a parent and future sexual partner[18] by demonstrating nesting, courtship, and other reproductive behaviors they would normally express to a potential conspecific mate. Yet, if they are taken between 10 to 14 days of age they may not accept the human as a future sexual partner,[18] may not display sexual behaviors toward humans, and may or may not allow semen collection or artificial insemination. One investigator recommends taking eyass Cooper's hawks from the nest at 7 to 10 days to be ideal for imprinting for falconry,[15] whereas another suggests taking young Cooper's hawks between 12 and 18 days of age.[19] Cooper's hawks taken after 18 days rarely develop the "tameness" falconers desire and may present what appears to be unexplainable fear or aggressive responses toward the falconer, trainer,

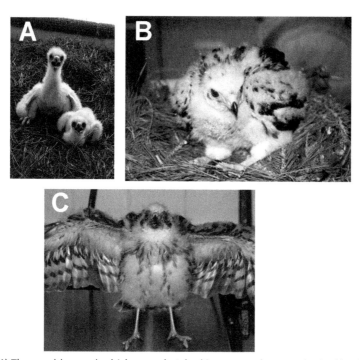

Fig. 1. (A) These golden eagle chicks were hatched in managed care and raised by their parents. Should the chicks need to be removed from the nest at this age, it is extremely important to limit human interactions that would cause the chicks to become malimprinted on humans. (B) As part of the imprinting process for use in falconry, this juvenile North American goshawk (approximately 2 weeks of age) is carried in an open nest box to allow it to become well socialized to people (both familiar and unfamiliar), animals (dogs), and various objects and sounds during the day. (C). This fledgling, female, sharp-shinned hawk is exhibiting an appropriate fear response toward a human. (*Courtesy of* M. P. Jones, DVM, Knoxville, TN.)

or handler.[19] These responses are the result of neophobia, which sets in after the sensitive period has passed.[20] This is a normal and important survival strategy for an adult bird, which should now show a fear response of new things as a means of survival rather than an openness to new things to learn about its environment as it did when it was in the sensitive period. It is not impossible to train a more mature bird, but it is less challenging when the bird is still open and receptive to new experiences during the sensitive period.

Most of the literature involving imprinting of raptors seems to focus on diurnal birds of prey. Nocturnal birds of prey (owls) are different in that they do not become imprinted to humans until later during fledgling development because their cues for identification to a species or object are determined more by sight and to a lesser degree sound.[18] McKeever suggests that the sensitive time lasts from 14 to 21 days up to 42 days.[21]

Imprinted raptors are also used in breeding situations, when at an appropriate age, the raptor accepts the human surrogate parent as a mate. Male raptors that are imprinted on humans can be trained to "copulate" and ejaculate onto a "hat," a mounted specimen or some other instrument specifically designed for semen collection.[22] Female raptors can be trained to voluntarily accept insemination from the surrogate mate (human). Consistent social interaction with the raptor is necessary to achieve the formation of pair bonds with humans. The process may take years, beginning with early stages of imprinting to the age of sexual maturity. Imprinted raptors used for falconry, which experience daily socialization with a particular human, will commonly form pair bonds with humans. It has been reported that raptors imprinted to humans are not suitable for natural breeding unless they are socialized with members of their own species at the same time; a process often termed dual imprinting. The aim is to have a bird that is acceptably comfortable around humans, easily recognizes its own kind, and yet does not present the undesired behaviors of demand vocalizations, aggressive behavior and other examples described later. Despite the thought that imprinted raptors may not be suitable for natural breeding it may still be possible to use an imprinted bird because courtship and sexual behavior are modal action patterns, as previously mentioned. One falcon breeder notes that human-imprinted falcons may breed naturally if they are placed with a mate and isolated from people; however, it may take some time and there is the potential for injury to the other falcon if the imprinted bird is a female (Bill Meeker, personal communication, 2020).

Influencing Behavior

Birds of prey like any other animals, are learning based on the principles defined by the science of behavior analysis. This science that focuses on behavior changes demonstrates that any organism's behavior can be influenced by environmental antecedents and consequences. This means all behavior birds present, whether it is desired or undesired by the caregiver, is governed by naturally occurring principles that influence behavior.

Savvy falconers and trainers who are well versed in the use of behavior analytical principles such as operant and classical conditioning, including counterconditioning, extinction, systematic desensitization, and differential reinforcement, can understand how to reach desired behavior goals and address behavior problems. For example, a hawk chooses to fly and hunt when the environmental antecedents indicate an opportunity for reinforcement exists, such as a human beating bushes with a branch. If this results in catching a rabbit, the bird is likely to participate again in the future. This is an example of positive reinforcement. A screaming bird can learn that loud vocalizations result in desired outcomes such as companionship or food. This too is positive reinforcement. However, it may be maintaining a behavior undesired by the caregiver. A potentially better option is to offer food or companionship before screaming and try to gain more insights into the antecedents for vocalizations and the desired consequences.

Other principles and procedures are useful for addressing challenges such as preventing fear responses. Gradually exposing an animal to something in a manner that does not evoke a fear response, paired with desired items (such as food) can be successful for introducing new items or experiences such as scales, people, perches, equipment, and medical instruments. In addition, undesired fear responses (and undesired aggressive behaviors) are often maintained by negative reinforcement. This same principle can be used to create desired responses. This application has been referred to as the constructional approach introduced by Israel Goldiamond[23] in the 1970s as a least intrusive procedure. When negative reinforcement is used in the constructional approach, the aversive stimulus is presented so that it barely creates an observable response (eg, the bird looks at the stimulus) or in some cases no response at all. The stimulus is removed at the moment the animal presents a desired response such as calm body language (eg, preening, looking at other stimuli, tucking a foot up into the body, rousing, feaking). Criteria can then be increased, for example, the distance between the stimulus and the bird is decreased with each approximation. Eventually, the bird learns to present calm and relaxed body language in the presence of the stimulus. Usually at this step in the process the bird is receptive to positive reinforcement procedures. This procedure has been used by the author to introduce people, towels for restraint, syringes, stethoscopes, and other novel objects. This benign use of this principle can be highly effective and a least intrusive procedure of providing the animal control over the aversive stimulus by presenting relaxed body language. It is especially appropriate when food is not the consequence the animal is seeking. This also demonstrates why it is important to not add labels of morality of good and bad to positive and negative reinforcement, but to remember they mean to add or remove a stimulus to increase behavior.

STAGES OF MATURATION

Fox describes the stages of maturation in raptors in the following sequence:[12]

- The newly hatched chick is offered food by parents.
- The chick begs for food from the parents.
- The newly fledged chick chases parent(s) for food, when satisfied it plays and chases objects resembling prey, but does not catch live prey.
- The chick physically attacks parents for food.
- The parent(s) drops dead prey for the chick which "chases" and catches it. The chick's search image is reoriented from the parents to the prey.
- The parent drops live prey which reinforces connection of pursuit with food.
- The chick has increasing difficulty in obtaining food from its parents and is left unattended for longer periods of time, it becomes more successful in catching its own live prey and begins to stray away from the nest area, self-hunting.
- The chick is completely weaned and independent.

Both sexes of recently fledged raptors will remain in the near vicinity of their nest for a period until dispersal. The sexually dimorphic and smaller males tend to develop more quickly behaviorally, become more proficient hunters quicker than their female siblings, and are more likely to disperse sooner than the females.[24]

In several raptor species, there may be an extended post-fledging period before complete independence that allows the raptor to mature, learn, and develop its hunting skills, while still receiving the benefit of extended parental care.[25–27] In some species such as eagles, this extended learning opportunity may take years to complete. However, if not handled carefully in managed care situations, it can lead to many undesired behaviors that may persist for the life of the bird of prey.[27,28]

Sociability

Most raptor species lead solitary lives except during periods of migration, courtship, and nesting periods. Species that are considered truly gregarious include Old World vultures, kestrels, caracaras (*Caracara* sp), and some species of eagles and hawks.[9,27,29–33] One of most notable examples of social structure among birds of prey is that of the Harris's hawk (*Parabuteo unicinctus*) of the Southwest United States, Central America, and even into some parts of South America.[26,27,33–38] This species demonstrates both cooperative hunting and breeding strategies in which critical advantages for members of the group are gained through prey-sharing and extended parental care for young Harris's hawks.[27]

The degree of sociality and group size may vary among Harris's hawk populations in the United States.[33,34,36,37] One study describes an interesting linear hierarchy that exists between Harris's hawks based on group observations in Arizona. Briefly, observed hawks were categorized as alpha, beta, or gamma hawks (most dominant to least dominant) based on interactions between dominant and subordinate hawks and frequency of supplanting behavior.[33,35] Supplanting described dominance behavior in which a more dominant hawk forces another to leave its perch as the first hawk approaches.[33] The most dominant hawk in these groups was always an adult female.[33]

Harris's hawk groups will cooperatively hunt prey as well as assist in the care of the current year's nestling. Cooperative hunting has its advantages in that much larger prey can be captured than by a single hawk allowing more for all group members.[34–36] This social behavior also provides increased opportunities to learn. A similar cooperative hunting behavior is seen in Harris's hawks used for falconry making this species a favorite among falconers who enjoy the social nature and comradery afforded by hunting together simultaneously.

Most birds of prey are territorial in nature rather than highly social. Species such as the California condor (*Gymnogyps californianus*), Mississippi kites (*Ictinia mississippiensis*), and ospreys (*Pandion haliaetus*) have been reported as weakly territorial,[9] whereas others consider ospreys to be very aggressive around the nest. Most other species exhibit variable territoriality. Goshawks, great horned owls, peregrine falcons, and prairie falcons are notoriously territorial and will vigorously defend their breeding territory and nest site against any intruders (including humans). In managed care, a raptor may claim a particular perch or area out of fear or an attempt to defend it against "human" or other intruders entering its enclosure or occupied space.

Creating Motivation

Training a bird of prey to work cooperatively with a falconer or handler is an involved process. Some important elements of this process are understanding how motivating operations work and using principles of behavior analysis to influence behavioral responses. The more falconers and trainers understand these components of behavior science, the less likely the reliance on intrusive methods that may be considered less conducive to positive animal welfare, such as creating excessive states of food deprivation.

By using strategies such as small approximations, sensitivity to animal body language, giving birds choice and control, building in strong reinforcement histories for behaviors, as well as adding variety in reinforcers, falconers and trainers can create highly motivated animals and behaviors (**Fig. 2**).

Traditional approaches have focused on keeping birds within specific weight ranges and micromanaging the amount of food offered to maintain the animal within that weight range. The problem with this approach is the number on the scale is not necessarily correlated to the animal's motivation for presenting behavior. A typical response to poor performance in this model is to reduce the animal's weight until a desired response is presented. However, this can lead to a variety of problems, especially if the weight reduction is excessive. These include the following: adjunctive behaviors (such as water gorging and pica), feather damaging behavior, aggressive behavior toward humans when food is present, excessive vocalization, persistent juvenile behaviors into adulthood, stunted growth if food was micromanaged during periods of development, and increased motor activity in anticipation of food. These can also be triggered by withholding just a small amount of food, if the reduction was excessive in the past.

It is important to understand that a bird's interest in acquiring food can be influenced by many factors without deprivation. One of the most important is using training

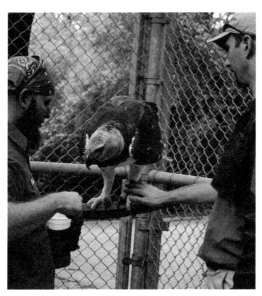

Fig. 2. Zookeepers at the Dallas Zoo train a female Harpy eagle (*Harpia harpyja*) to be comfortable with touch. This facilitated regular health checks as well as reducing stress for capture and restraint. The bird was also trained for voluntary application of anklets and jesses for transport on the glove for educational presentations. A video of the training is available at https://youtu.be/IeP1CBrkJtc. (*Courtesy of* B. Heidenreich, Austin, TX.)

strategies as mentioned. Falconers can also manage how and when food is delivered. For example, doing preference assessments, considering nutrient-dense high-caloric food items compared with items that are less dense, how much time has passed in between feeds, how much food was fed in the previous session are all considered components of food management that do not rely on micromanaging the bird's weight to influence motivation.

It is still advisable to monitor a bird's weight to ensure optimum health and welfare as well as palpate the keeled sternum and pectoral muscle to evaluate body condition. Birds that engage in adjunctive behavior can weigh "normal" due to ingestion of foreign bodies.

BEHAVIORAL PROBLEMS

Behavioral problems such as feather damaging behavior, excessive vocalizations, and aggression are frequently reported in psittacine species. These problems also occur in birds of prey but are either reported infrequently or not as well documented. Ultimately, many behavioral problems in raptors in managed care are commonly a direct result of improper handling and lack of understanding of behavior analytical principles and their practical application. It is important to remember that changes in behavior may be an indication of the presence of disease in a raptor and should be evaluated appropriately.

Infantile Behavior

Infantile behavior (eg, food begging, crouched posturing, open wing fluttering, and juvenile vocalizations) is seen more commonly in juvenile raptors in managed care, although birds of prey of all ages may exhibit this behavior, including adult raptors that have recently come into managed care. Once the behavior has been triggered by environmental stimuli and/or context, it can then get inadvertently reinforced, which may create a behavior that is very resistant to extinction, meaning it persists, sometimes for long duration depending on the reinforcement schedule and other contributing factors at play.

Food Begging

Food begging is commonly seen in malimprinted raptors that are responding in hunger to their surrogate human parent, as well as nonimprinted or wild raptors that have recently been introduced to managed care. In many instances, birds that are being treated for medical or surgical problems or maintained in rehabilitation centers may revert to juvenile behaviors once they learn humans are their source of food.[39] This seems particularly true of juvenile red-tailed hawks that revert to food begging and exhibit other body language that correlates to calm and relaxed behavior and no longer presents fear responses toward humans. This transformation from a completely wild hawk to an observably tame hawk may take only a few days of captivity. However, once the hawk begins to lose fear of the human, one must be cautious when feeding such a raptor. These hawks will exhibit behaviors similar to what would be expressed toward humans as they would toward a parent, sibling, or competitor and attempt to snatch the food directly from the hand that feeds them. This can create a condition that can trigger an aggressive response toward humans when offering food. Aggressive behavior can be avoided by keeping birds relatively satiated, offering food away from perceived territories, disassociating food directly with humans (offer food on a stump or glove), observing the bird with peripheral glances instead of staring straight on, and avoiding standing over birds. Careful observation of bird body language and connection to actions that trigger undesired responses can help increase handler sensitivity to avoid triggering aggressive behavior. Furthermore, it is important to consider the contextual elements (factors) that influence aggressive behaviors and determine if these elements are contributing factors. These contextual elements may include, but are not limited to, season, age, territorial behavior and social behaviors, environmental changes, neophobia, and even reinforcement history, punishment history, or shaped anticipatory behaviors.

Mantling

Mantling is a natural behavior exhibited by most birds of prey when they have captured prey or taken possession of a food item. When mantling, the raptor adopts a hunched posture with wing and tail feathers spread out to conceal its prey and to prevent other raptors or competition from stealing it. Often, the feathers on the nape are raised as well. In addition to serving as a method to protect its meal, mantling may be exhibited as part of social behavior.[40] Perhaps the most interesting proposed function of mantling is to "corral" the captured prey, confusing it, and thereby preventing an easy escape should it break free from the raptor's talons.[12,41] While mantling is a natural behavior it can be taken to an extreme and become a problem, often a precursor to aggressive behavior. Excessive mantling typically involves the raptor spreading its wings and tail and at times actually laying down on the ground, glove or perch to cover its meal. Causes of excessive mantling include coercive handling of a falconry bird while it is on a kill, sharp reductions in the amount of food offered to a bird of prey, sharp reductions in the weight of the bird causing it to be too hungry, attempts to take a kill or other food away from the raptor, or standing over a bird while it is eating. Fortunately, in young raptors mantling tends to become less intense as the bird matures but can easily return with improper handling as described previously.[18] One way to prevent excessive mantling by a raptor is to never take food from it; it is allowed to consume whatever it catches or whatever is offered until it is satiated or is offered a substitute portion. The raptor is able to satisfy itself and has had every opportunity to eat everything it was given.

Excessive Vocalizations

Excessive vocalizations or vocalizing for prolonged periods, often hours, is not un-common to many species of birds, including psittacines and raptors. Vocalizing is a normal behavior that is often demonstrated by juvenile raptors in relation to parent birds, but also a normal part of the daily activity of forming/maintaining relationships in social situations. Young raptors will vocalize in recognition of their parents and in anticipation of being fed. In managed care, juveniles and older raptors that recognize the human handler as the source of food or potential mate, may vocalize. All species of raptors in managed care can exhibit this behavior. The problem is intensified by the rather loud and continuous vocalizations that some raptors can emit; falcons (both small and large species) and larger accipiters, in particular, can be extremely loud and incessant even when the handler is not in sight.

Demand vocalizations is a difficult problem to manage, as it is one that is easily (and often unintentionally) reinforced in an effort to get the bird to cease vocalizing. For example, feeding a raptor that is vocalizing out of hunger may get it to stop for a short time; however, it will only reinforce the behavior. This is especially true if all interactions with the raptor are oriented around feeding it. Using applied behavior analyses princi-ples in such cases will once again provide appropriate management options such as increasing non–food-oriented time with the hawk to signify that your presence does not always mean that food will be offered. There is also some thought juvenile raptors that are unsuccessful catching prey may scream out of frustration.[16]

Using aversives such as shouting in an attempt to punish the undesired vocaliza-tions or removing attention are unlikely to be effective and have fallout of damaging the relationship between the falconer and the bird. It is far more successful to set the bird up for success and reinforce the desired behavior.

As raptors mature, most demand vocalizations will diminish or stop all together un-less inadvertently reinforced, although this may take some time. Providing falconry birds with plenty of opportunity to chase and successfully catch prey may dramatically influence the degree and duration of the demand vocalizations and help orient the raptor away from the human as its food provider. The sooner the young raptor is catching prey the less likely it is to vocalize for desired consequences and remain ori-ented to the falconer or trainer as the sole source of food and continue through its normal maturation process.

Imprinting and Courtship

At times, female raptors in managed care that are imprinted on humans will revert to juvenile or infantile behaviors more readily than males because juvenile behavior pat-terns form a larger part of the female's courtship behaviors.[15] Females adopt juvenile behaviors including begging for food, screaming, and other displays as a part of pair bonding when attempting to get the male to pass food to them.[15] These same behav-iors may be displayed to a human to which a raptor has been imprinted and some type of pair bond has developed between raptor and human.

Undesired Aggressive Behavior

Although a raptor has the ability to present aggressive behavior, just like any other behavior, it is expressed under certain contexts. It is important to note there are trends that can be observed with raptors that seem to be consistent. Many raptors present aggressive behavior when an intruder enters a space in which the bird lives and can include the mews, a perch, or other locations. It is also common for birds of prey to present aggressive behavior in the presence of food (or a conditioned reinforcer such as a lure), in particular if they are quite motivated to eat and had prior experiences in which food or the lure were taken away while the bird was still quite engaged with it. Looking directly at a bird of prey while it is engaged with food can also cause aggressive responses. Aggressive responses can also be more likely to be presented if a bird is imprinted on humans or behaves (due to training) as if it were an imprint. What is inherited is not the behavior but a susceptibility to reinforcement.[42] And because aggressive responses are behaviors, they are influenced by learning. This means aggressive behavior can be reduced or increased depending on the choices of the trainer, including to adjust the environment, that is, the antecedents of aggressive behavior. If the stimuli cannot be removed, the environment can be arranged to reduce or remove antecedents for aggressive behavior and desired responses can be reinforced under less stimulating conditions. The stimuli that trigger aggressive behavior can be gradually increased as the bird learns the correct response. Eventually the bird can be trained to give desired responses under more stimulating conditions.

Aggressive body language

Raptors commonly exhibit defensive or aggressive body language and vocalizations before initiating physical contact (**Fig. 3**). Species such as large owls, hawks, or eagles can cause serious bodily harm if aggression results in physical contact. When frightened or aggressive, raptors may assume threat postures to make themselves appear larger, and perhaps more intimidating to would be predators. Threatened or aggressive owls will hunch forward, open, arch, and spread their wings away from the body, fluff their body feathers outward, and raise the feathers along the nape. This posture can often be accompanied by a rocking back and forth motion while shifting weight from one leg to the other and staring directly at the offending object or person.

If the stimulus is presented that creates an extreme fear response that causes the bird to be pushed past threshold, with no avenue for escape available, the bird may flip onto its back with its feet held upward and in a position ready to protect itself or charge the offender. Owls, such as great horned owls and barred owls, tend not to adopt this posture but prefer to exhibit behaviors described earlier.

Several vocalizations may accompany aggressive behavior in raptors. Certainly, some raptors may not vocalize at all before aggression. Harris's hawks typically produce a low drawn out croak or a high-pitched "twittering" to indicate that something is upsetting them. Owls such as great horned owls, screech owls, and barred owls will hiss and loudly click the upper and lower beaks together (bill clapping), accipiters may repeatedly produce a "kek-kek-kek" vocalization in rapid succession, and falcons my scream and hiss to indicate their displeasure.

Intraspecific aggression

Intraspecific aggressive behavior is of considerable concern owing to the sometimes-extreme reverse sexual dimorphism (the male is usually a third smaller than the female) seen in most raptor species. A prime example of this aggression can be seen in goshawks in managed care during the breeding season. There may be considerable risk of injury, death, and even consumption, when introducing a smaller male to a female

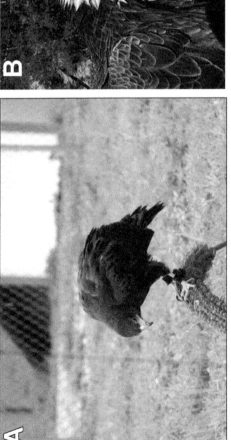

Fig. 3. (A) This male Harris' hawks is exhibiting aggression toward an unfamiliar human (author) in the weathering yard. Getting too close to this hawk would likely lead to an attack. (B) Resource guarding (food) and aggressive posturing by an adult, male bald eagle. Note the hunched posture and raised hackles as this picture was taken. ([A] Courtesy of M. P. Jones, DVM, Knoxville, TN; and [B] Courtesy K. Dotson, Pigeon Forge, TN.)

for breeding. Often, the male is provided avenues of visual and physical escape or the female's flight capabilities are temporarily diminished to reduce injury and prevent capture of the male.

Certainly, new arrivals may experience aggression leading to trauma as they navigate interactions with conspecifics, especially when food is made available. One way to solve this issue is to rearrange the exhibit or enclosure before adding new birds and provide multiple areas for raptors to separate themselves from others in the enclosure. If a pair is formed, that pair will need to be removed from the group.

In free-ranging, social raptors like Harris's hawks, a dominance hierarchy affects relationships within and between individuals in a group (see the Sociability section). Aggression is uncommon between Harris's hawks of the same group or breeding unit. In managed breeding situations, Harris's hawk breeders allow young hawks to learn proper social etiquette through prolonged interaction with adults and siblings[26,41] similar to what would be experienced in their wild conspecifics. By allowing the young to remain with the parents for 12 to 20 weeks before sending them to falconers, the young hawks learn to be submissive (ie, flying to another perch or side-stepping the adult as it approaches) toward adults.[26] Food begging can be a submissive behavior. In these situations, the adults will "punish" the young hawks when they exhibit inappropriate behaviors such as fighting with siblings and other immature hawks, not moving away when an adult approaches, leaping over or bumping into an adult, or knocking a parent off of its perch. In response, the adults may start with threat postures or alarm vocalizations, and escalate to foot stomping on the perch, foot holding, striking the young hawk with an open foot, plucking a contour feather from the shoulder or breast, or biting the bare skin of the face.[26] If the young hawk repeats the same behavior, the parents may strike the young bird forcibly from a perch with both feet or chase the young hawk around the chamber while alarm-calling and repeatedly striking it.[26] When Harris's hawks are removed from parents and raised in isolation, they often lack the training their parents would have provided. This may lead to a potentially dangerous situation when they are hunted in a cast (group) with other Harris's hawks that are unfamiliar with each other. In most group hunting situations with falconry birds, dominance displays such as supplanting, when one hawk forces another to leave its perch as the first hawk approaches,[33] may only lead to brief physical contact between hawks. In some, this may lead to more intense contact resulting in physical injury. It is interesting to note that some species that are considered very aggressive to conspecifics (eg, goshawks or red-tailed hawks) have been flown and hunted together in casts by falconers with little to no aggression.

Siblicide, also referred to as Cainism, fratricide, or even brood-reduction, has been reported in a number of species of birds of prey and is especially common in eagles.[16,43-46] Siblicide is characterized as obligate where the second hatched nestling routinely dies as a result of aggression from its nest mate, or facultative, where the second hatched chick occasionally dies as a result of aggression from the other chick.[47] Several factors contribute to the occurrence of siblicide including time between hatching, difference in hatching weight, sex and hatching sequence, and parent provided resource competition. The death of the subordinate chick may occur as a result of injury, starvation, and even falling from the nest to escape.[26] Surprisingly, the adults appear to make no attempt to stop this activity or even interfere with this process.[16] Siblicide may also be an adaptive strategy that benefits the surviving offspring and parents.[43] One study demonstrated that the remaining nestling in experimentally reduced brood enjoyed a net benefit in food intake, despite a drop in bulk food delivers by their parents.[45] In this study, 15 brood manipulations involving 11 species, including kestrels and eagles, occurred, and in all cases (eight) in which the food supply was accurately measured, the biomass received per individual nest-ling increases by 33% to 313%.[45] Of course, in managed care, human intervention may be necessary to prevent injury or death to younger, smaller siblings.

Interspecific aggression toward other avian species

Interspecific aggressive behavior usually involves conflict within a managed care sit-uation, because modal action patterns might be triggered by a particular stimulus. For example, placing different species together in the same aviary can lead to injury, espe-cially if evasive behaviors used by one species, or an awkward landing on a perch, trig-gers predatory behavior in another. A raptor that has no avenue of escape will most likely use aggressive behavior in an effort to defend itself from other raptorial species. Quite often the only way to prevent or resolve aggressive behavior is to remove incom-patible birds from the enclosure.

Interspecies predation does occur in free-ranging raptors. For example, increased predation of American kestrels by larger species such as peregrine falcons or Coo-per's hawks has reportedly contributed to the decline of American kestrels in some re-gions.[48] Certainly, many falconers in the western United States have lost their falcons to predation by free-ranging golden eagles (*Aquila chrysaetos*).

Interspecific aggression toward humans

Aggressive behaviors may be directed at humans and are expressed when the right trigger(s) is present. Footing (grabbing), aggressive displays, or flying into the face of the handler/trainer may be triggered unknowingly by improper handling, improper socialization, food restriction and hunger, and territoriality or resource guarding. Furthermore, an aggressive response may also be cumulative as multiple factors, un-related events or similar events may (unrecognized by the falconer/handler) build on themselves. For example, most falconers, handlers, or trainers will allow the raptor to eat what is offered to it on the glove or perch and never try to take a portion or add to what was offered. When sleight of hand is attempted to add or remove food, the raptor may grab the ungloved hand containing food to either prevent food from be-ing removed or in anticipation of food being added. This reaction may then become a reinforced behavior that is repeated.[39] Some species (eg, accipiters) are more easily triggered by conscious and unconscious mistakes or behaviors from their handler, especially if they are malimprinted.

Familiarity, especially in imprinted raptors, may also lead to aggression, as the raptor tends to treat the handler as a competition and has no fear response that might cause the bird to redirect its aggressive tendencies.[39] Interestingly, even the gregar-ious and somewhat easily trained Harris's hawk may become aggressive toward humans.

Free-ranging raptors generally try to avoid human contact and urban areas; howev-er, they can and will attack humans if necessary. These attacks are common in the spring when raptors are defending their nest and surrounding territory from intruders. Goshawks, especially the female, prairie falcons, peregrine falcons, great horned owls, and even the diminutive screech owls (*M asio*) will defend their nest/territory vigorously against any intruder.[49,50] Aggressive behaviors, depending on the size and temperament of the raptor, may range from being mildly annoying to resulting in serious injury. Rehabilitated and released raptors that have not been properly so-cialized are malimprinted, or lack appropriate hunting skills may show aggressive be-haviors. When unsuccessful capturing prey, these raptors may show aggressive behavior or harass unsuspecting individuals for food. These confrontations can be especially disturbing if a larger bird of prey such as a bald eagle (*Haliaeetus leucocephalus*) is involved. In all instances of aggression, it is important to make a strong effort to identify triggers and develop a training program to remove or reduce the undesired behavior.

Resource Guarding and Territorial Behavior

Establishing and protecting breeding or foraging territories is a natural tendency of most, if not all, birds of prey. Generally, territory size is large enough to meet the nesting, foraging, and breeding activities necessary to reproduce.[41] When space is limited, territories may vary in size or even overlap. Aggression may occur in a communal/mixed group aviary. Territoriality within a communal enclosure, especially if a pair is formed is especially dangerous to other members of the group. The potential for physical aggression may increase when food is made available. Once a territory is defined, it is rarely abandoned or forgotten over time.

Free-ranging raptors must establish and defend their territories to survive and reproduce. In managed care, raptors may display aggression that is sometimes described by humans as territorial or resource guarding, as it occurs in an area in which a hawk was previously or currently fed and may include an entire enclosure or certain areas within the enclosure. However, aggression in aviaries is often a learned behavior, highly efficient to provide faster delivery of food and reducing the time of human presence. Fear of humans can also be involved as wild birds quickly learn that escape is not possible in an enclosed area and that aggression is the most functional behavior to move people away. Therefore, aggression in an enclosed area should not always be interpreted as normal territorial behavior, but rather include other differentials that might help manage the problem more effectively.

In free-ranging raptors, the male often establishes, reestablishes, and maintains a territory, although both sexes may exhibit territorial behavior.[41] These behaviors, which may include aerial displays singly or in tandem, conspicuous perching, and vocalizations, occur near the nest site or territory. In the context of inappropriate resource guarding or territorial displays of raptors in managed care, usually body language and vocalizations indicative of aggressive behavior are displayed when the territory is approached. These displays of aggressive behavior may or may not lead to physical contact depending on environmental stimuli, reinforcement history, contextual elements, such as reproductive state.

Management of territorial behavior involves determining the site or cause of the behavior. If it is associated with food, it may help to avoid feeding the hawk in that area. Some species, in particular the accipiters, are well known for developing aggressive behavior in response to territorial behavior and resource guarding. For example, malimprinted Cooper's hawks exhibit aggressive displays that include side-to-side, snakelike movements of the head and neck, excessive mantling, turning their back to the handler (even while on the glove) while looking over their shoulders, and feigning attacks to name a few. Ultimately, these displays will lead to physical contact (grabbing or footing) if the problem is not identified and resolved. Careful observation of antecedents, consequences for aggressive behaviors, prior handling procedures, awareness of social relationships to humans, seasonal occurrence of the behavior, and the bird's relationship to food may help to identify causes of territorial behavior and/or resource guarding behavior as well as develop a plan for resolution.

Feather Damaging Behavior

Feather damaging behavior is well documented in many avian species where etiologies range from infectious and noninfectious diseases to behavioral problems. However, feather damaging behavior and self-mutilation are reported with less frequency in raptors. When these behaviors occur, they are often seen in birds that have been in managed care for an extended period, those placed in extremely stressful situations (eg, near noisy urban development or barking dog), or those that are isolated and deprived of social interaction with conspecifics or humans. Etiologies of feather damaging behavior are similar to those in other species including, but not limited to, noninfectious diseases (eg, hepatic, renal, cardiovascular, or neoplastic diseases), infectious and inflammatory diseases, orthopedic or soft tissue trauma, lack of enrichment, lack of exercise, reproductive frustration, or redirected aggression. All raptors in managed care may exhibit feather damaging behavior; however, feather damaging behavior seems to be more common in captive bred Harris's hawks than other species. It would seem that Harris's hawks need more environmental enrichment and social interaction, especially with conspecifics, while in managed care.

Usually, the feather damaging behavior is noted on the legs in the femoral and tibiotarsal regions, the pectoral regions (**Fig. 4**) as well as around the shoulder region and dorsal antebrachium. Usually, the primary and secondary flight feathers are left undamaged.

It would make sense that self-mutilation is infrequently reported in wild raptors as they have no need to express this behavior or are unlikely to survive. However, wild birds will mutilate themselves while in managed care. Most commonly, the cause

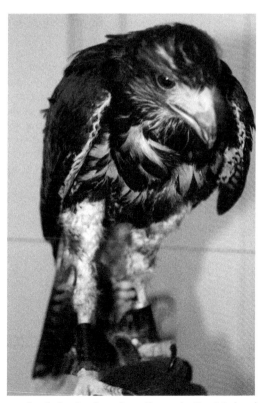

Fig. 4. Feather destructive behavior in a juvenile, male Harris's hawk. Note the loss of feathers in the tibiotarsal and caudal pectoral regions. (*Courtesy of* M. P. Jones, DVM, Knoxville, TN.)

may be associated with trauma to an appendage or iatrogenic causes. Interestingly, one author (MPJ) has observed self-mutilation in free-ranging screech owls and a red-tailed hawk (**Fig. 5**) brought into managed care for wing injuries and following placement of external coaptation (Figure-8 bandage) on their injured wings. Merlins (*F columbarius*) and American kestrels have been known to mutilate their own feet.

Although the motivation for behavior problems may be difficult to determine in raptors, the principles of management of feather destructive behavior or self-mutilation are essentially the same as other species. The goal is to try to identify and treat the underlying cause. Initially, a detailed history, a thorough physical examination, and a complete behavior analysis may diagnose the concern and limit the necessity of additional tests. As well, observation of the behavior by video taken by the handler/agent may be necessary should the raptor not demonstrate the behavior in front of a "stranger." Laboratory diagnostics (complete blood count, biochemical analysis) will help to strengthen the minimum database if necessary. Ancillary diagnostic tests may include fecal examination, radiographs, skin and feather pulp cytology, skin biopsy, histopathologic examination and appropriate culture and sensitivity test of affected areas of skin. If the results of the diagnostic tests are sufficient to explain the clinical signs, then consider treating appropriately. If they are not, then consider behavioral causes for feather damaging behavior or self-mutilation and consider consultations with a team of avian and veterinary behaviorists. At this time, data regarding pharmacologic intervention for feather destructive behavior or self-mutilation is limited. Hormonal treatment (GnRH agonists) has been used successfully in a male broad-winged hawk with seasonal behavioral abnormalities including feather damaging behavior and excessive masturbation (Desmarchelier, personal communication, 2020)

Management of behavioral cases of feather damaging behavior or self-mutilation is complex. Many behavioral problems are acute manifestations of chronic conditions and it may require long-term management to achieve resolution. Treatment should center around identifying environmental conditions that led to development of the undesired behavior. Mutilation wounds should be cleansed and dressed appropriately. Environmental factors should be evaluated for those species that are easily stressed (eg, screech owls and small accipiters). These should have a quiet environment and the opportunity to escape the gaze of predators (eg, larger raptors, humans) while in managed care. Screech owls in particular may benefit from having a hide box placed in their enclosure or the entire front of the enclosure may be covered.

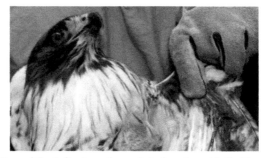

Fig. 5. Self-mutilation of the left wing of an adult, female red-tailed hawk. The hawk mutilated the distal wing following application of external coaptation for a pronounced wing droop and suspected brachial plexus avulsion. (*Courtesy of* M. P. Jones, DVM, Knoxville, TN.)

For falconry birds or other raptors in long-term managed care, enrichment should be provided to improve their welfare. Enrichment may take many forms. For example, during long periods of inactivity, falconry/educational birds may be given the opportunity to "forage," chase prey (ie, luring), play with toys, exercise, bathe (sun and water), given controlled exposure to the elements, or learn new activities through operant conditioning. Social species such as Harris's hawks may also benefit from social enrichment and housing with other Harris's hawks. Enrichment requirements can vary greatly between species and individuals and are best evaluated on a case by case basis. The Association of Zoos and Aquariums Raptor Taxon Advisory Group has collected resources and enrichment ideas that can be provided for birds in managed care. These are easily accessed at: https://www.raptortag.com/enrichment.html.

SUMMARY

Birds of prey are intelligent species displaying highly complex behaviors in the wild such as foraging, courtship and nest building, migration, bathing, or preening, and even prey selection or preference. The behaviors are influenced by learning. Training birds of prey requires an understanding of how motivating operations work and how to use principles of behavior analysis to influence behavioral responses. Traditional approaches to behavior management focused on keeping birds within specific weight ranges and micromanaging the amount of food offered to maintain the animal within that weight range. However, this can lead to a variety of problems including adjunctive behaviors, feather damaging behavior, aggression, excessive vocalizations, and persistent juvenile behaviors into adulthood. Falconers, trainers, and handlers who have an understanding of the use of operant conditioning, classical conditioning, as well as other behavior analytical principles can understand how to reach desired behavior goals and address behavior problems. The more falconers and trainers understand these components of behavior science, the less likely the reliance on intrusive methods that are less conducive to positive animal welfare.

CLINICS CARE POINTS

- Gradually exposing a raptor to something in a manner that does not evoke a fear response, paired with desired items (such as food) can be successful for introducing new items or experiences such as scales, people, perches, equipment, and medical instruments.
- Creating motivation through traditional approaches to weight management focus on keeping birds within specific weight ranges and micromanaging the amount of food offered. However, a raptor's interest in acquiring food/motivation can be influenced by many factors without deprivation.
- Using aversives such as shouting in an attempt to punish the undesired vocalizations or removing attention are unlikely to be effective and have fallout of damaging the relationship between the falconer/trainer and the raptor. It is far more successful to set the bird up for success and reinforce the desired behavior.
- While data regarding application of pharmacologic intervention for feather destructive behavior or self-mutilation is limited in raptors, hormonal treatment with GnRH agonists may be useful in some circumstances.

DISCLOSURE

The authors have nothing to disclose.

REFERENCES

1. Barlow GW. Modal action patterns. In: Sebeok TA, editor. How animals communicate. Bloomington (IN): Indiana University Press; 1977. p. 98–134.
2. Svartberg K, Forkman B. Personality traits in the domestic dog (*Canis familiaris*). Appl Anim Behav Sci 2002;79:133–55.
3. Ilska J, Haskell MJ, Blott SC, et al. Genetic characterization of dog personality traits. Genetics 2017;206:1101–11.
4. Massen JJM, Antonides A, Arnold AMK, et al. A behavioral view on chimpanzee personality: exploration tendency, persistence, boldness, and tool-orientation measured with group experiments. Am J Primatol 2013;75:947–58.
5. Dutton DM. Subjective assessment of chimpanzee (*Pan troglodytes*) personality: reliability and stability of trait ratings. Primates 2008;49:253–9.
6. MacKay JR, Haskell MJ. Consistent individual behavioral variation: the difference between temperament, personality and behavioral syndromes. Animals (Basel) 2015;5(3):455–78.
7. Gosling SD. From mice to men: what can we learn about personality from animal research? Psychol Bull 2001;127:45–86.
8. Herborn KA, Macleod R, Miles WTS, et al. Personality in captivity reflects personality in the wild. Anim Behav 2010;79:835–43.
9. Weidensaul S. Behavior. In: Raptors: the birds of prey. New York: Lyons and Burford Publishers; 1996. p. 86–93, 94-106.
10. Eastham CP, Nicholls MK. Morphometric analysis of large Falco species and their hybrids with implications for conservation. J Raptor Res 2005;39:386–93.
11. McCabe BJ. Visual Imprinting in birds: behavior, models, and neural mechanisms. Front Physiol 2019;10:658.
12. Fox N. Development and behavior. In: Understanding the bird of prey. Blaine (WA): Hancock House Publishers; 1995. p. 176–95.
13. Immelman K. Ecological significance of imprinting and early learning. Annu Rev Ecol Syst 1975;6:15–37.
14. Bildstein KL. Raptors: the curious nature of diurnal birds of prey. ProQuest Ebook Central. Ithaca (NY): Cornell University Press; 2017. p. 67–82. Available at: http://ebookcentral.proquest.com/lib/utk/detail.action?docID=4857218.
15. McDermott M. Problems. In: The imprint accipiter. Cedar Hill (MO): Michael McDermott, Publisher; 1998. p. 143–68.
16. Heidenreich M. Management of raptors in captivity. In: Birds of prey: medicine and management. Malden (MA): Blackwell Science, Inc.; 1995. p. 5–23, 35–61.
17. Koehler A. Captive breeding of some raptors. Raptor Res News 1969;1:3–18.
18. Jones CG. Abnormal and maladaptive behavior in captive raptors. In: Cooper JE, Greenwood AG, editors. Recent Advance in the Study of Raptor Diseases, Proceedings of the International Symposium on Diseases of Birds of Prey. West Yorkshire: Chiron Publications; 1980. p. 53–9.
19. McElroy H. Hand raising the Cooper's hawk from the early stages of withdrawal. In: Desert hawking II. Yuma (AZ): Cactus Press; 1977. p. 9–14.
20. Greenberg R, Mettke-Hofman C. Ecological aspects of neophobia and neophilia in birds. Curr Ornithol 2001;16:119–78.
21. McKeever K. Care and rehabilitation of injured owls. 4th edition. Lincoln (ON): WF Rannie Publishing; 1987.
22. Boyd LL, Schwartz CH. Training imprinted semen donors. In: Weaver JD, Cade TJ, editors. Falcon propagation: a manual on captive breeding. Boise (ID): The Peregrinefund, Inc.; 1991. p. 24–30.

23. Goldiamond I. Toward a constructional approach to social problems: ethical and constitutional issues raised by applied behavior analysis. Behav Soc Iss 2002;11: 108–97.

24. Bildstein KL. Causes and consequences of reversed sexual size dimorphism in raptors: the head start hypothesis. J Raptor Res 1992;26:115–23.

25. Bustamante J. The post-fledgling dependence period of the black-shouldered kite. J Raptor Res 1994;27:185–90.

26. Coulson J, Coulson T. Natural history of Harris's Hawk. In: The Harris' hawk revolution. Pearl River (LA): Parabuteo Publishing; 2012. p. 11–64, 459–544.

27. Bednarz JC, LIgon JD. A study of the ecological bases of cooperative breeding in the Harris'Hawk. Ecology 1988;69:1176–87.

28. Wood PB, Collopy MW, Sekerak C. Postfledging nest dependence period for bald eagles in Florida. J Wildl Mange 1998;62:333–9.

29. Whitacre DF, Burnham WA. Ecology and conservation of Tikal's raptor fauna. In: Whitacer DR, editor. Neotropical birds of prey: biology and ecology of a forest raptor community. Ithaca (NY): Cornell University Press; 2012. p. 328–99.

30. Harel R, Spiegel O, Getz WM, et al. Social foraging and individual consistency in following behaviour: testing the information centre hypothesis in free-ranging vultures. Proc Biol Sci 2017;284:20162654.

31. Donázar JA, Feijóo JE. Social structure of Andean condor roosts: influence of sex, age, and season. The Condor 2002;104:832–7.

32. Thiollay JM. Foraging, home range use and social behaviour of a group-living rainforest raptor, the Red-throated Caracara Daptrius americanus. Ibis 1991; 133:382–93.

33. Dawson JW, Mannan RW. Dominance hierarchies and helper contributions in Harris' Hawks. Auk 1991;108:649–60.

34. Clark WS. Group size of Harris' hawks (Parabuteo unicinctus) in south Texas. Wilson J Ornithol 2017;129:364–8.

35. Coulson JO, Coulson TD. Reexamining cooperative hunting in Harris's Hawk (Parabuteo unicinctus): large prey or challenging habitats? Auk 2013;130:548–52.

36. Bednarz JC. Pair and group reproductive success, polyandry, and cooperative breeding in Harris' Hawks. Auk 1987;104:393–404.

37. Dwyer JF, Bednarz JC. Harris's hawk (Parabuteo unicinctus). The Birds of North America online. 2020. Available at: https://birdsoftheworld.org/bow/species/hrshaw/cur/introduction. Accessed June 17, 2020.

38. Coulson JO, Coulson TD. Group hunting by Harris' hawks in Texas. J Raptor Res 1995;29:265–7.

39. Jones MP. Raptors: paedlatrics and behavioural development and disorders. In Chitty J, Lierz M, editors. British small animal veterinary association (BSAVA) manual of raptors, pigeons, and passerine birds. Gloucester: BSAVA; 2008. p. 250–9.

40. Rottraut I. Influence of social behavior on prey-catching in barn owls. Bird Behav 1990;9:7–13.

41. Johnsgard PA. Comparative behavior. In: Hawks, eagles & falcons of North America. Washington, DC: Smithsonian Institution Press; 1990. p. 39–58.

42. Skinner BF. Contingencies for reinforcement. A theoretical analysis. New York (NY): Appleton-Century-Crofts; 1969.

43. Mock DW, Drummond H, Stinson CH. Avian siblicide. American Scientist 1990; 78:438–49.

44. Meyburg BU, Pielowski Z. Cainism in the greater spotted eagle (Aquila clanga). Bull Birds Prey 1991;4:143–8.

45. Simmons RE. Siblicide provides food benefits for raptor chicks: re-evaluating brood manipulation studies. Anim Behav 2002;6:F19–24.

46. Hernández-Matías A, Real J, Parés F. Siblicide in Bonelli's eagle (*Aquila fasciata*). J Raptor Res 2016;50:125–8.

47. Edwards TC, Collopy M. Obligate and facultative brood reduction in eagles: an examination of factors that influence fratricide. Auk 1983;100:630–5.

48. Ely TE, Briggs CW, Hawks SE. Morphological changes in American kestrel (*Falco sparverius*) at continental migration sites. Glob Exol Conserv 2018;15:e00400. Available at: https://www.sciencedirect.com/science/article/pii/S2351989417302640. Accessed June 17, 2020.

49. Sproat TM, Ritchison G. The antipredator vocalization of adult Eastern Screech owls. J Raptor Res 1994;28:93–9.

50. Parker JW. Raptor attacks on people. J Raptor Res 1999;33:63–6.

Clinical Reptile Behavior

Lionel Schilliger, DVM, DECZM (Herpetology), DABVP (Reptile and Amphibian Practice)[a],
Claire Vergneau-Grosset, DVM, IPSAV, CES, DACZM[b],*,
Marion R. Desmarchelier, DVM, DACZM, DECZM (ZHM), DACVB[c]

KEYWORDS

- Snake • Lizard • Chelonian • Tortoise • Turtle • Behavior
- Environmental enrichment

KEY POINTS

- Owners and veterinarians less familiar with reptiles may misinterpret reptile behaviors. Understanding the natural history of different species is key to interpreting their behavior in captivity.
- Common reasons for behavioral consultations include hyperactivity, self-mutilation, frequent biting, abnormal repetitive behaviors, and postural abnormalities.
- Abnormal behaviors identified by owners can be normal, but inappropriate, or abnormal and secondary to environmental or medical causes.
- Aggression can be induced by various factors, such as fear, pain, resource guarding, or sex hormones. Appropriate management begins by identifying the cause.
- Addressing behavioral issues involves understanding the root cause, implementing relevant environmental modifications, developing a behavior modification plan, and choosing medication when appropriate.

 Video content accompanies this article at http://www.vetexotic.theclinics.com.

Reptile behavior is complex and varies widely among the approximately 11,000 species included in the nonavian reptile class.[1] It is estimated that more than 5 million reptiles were kept as pets in 2007 in the United Stated alone.[2] North America is the biggest consumer market for companion reptiles worldwide, with a 22% increase in the number of animals exchanged since 2002.[3] Although pet reptiles are becoming more common in households, their behavior could be misinterpreted by owners less familiar with reptile physiology and natural history. Reptile behavior is increasingly being studied from complex cognition[4] to adaptation to spaceflight conditions, where

[a] Clinique Vétérinaire du Village d'Auteuil, 35 Rue Leconte de Lisle, Paris 75016, France; [b] Service de Médecine Zoologique, Department of Clinical Sciences, Université de Montréal, 3200 rue Sicotte, Saint-Hyacinthe, Québec J2S 2M2, Canada; [c] Department of Clinical Sciences, Université de Montréal, 3200 rue Sicotte, Saint-Hyacinthe, Québec J2S 2M2, Canada
* Corresponding author.
E-mail address: claire.grosset@umontreal.ca

Vet Clin Exot Anim 24 (2021) 175–195
https://doi.org/10.1016/j.cvex.2020.09.008
1094-9194/21/© 2020 Elsevier Inc. All rights reserved.

vetexotic.theclinics.com

thick-toed geckos were shown to be able to remain attached to surfaces during weightlessness.[5] Although the fascinating topic of reptile behavior cannot be summarized in a single article, the objective of this article is to help practitioners differentiate normal from abnormal behaviors in reptiles commonly encountered in veterinary consultation. Thus, crocodilians, venomous reptiles, and tuataras will not be discussed in this article. Another goal is to assist practitioners in addressing common owner complaints regarding reptile behaviors. These may include behaviors associated with inappropriate husbandry where veterinarians should be able to advise the owner appropriately.

NORMAL REPTILE BEHAVIOR
In Captive Settings

Knowledge of what constitutes normal behavior is required to identify abnormal behavior. Because reptiles are ectotherms, their physiology and behavior are influenced by their environment, as evidenced by the dramatic changes in their locomotor, reproductive, and feeding behavior under differing environmental conditions.

Reptile location in a terrarium is strongly influenced by available ultraviolet light (UV) and environmental temperature. For instance, captive juvenile leopard geckos (*Eublepharis macularius)* favor behavioral thermoregulation rather than hiding from potential predators.[6] When exposed to excessive temperatures, bearded dragons and spiny tailed lizards (*Uromastyx* spp.) keep their mouth open and breath with short, shallow respirations (polypnea), which should be differentiated from true dyspnea. Temperatures outside of the preferred optimal temperature zone can also induce brumation or estivation, especially in tortoises of the genus *Agrionemys* spp. Brumation and estivation are associated with decreased activity, which should not be interpreted as lethargy. Snakes spending an extensive amount of time in their water bowls might be kept in conditions with excessive temperature, but should also be examined to detect mites, as bathing is a common response to mite infestation. Chameleons rely heavily on access to UVB light, and studies have shown that they exhibit light-seeking behavior according to individual vitamin D requirements.[7] When stressed, certain reptiles also change body posture; bearded dragons flatten their body dorsoventrally, while chameleons tend to flatten laterally, vibrate, and stay close to vertical elements. Whenever juvenile bearded dragons (*Pogona vitticeps*) encounter conspecifics or are approached by handlers, they may display circling motions of the forelimbs, which is a common behavior in this species (Video 1).

Reptiles were once believed to have a low degree of sociality and parenteral care; however, this hypothesis is increasingly questioned by recent findings. Chelonians can learn visual cues by observing conspecifics,[8] and skinks can participate in complex social organization.[9] Reptiles display a wide diversity in maternal care, such as egg brooding in ball pythons (*Python regius*), protective maternal behavior toward hatchlings among prehensile-tailed skinks (*Corucia zebrata*), and even sharing shelters with conspecifics among certain lizards (**Fig. 1**). Conspecific interactions among reptiles typically increase during breeding season, as evidenced by complex nuptial parades in anoles (*Anolis* spp.).[10] Madagascar boas (*Acrantophis madagascariensis*) fight using their spurs, while male box turtles (*Terrapene* spp.) will sometimes place their hind limbs between the carapace and plastron of the female during mating to prevent the female from closing her shell.[11]

Reptiles communicate through visual and vocal signals, as well as through pheromones. Among visual signals, color changes and dewlap expansion (throat fan) in anoles and frilled lizards *(Chlamydosaurus kingii)* (**Fig. 2**) can be impressive, and

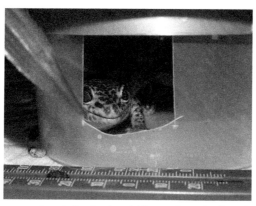

Fig. 1. Example of a gregarious behavior in which a male and a female leopard gecko (*Eublepharis macularius*) share the same shelter despite being provided multiple hiding places at the same temperature. (*Courtesy of* C. Vergneau-Grosset, DVM, Saint-Hyacinthe, Canada.)

they are typically displayed by males to attract females.[10] Male anoles with heavy mite burden display less frequently and progressively lose dewlap coloration.[10] Many species, including male green iguanas (*Iguana iguana*) and anoles display head bobbing and flex/extend their arms (push-ups) as an intimidation signal or to indicate territoriality.[12] The throat of bearded dragons darkens in situations of agonistic behavior toward a conspecific. When occurring in individually housed animals, it is often caused by their reflection on glass surfaces. Green iguanas and bearded dragons can approach competitors with a slight head tilt, not to be mistaken for a vestibular syndrome. Chameleons can change light reflections on their skin by rearranging melanosomes within their skin chromatophores in order to change their color. Changes in colors are sudden and indicate differing physiologic or behavioral changes. For instance, female veiled chameleons (*Chameleo calyptratus*) show typical colors during folliculogenesis characterized by blue and orange spots. Pregnant female chameleons will also show a typical color pattern (**Fig. 3**). In male veiled chameleons, mathematical models have shown a correlation between the brightness of the body stripes and head

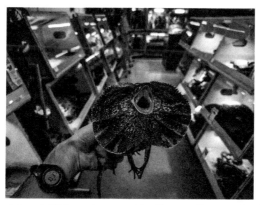

Fig. 2. Frilled-necked lizard (*Chlamydosaurus kingii*) spreading out its frill and gaping its mouth when frightened, displaying bright orange scales. (*Courtesy of* K. Daoues, Paris, France.)

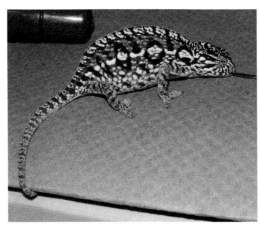

Fig. 3. Example of a pregnant female chameleons (*Chamaeleo calyptratus*) showing a typical color pattern. (*Courtesy of* C. Grosset, DVM, Saint-Hyacinthe, Canada.)

color, and the likelihood of engaging in fights.[13] Skin color in reptiles can also be affected by nutritional factors and environmental temperature. For instance, lizards on a diet high in carotenoids will display brighter red-orange colors.[14]

Certain visual signals that require UV vision are not detectable to the human eye.[15] Many reptiles possess UV vision, including members of the Iguanidae, Gekkonidae, and snakes.[16] Hence, certain male lizards will copulate with females only when they harbor a receptive pattern, which is only visible under UV light.[16] Thus, lack of breeding success should not be necessarily interpreted as a behavioral problem, as visual deficits or inappropriate cues can interfere with mating.

Reptiles also communicate through vocal signals. For instance, tokay geckos (*Gekko gecko*) are able to adjust their vocalization to the surrounding noise intensity, indicating a sophisticated degree of communication ability.[17] Repeated calls are normal in this species and should not be misinterpreted for distress by owners (Video 2). Reptiles also perceive pheromones via their vomeronasal organ and perform repeated tongue flicks when exploring a new environment.

Normal feeding and drinking behaviors can sometimes raise questions from owners. Chameleons are unable to drink from bowls as they lick water off of leaves in the wild; therefore, a drip system or spraying water on plants is necessary in captivity. Unusual, but normal, feeding behaviors include juvenile green pythons moving their tails as a lure to catch prey. Geckos frequently eat their molt (**Fig. 4**). Whether this behavior is related to protein recycling, a defense mechanism against predators, or both remains unknown. Wood turtles (*Glyptemys insculpta*) stomp their feet to create vibrations to mimic rain in an effort to lure earthworms to the surface.[18] Lithophagy (ingestion of soil and substrate) is considered normal in many tortoises and might be a way to acquire mineral nutrients.

During Handling, Physical Examination, and Medical Procedures

During clinical examination, reptiles will behave in various fashions depending on the taxa involved. Tortoises tend to lie motionless on the examination table and retract completely into their shells as a means of self-defense. Large African tortoises (leopard tortoises [*Stygmochelys pardalis*]) and African spurred tortoises (*Centrochelys sulcata*) possess a powerful retraction reflex, and the clinician must be careful

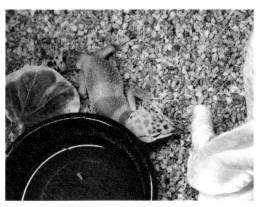

Fig. 4. A carrot-tail leopard gecko (*Eublepharis macularius*) after ingesting its molt. The remaining molt is visible on its head. (*Courtesy of* C.Grosset, DVM, Saint-Hyacinthe, Canada.)

when positioning his or her hands around the head, neck, and limbs, especially at the level of the prefemoral pits and the axillofacial depressions. In a testament to their strength, these species can sometimes only be properly examined under sedation. Smaller species can also display a retracting reflex (Burmese star tortoises [*Geochelone platynota*] and Indian star tortoises [*Geochelone elegans*]). Some species can enclose themselves within their shell by use of a cranial hinged plastron (eg, Madagascarian spider tortoises [*Pyxis arachnoides*]), dual cranial and caudal hinged plastrons (eg, box turtles [*Terrapene* sp., *Cuora* sp.]), or a hinged caudal carapace (eg, Bell hinge-back tortoises [*Kinixys belliana*], forest hinge-back tortoise [*Kinixys homeana*]).

In contrast, nonapathetic aquatic turtles tend to be active and move quickly on the examination table. When handled, they usually thrash around and can inflict severe scratches or bites wounds (**Fig. 5**). Like tortoises, they often urinate on the consultation table if stressed. Some species (eg, African helmeted turtle [*Pelomedusa subrufa*]) can expel malodorous cloacal glands secretions when stressed.

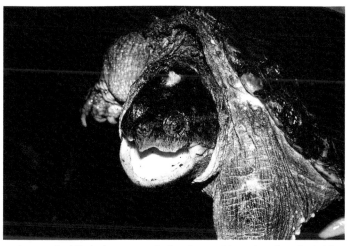

Fig. 5. Snapping turtle (*Chelydra serpentina*) trying to bite when handled. (*Courtesy of* L. Schilliger, DVM, Paris, France.)

Large lizards (eg, green iguanas, monitor lizards [*Varanus* sp.], tegus [*Tupinambis* sp.]) can bite, tail whip, or inflict serious scratches in self-defense. Inflation of the body, opening the mouth, unfolding the gular dewlap (where present), standing in an elevated position, and jerking head movements are displayed to intimidate predators or rivals, or impress a potential mate (Video 3). The green iguana often adopts a U-shaped position on the examination table, presenting its head and tail in readiness to attack. Iguanas tend to attempt escape; a firm restraint is therefore crucial by holding both forelimbs against the thorax and both hindlimbs against the tail. Bearded dragons (*P vitticeps*, *P henrylawsoni*) are generally docile and can be handled easily, without biting or trying to escape. They can become cataleptic and immobile when held in a supine position, but will revert to a normal state once replaced into the prone position. This behavior, associated or not with the oculocardiac reflex, can be exploited to facilitate clinical examination. However, there are few data on the impacts of this procedure (oculocardiac reflex) on the stress of the animals. It is unknown whether the oculocardiac reflex eliciting vagal stimulation can be part of a fear-free examination, or whether applying ocular pressure is actually uncomfortable. Male chameleons sometimes adopt a defensive posture and can inflict a painful bite (eg, veiled chameleons). Some species (eg, leaf chameleons [*Brookesia* sp.], Oustalet chameleons [*Furcifer oustaleti*]) vibrate when handled, similar to that of a phone vibrator, which should not be a cause of concern.

When seized from behind the helmet, chameleons and some other species (eg, geckos) tend to open the mouth, which facilitates examination of the oral cavity (**Fig. 6**). Some lizards (eg, crested geckos [*Correlophus ciliatus*], day geckos [*Phelsuma* sp.]) display an autotomy reflex by breaking off their tail at the level of predetermined fractures on the coccygeal vertebrae (**Fig. 7**). Vibration of the tail precedes this action, in which case the animal should be quickly released to prevent an amputated tail and a disgruntled owner. The tail can also break off when a thrashing lizard is held firmly by the tail. Day geckos can spin during handling and remove a part of their skin, exposing underlying subcutaneous tissues. Geckos belonging to the genus *Geckolepis* spp. can shed their skin, which is a natural response against predation.

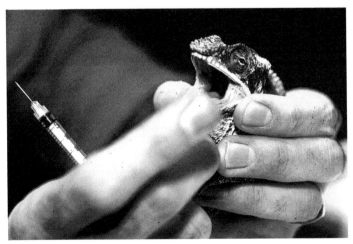

Fig. 6. When seized from behind the head, some lizards (such as chameleons and geckos) tend to open the mouth, which facilitates examination of the oral cavity. (*Courtesy of* L. Schilliger, DVM, Paris, France.)

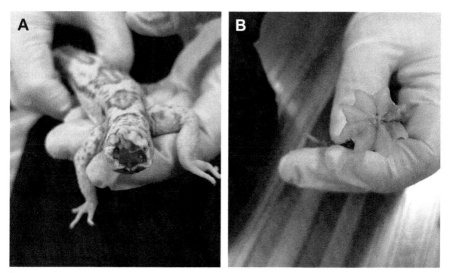

Fig. 7. Autotomized tail in a leopard gecko (*Eublepharis macularius*). (*A*) Individual with a recently autotomized tail. (*B*) Autotomized distal tail (spontaneous movements may be present on the separated tail for a few seconds). (*Courtesy of* C.Grosset, DVM, Saint-Hyacinthe, Canada.)

Surprisingly, intraspecific aggression, and not predation, has been shown to be the major cause of tail loss in 2 gecko species on Mediterranean islands.[19] Some geckos utter a loud barking cry when seized (eg, tokay gecko [*G gecko*]). Other species-specific behaviors include that of the girdled lizard (*Ouroborus cataphractus*), which seizes its own tail in its mouth to take the appearance of an armadillo (**Fig. 8**), or the horned lizard (*Phrynosoma* sp.), which can eject blood from ocular and periocular blood vessels up to 1 m in distance.

The behavior of snakes is family-specific. Colubrids are usually lively and seek to escape as soon as their cage is opened. During handling, they will incessantly seek

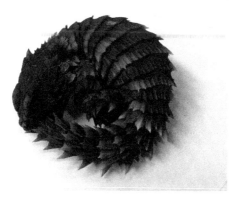

Fig. 8. Girdled lizard (*Ouroborus cataphractus*), seizing its tail in its mouth to take the appearance of an armadillo. (*Courtesy of* C. Paillusseau, DVM, Paris, France.)

to escape the person's grasp. Some species (eg, aquatic colubrids) secrete malodorous musk scents from their cloacal glands. Boids are more indolent when the transport bag or box is opened and tend to remain within the container. The constrictor boa (*Boa constrictor*), the Burmese python (*Python molurus bivittatus*), the reticulated python (*Malayopython reticulatus*), the green tree python (*Morelia viridis*), and the emerald tree boa (*Corallus caninus*) are among the many boids that can bite in self-defense. On the other hand, the ball python is rarely aggressive and adopts a rather peculiar behavior when stressed; it wraps itself into a ball, its head buried into the rings formed by its body. Boids and colubrids can produce a loud noise during handling because of quick ejection of the air from the lung through the small tracheal opening. Most snakes handled shortly after a meal will regurgitate in response to stress and the attempt to escape. Autotomy is also described in African colubrids belonging to the genus *Psammophis* spp., *Natriciteres* spp., and *Hapsidophrys* spp.[11]

When handling venomous snakes, it goes without saying that particular care must be taken to avoid being bitten. Rattlesnakes will shake their rattle at the end of their tails to warn predators. Cobras flatten their necks in the shape of a cap and stand up on their curved body before projecting themselves forward to bite. Some nonvenomous snakes mimic this behavior, notably the North American colubrids (*Lampropeltis* sp. and *Pantherophis* sp.), which shake the end of their tail when cornered. Hognose snakes (*Heterodon* sp.) flatten their neck by adopting a typical cobra position to confuse predators and can also display astonishing thanatosis when threatened. The thanatosis display consists of convulsions in the supine position and then mimicry of a state of apparent death with the mouth open, extruded tongue, and expressing a putrid odor from cloacal glands. This behavior is also well described in the grass snake (*Natrix helvetica*). Tail display in also a prey-predator defensive mechanism that can be observed in the South American hognose snake (*Xenodon durbignyi*) (**Fig. 9**).

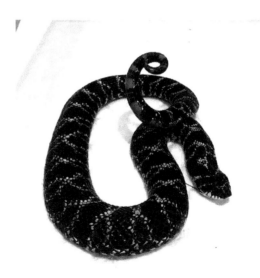

Fig. 9. Tail display in a prey/predator defensive mechanism in a South American hognose snake (*Xenodon durbignyi*). (*Courtesy of* C. Paillusseau, DVM, Paris, France.)

When placed back into a cotton transport bag, most snakes will typically seek to exit it immediately. It is, therefore, advisable to tighten the bag around the forearm of the arm holding the snake before releasing the snake into the bag.

Behavioral Considerations During Hospitalization

Although reptile behavior is species-specific, the flight reflex is near universal across species. Turtles and tortoises constantly attempt to escape their terrarium, especially when kept in a cramped space. Some species of snakes (eg, *colubridae*) will exploit every opportunity to escape, including the smallest opening in their terrarium, while larger and more powerful snakes are able to slide open unlocked terrarium doors. Some species of lizards (eg, *Physignathus cocincinus*) will rub their rostrum against transparent terrarium panes during the entire period of their hospitalization, resulting in self-administered rostral wounds (**Fig. 10**).[20] In such species, terrariums with transparent panes should be avoided.

To avoid behavioral abnormalities in hospitalized reptiles, it is important to have a dedicated room heated to 28°C for most species. Nonreptile patients, such as dogs, cats, ferrets, rats, or rabbits must be kept in a separate room as they are reptile predators or preys, and their presence can cause psychological stress and trigger a dramatic flight reflex. Similarly, reptile patients should not be in eyesight of other predatory reptiles (eg, lizards and snakes). Each terrarium should be equipped with a separate hotspot to create a warmer zone heated at the species' maximal preferred temperature (typically 32°C). Shade-dwelling species should be offered the appropriate amount of filtered light and UVBs. It has been shown that UVAs can trigger agonistic behaviors in certain lizards (eg, green anole [*Anolis carolinensis*]).[21] Dietary supplements can also affect animal behavior; in 1 study, basking time (necessary in the production of pre- and provitamin D3) decreased as vitamin D3 supplementation was increased.[7] Similarly, exposure to natural sunlight can increase aggression levels in some species by increasing testosterone levels (eg, green anole [*A carolinensis*]).[22]

A hiding place should be present in every terrarium to allow the reptiles to hide from visual stressors. In the case of gestating females, a laying box must always be

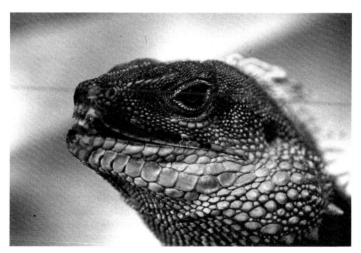

Fig. 10. Self-administered rostral wounds in a Chinese water dragon (*Physignathus cocincinus*) after rubbing his rostrum against transparent terrarium panes. (*Courtesy of* L. Schilliger, DVM, Paris, France.)

provided (eg, humid sand); this is especially crucial in the case of patients with egg retention, where a suitable laying box can help trigger oviposition. Lizards and turtles ingest terrarium substrate when alimentary fibers or minerals are deficient in the diet, and reptiles should be monitored when offered nesting material. Snakes sometimes ingest pads or paper towels if they can smell traces of prey animals.

MAIN PRESENTATIONS FOR BEHAVIORAL PROBLEMS IN PRACTICE
Restlessness and Hyperactivity

Restlessness and hyperactivity are commonly related to overheating, which increases thermodependent metabolism and activity levels. Agitation, as evidenced by continuously seeking to escape the terrarium, should first prompt verification of the terrarium's temperature setting. Overcrowding, cohabitation with a territorial or aggressive specimen, sexual arousal, and severe hunger can also cause hyperactivity.

In female aquatic and terrestrial turtles, restlessness can also be suggestive of imminent oviposition; a laying box should be immediately provided to avoid egg retention. Restlessness can also be observed in stressed or wild-caught snakes.

Self-Mutilation

Self-mutilation in reptiles can have various causes. Lizards indefatigably rubbing their rostrum on transparent panes of a terrarium can become a compulsive repetitive behavior (especially in water dragons), which can result in severe rostral trauma, eventually leading to maxillary and mandibular osteomyelitis (see **Fig. 10**). This behavior can also be caused when lighting from inside the terrarium creates a reflective surface on the glass, causing the lizard to confuse its reflection with a congener (especially chameleons and green iguanas). In this instance, it is recommended to apply plasticized films onto the glass or plastic panes to reduce reflections. Stressors within the terrarium that triggers the animal's flight reflex can also cause rubbing of the rostrum against the terrarium.

Autotomy is a behavioral reflex that involves self-amputation of the tail to escape a predator's grasp or cause a diversion that allows for escape (see **Figs 7 & 12**). It is seen in the *Cordylidae, Dactyloidae, Dibamidae, Gerrhosauridae, Gymnophthalmidae, Lacertidae, Leiocephalidae, Liolaemidae, Opluridae, Shinisauridae, Sphenodontidae, Xantusiidae* families, as well as some species within the *Agamidae, Iguanidae*, and *Teiidae* families.[11] Geckos of the genus *Correlophus* sp. can also remove their stitches after surgery, which is a form of self-induced trauma.

Thermal burns are a form of unintentional self-mutilation that arises when thermal gradients are not respected (eg, excessive hot spot or excessive cold spot), leading reptiles to remain stuck on a heat source from which they suffer severe burns.

Aggression

Interspecific and intraspecific aggressions are commonly seen in pet reptiles. Biting is the most common manifestation of aggression toward people. Aggression is a natural behavior with many different functions for reptiles. Predatory aggression is the silent and rapid aggression leading to the death and ingestion of a prey. Territorial aggression is displayed toward conspecifics and other intruders when defending a certain area, usually to defend limited resources, including females.[23] Not all reptile species are territorial in the wild. Intraspecific aggression also occurs during the breeding season between males fighting for females. Finally, fear-based aggression occurs when a reptile feels threatened and chooses fight instead of flight.[24]

All of these types of aggression can be seen in captivity in normal expected contexts or as displaced inappropriate behaviors. Reptiles rely heavily on smell and pheromone detection to hunt prey. Therefore, it is advisable not to handle rodent bedding or live prey before accessing a carnivorous reptile enclosure, as this could result in an accidental predatory aggression. To condition reptiles to feed only in certain areas and improve owner's safety, some individuals benefit from being fed exclusively outside of their terrarium, in a different tank. Territorial aggression is often overdiagnosed when a reptile bites the hand that is entering the terrarium. Although this is an appropriate differential diagnosis in this context, most reptiles actually bite because of fear of the upcoming handling and potential previous negative experiences in a similar situation. To avoid this situation, owners should be educated to not handle snakes during or prior to molt. Learning the reptile body language is also key to bite prevention, as warning signs are often ignored by the owners. For instance, corn snakes usually display vibrations of the distal part of the tail before biting. Many snakes will display an S shape with their neck before striking. Bearded dragons may develop a black gular region prior to biting. Green iguanas may display head bobbing or a tail flick before swiping with their tail or biting. Chameleons may take a darker color and open the mouth (**Fig. 11**). Reviewing videos of the behavior problems with the owners might help target some individual fearful behaviors. Appropriate handling to improve reptile comfort should also be taught to owners, such as handling the reptile with 2 hands, never letting the caudal part of the body hang down, and refraining from holding the snake forcefully behind its head. Pain-related aggression occurs in reptiles. One of the authors (CVG) has seen this occur in a carpet python presented with a pancreatitis. Therefore, potential causes of pain should be investigated when a reptile is presented for an acute onset of repetitive biting. Intraspecific aggression is normal when testosterone increases during the breeding season in many species. It is important to research the species natural history to avoid inappropriate social groupings. For instance, intact adult male leopard geckos should never be kept in the same terrarium.[25] Intraspecific biting may also be misinterpreted by owners, especially during mating behavior, which often involves female neck biting by the male.[26] Aggression behavior linked to sex hormones could be redirected toward people as is commonly seen in mature male green iguanas. Only an accurate identification of the type of

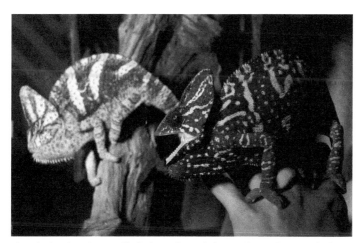

Fig. 11. Color darkening in a veiled chameleon (*Chamaeleo calyptratus*). (*Courtesy of* L. Schilliger, DVM, Paris, France.)

aggression allows for appropriate management of the situation. Treating fear aggression like territorial aggression could result in a vicious circle of increased fear and bite intensity.

Repetitive Behaviors

Owners may consult for repetitive behaviors observed in their reptiles. Again, practitioners should attempt to different normal from abnormal behavior. Reptiles trying to escape an inadequate environment may move back and forth in front of a window in an attempt to find an exit from the terrarium. Pregnant females trying to dig a nest may also attempt to dig frenetically even if no substrate is present in the habitat. In these cases, repetitive nonproductive behaviors are the result of a suboptimal captive environment.

Alternatively, certain repetitive movements may reveal underlying medical problems. For instance, chelonians displaying rhythmic limb movements may in fact be dyspneic. Abnormal repetitive movements can also be associated with stress. Similar to what is described in mammals, it is documented that certain prenatal factors, such as egg incubation temperature, can predispose individual lizards to developing stereotypic behaviors.[27]

Postural Abnormalities

Reptiles may be presented for postural abnormalities. In this case, strictly behavioral abnormalities should be differentiated from medical problems.

Turtles floating with 1 side tilted toward the surface may have asymmetrical lung lesions or dilations of the gastrointestinal tract by gas.[28]

Neurologic signs should be differentiated from musculoskeletal problems, behavioral signs, and developmental abnormalities. Certain selected reptile morphs will often display neurologic abnormalities affecting their locomotion and body posture. This is the case of spider ball pythons and jaguar carpet pythons (*Morelia spilota*), which develop a wobble syndrome of genetic origin characterized by head tremors, incoordination, and lack of righting reflex.[29]

Head tilt may be of behavioral or neurologic origin in certain lizards. If the origin is behavioral, this sign will be intermittent. Opisthotonus should be differentiated from dyspnea in snakes; indeed, snakes in respiratory distress may keep their head and cranial part of the body toward the ceiling and wave it back and forth laterally. This behavior may be an attempt to clear the upper airways as mucus may fall toward the lung with gravity. In case of compensatory behavior associated with dyspnea, respiratory sounds may be heard; open mouth breathing may be present, and gular breathing may be visible. Differential diagnoses for this behavior include true opisthotonus, which may be caused by pathogens affecting the central nervous system, or thiamine deficiency.

Lack of righting reflex should be differentiated from catalepsy, a state where reptiles retain rigidity and may not return to sternal position. Catalepsy or thanatosis is a physiologic mechanism described in certain ophidian species such as grass snakes (*Natrix natrix*) or hog-nosed snakes (*Heterodon* spp.).[30] This behavior is thought to be a defense mechanism discouraging predators from attacking the snake.

Loss of Appetite Related to Improper Diet or Husbandry

Partial or complete anorexia in reptiles can be the result of a poor quality diet, inadequate environmental conditions, or pain.[31] Failure to meet nutritional requirements, such as feeding animal tissue to a herbivore or plant material to a carnivore, or providing species-inappropriate prey can induce eating and drinking disorders. It should be noted that for many species, dietary preferences change with age, especially among omnivores, such as bearded dragons. Feeding behavior has been shown to be a marker of postoperative pain in snakes.[31]

Similarly, abnormally low or high ambient temperature or hygrometry can affect drinking behavior. Species-specific hydration behavior should be taken into account for every species. For example, chameleons drink only water that is beading on surfaces (eg, rocks or leaves), and the absence of a dripper or misting system in a chameleon terrarium can cause dehydration.

Pain-Related Behavioral Issues

Recognizing and characterizing pain in animals are often difficult (**Table 1**). In comparison to higher vertebrates commonly seen in veterinary practice, reptiles are even less able to provide interpretable information on the intensity and character of nociception.[32] According to the International Association for the Study of Pain, pain is defined as an unpleasant sensory and emotional experience associated with actual or potential tissue damage, or described in terms of such damage.[33] This definition includes a central modulation of pain that is not confirmed in reptiles devoid of neocortex. Therefore, the term nociception is more rigorous in certain reptiles, while pain can be used in chelonians who have a neocortex. Identifying nociception in reptiles thus requires careful observation to discriminate normal behavior from behavior possibly indicative of discomfort (**Figs. 12** and **13**).[34] Feeding delay may be an interesting indicator of nociception in snakes.[31] However, certain changes can be subtle in reptiles. For more information about nociceptive signs and antinociception in reptiles, readers should refer to other reviews.[35,36]

ADDRESSING BEHAVIORAL ISSUES

Reptiles are rarely presented to veterinarians primarily for a behavioral issue, but rather to address the observed consequences of an inappropriate behavior. This

Table 1
Behavioral signs of nociception and pain in reptiles

The Following Clinical Signs May Be Related to Pain in Reptiles:		
Snakes	**Chelonians**	**Lizards**
Reduced appetite, delayed striking	Reduced appetite	Reduced appetite
-	Closed eyelids	Closed eyelids
-	Head and neck stretched in and out of the shell	Elevating and extending their head
Biting when handled	Biting when handled	Biting when handled
-	Lameness	Lameness
Abnormal posture	Abnormal posture	Abnormal posture
-	-	Color changes
Abnormal respiratory movements	Abnormal respiratory movements	Abnormal respiratory movements
Restless, agitation during handling	-	-
Body less coiled at the site of pain	-	Arching the back Avoid ventral recumbency

Data from Refs.[31,32,34–36]

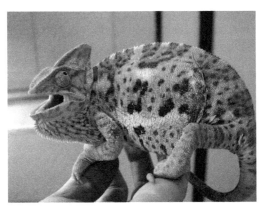

Fig. 12. Spayed female veiled cameleon (*Chamaeleo calyptratus*) displaying pain and discomfort (trying to bite) when handled. (*Courtesy of* L. Schilliger, DVM, Paris, France.)

might be because some owners are not able to recognize behavioral abnormalities, do not know veterinarians can provide them with solutions to these issues, or because reptiles do not display abnormal behavior as much as domestic species do. Pet reptiles have not been domesticated; therefore, selection of aberrant behaviors or neurotransmitter diseases is less likely to have occurred. In parallel, genetic diversity is generally preserved, and inbreeding is less likely to affect the behavior of captive reptiles. However, captive environment and life as pets can have some significant effects on reptile mental health. Reasons for behavior consultations include interspecific aggression (toward people or other species), intraspecific aggression, and self-mutilation as already mentioned. Every patient with behavioral issues will benefit from a systematic approach to reach an accurate diagnosis and then choose the most appropriate management plan.[37] This approach includes getting a thorough history, a behavioral analysis, and a medical evaluation.[37] When potential causes are identified for the problem behavior, a combination of behavior modification, environmental adjustments, and/or medication can be appropriately implemented.

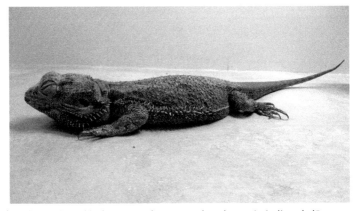

Fig. 13. Closed eyelids and lethargy can be signs related to pain in lizards (*Pogona vitticeps*). (*Courtesy of* F. Gandar, DVM, Liège, Belgium.)

Getting to a Diagnosis Through a Systematic Approach

Failure to appropriately diagnose behavioral issues is often because of the absence of an organized approach that should be similar to that used for medical work-ups.[37] Every case should be considered unique even if the presentation appears similar; a water dragon can hurt its rostrum because the terrarium is too small, because of loud noises in the environment, or because a cat is jumping on the sides of the enclosure. Thus, the same behavior in the same species resulting in the same physical consequences can have various causes that will require different approaches. In order to establish a thorough list of differential diagnoses for the behavioral issue, the following 3 steps should be considered, in no particular order:

Taking a thorough history is an important part of every reptile consultation.

When addressing a behavioral issue, review of the diet and the environment is as critical as for any medical presentation.

Rearing situation, breeding history, previous social environment, complete medical history, and play, elimination, sleep, and exploratory patterns should be reviewed if applicable.

Many environmental modifications may be identified at that stage to help decrease the problem behavior and improve the overall animal health and welfare. And although rearing history cannot be changed for the current case, recognizing predisposing factors might help prevent similar cases from occurring in the future. It is known, for example, that incubation temperature can affect gecko behavior.[38] Behavior analysis will determine in which context the problem behavior occurs, what the triggers are, what the behavior looks like, and what the consequences for the animals are. This will allow one to adjust the environment to modify the problem situation, to remove environmental triggers if present, and to work on consequences. If the animal repeats the behavior, it is most likely reinforcing to the animal, in a way that can be obvious or sometimes difficult for practitioners to comprehend. This analysis will lead to the behavior modification plan, a key to the therapeutic success. Last, but not least, an exhaustive physical examination with appropriate diagnostics is essential to establish potential involvement of an underlying medical condition.

Behavior Modification in Pet Reptiles

Most behavior problems will be more effectively managed if a behavior modification plan is implemented. It is especially important in cases of aggression toward people. Identification of the context and the triggers of the aggression will allow for a better prevention of the aggression. For example, if a snake bites every time the owner puts his or her hand in the terrarium when the snake is hungry, the authors could recommend alternative ways to interact with the animal. The snake could be gently transferred with a hook into a container so the owner could clean the terrarium. Ideally, the snake could be trained to target and then to voluntarily transfer into another space where it could be fed or exercised while the cage is accessible to the owner.[39] Adjusting the diet and feeding in a different area could also be a good option. Cases of fear-based aggression should focus on allowing the reptile to escape the threat, removing the fearful stimulus as much as possible, and interacting in a positive way with the animal (ie, target training). Predictable interactions are also reassuring for reptiles and will decrease fear-induced behavior. Independent of the primary cause of the aggression, whether it was fear, territorial, testosterone-related, or predatory, the animal has learned that aggression functioned well to achieve its goal. Although one can often address the primary cause with drugs and environmental changes, only a behavior modification plan will teach the reptile which alternative behavior is more appropriate to reach the same reinforcing consequence. If one can provide it with an even more reinforcing consequence to this alternate appropriate behavior, it will most likely make the right choice for both parties. Target training is easily achieved in most chelonians and lizards, and although slightly more challenging, can also be used in snakes (Videos 4 and 5). Results can be reached within days with turtles and lizards and within a few weeks with most snakes. Excellent education groups and resources are available on the Internet and can provide training and support to an owner willing to start training his or her pets. Behavior modification techniques can also be useful for patients with specific medical conditions. With biomedical training, captive reptiles can be weighed, injected, trained for voluntary blood draws, and stand still for nail filing or wound care.[40] Food is the most common reinforcer used with reptiles (eg, insects, fruit purees, baby food, and nectar), but scratching under the neck for lizards or on the shell for chelonians can also be preferred by some individuals (Video 6). The reader is referred to the article about behavior modification in this issue for more information.[41]

Environmental Enrichment for Behavior Problems

Most reptiles presented in consultation benefit from environmental changes to improve their health. Additional adjustments can easily be implemented to enhance their behavior and welfare. Enrichment increases animal choice and control over their environment, and promotes species-appropriate behaviors.[42] Providing hiding places will help resolve fear aggression cases. Promoting exercise with enrichment items such as climbing walls, platforms, branches, and paper rolls is likely to reduce stress and boredom and will encourage normal behavior.[4] Offering appropriately sized terrariums is important, but inciting reptiles to display natural behaviors, even in the smallest quarantine containers, is critical (Video 7). Objects that are easily available can be used to enrich small snake enclosures (**Fig. 14**). Animals do not perform behaviors that serve no purpose. Behavioral thermoregulation is a key activity in reptiles. Reptiles need a thermal gradient and should not have to choose between a warm place or a place to hide. Providing resources and enrichment throughout an appropriate thermal gradient can, therefore, reduce stress and inappropriate behaviors.[11] Finding the right balance between safety, hygiene, and enrichment when choosing the substrate for a pet reptile can be challenging. If natural substrates like sand or

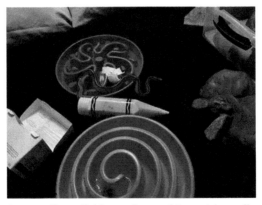

Fig. 14. Objects that are easily available can be used to enrich small snake enclosures, as shown with this Thai bamboo ratsnake (*Oreocryptophis porphyraceus coxi*). (*Courtesy of* L. Petrella, Calgary, Canada.)

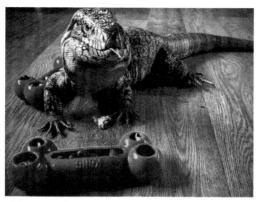

Fig. 15. Black and white tegu (*Salvator merianae*) using a dog food toy as enrichment. (*Courtesy of* J. Baldwin, Totton, UK.)

soil cannot be used on a regular basis in the terrarium, they could still be offered as enrichment under supervision. For example, lizards could be allowed to hunt in a sand box (Video 8). Feeding toys and food puzzles for dogs and cats can be used by reptiles (**Fig. 15**). Most plastic toys float and can be given to aquatic species. Socks provide great additional hiding places for snakes. Adapting the social environment is essential, as aggression is common when keeping a nonsocial species at unnatural high densities.[43] Many reptiles are relatively solitary as adults, but can be social and benefit from group housing when younger (eg, crocodilians and iguanas) or even for life (eg, geckos) (see **Fig. 1**; Video 2). Some species even exhibit stable social grouping and family systems (eg, Australian black rock skinks [*Eugernia saxatilis*] and great desert skinks [*E kintorei*]).[44]

Behavior-Influencing Medications

True anxiety disorders are uncommon in pet reptiles. The use of psychotropic drugs in an attempt to control normal behaviors displayed by reptiles placed in stressful situations, such as keeping multiple males without any possibility to escape, should not be recommended. Environmental changes should always be implemented when necessary. It is likely that aggression is in part regulated by monoamine neurotransmitters in reptiles as it is in other species.[45,46] However, the use of psychotropic drugs should be reserved to cases where the animal's welfare is affected by a condition impairing normal neurotransmission (ie, anxiety disorders) or only temporarily before environmental adjustments are made. These medications aim at restoring normal neurochemical balance in some neurotransmitter pathways, but are unlikely to be efficient to help animals with normal neurotransmitter function in an abnormal situation. By asking if most reptiles would behave in a similar way if placed in the same context, one can differentiate between an inappropriate, but normal behavior, and an aberrant behavior that could benefit from psychotropic medication. There is no information in the literature on the use of short-acting medication (ie, trazodone) that could be useful to relieve fear, anxiety, and stress during hospitalization and transport in reptiles. Further research is required in this area.

Normal elevation of blood testosterone appears associated with increased aggressive behaviors in males of various species.[47,48] Intraspecific aggression during the reproductive season has been favored by natural selection and can be redirected toward people in captivity. Although normal, these behaviors can be problematic and even dangerous in some species. If the individual is not part of a breeding program, its welfare can be affected by these seasonal increases in sex hormones as they encourage natural behavior that cannot take place and might create frustration, leading to redirected aggression toward owners. Chemical or surgical castration could, therefore, be considered.[49,50] Although more studies are required, timing of intervention appears to be important. Reduction of testosterone levels is best achieved if the treatment is applied before the initial increase.[48] Celioscopic and celioscopy-assisted orchiectomy has been safely used in several species, including chelonians and iguanas.[50,51] Deslorelin implants have shown promising results to reduce gonadotropin levels in some species in anecdotal reports (ie, bearded dragon and green iguanas),[52,53] but not in others (ie, yellow-bellied sliders [*Trachemys scripta*]).[54]

Observing reptile behavior proves captivating, as one can continuously learn more about species-specific behavior and individual preferences. A better understanding of their body language is the first step to make the right diagnosis, medical or behavioral. As knowledge improves on what is normal for them to do, clinicians are better equipped to recognize abnormal findings earlier in the process. Although the science of reptile welfare is still in its infancy, it has come a long way from keeping reptiles in barred environments to enriched flexariums promoting natural behaviors. Training reptiles with positive reinforcement is getting more and more popular in the owner community and is a great way to start communicating with pet reptiles in a language they can understand. All of these changes strengthen the reptile-owner bond and result in a better welfare for the pet and in an increased level of veterinary care.

CLINICS CARE POINTS

- Hyperactivity and self-mutilation may be associated with inappropriate environments in reptiles. Thus, taking a thorough history is strongly recommended.
- Biting may be associated with improper handling technique and/or pain, which should be investigated through a medical approach.
- Postural abnormalities are often a clinical sign of medical problem, and should be investigated with advanced diagnostic tests as needed.

DISCLOSURE

No conflict of interest to disclose.

SUPPLEMENTARY DATA

Supplementary data related to this article can be found online at https://doi.org/10.1016/j.cvex.2020.09.008.

REFERENCES

1. Uetz P, Hošek J. The reptile database 2019. Available at: http://www.reptile-database.org/. Accessed July 13, 2019.
2. AVMA. U.S. Pet ownership & demographics sourcebook. In: AVMA. 2012. Available at: https://www.avma.org/KB/Resources/Statistics/Pages/Market-research-statistics-US-pet-ownership.aspx. Accessed July 13, 2019.
3. Laidlaw R. Scales and tails: the welfare and trade of reptiles kept as pets in Canada. In: World Society for the Protection of Animals. 2007. Available at: https://www.zoocheck.com/wp-content/uploads/2016/06/Reptile_Report_FA.pdf. Accessed October 27, 2020.

4. Burghardt G. Environmental enrichment and cognitive complexity in reptiles and amphibians: concepts, review, and implications for captive populations. J Appl Behav Sci 2013;147(3–4):286–98.
5. Gulimova V, Proshchina A, Kharlamova A, et al. Reptiles in space missions: results and perspectives. Int J Mol Sci 2019;20:3019.
6. Craioveanu O, Craioveanu C, Miresan V. Plasticity of thermoregulatory behavior in leopard geckos (*Eublepharis macularius*, Blyth 1954). Zoo Biol 2017;36(4):273–7.
7. Ferguson GW, Gehrmann WH, Karsten KB, et al. Do panther chameleons bask to regulate endogenous vitamin D3 production? Physiol Biochem Zool: PBZ 2003; 76(1):52–9.
8. Davis KM, Burghardt GM. Training and long-term memory of a novel food acquisition task in a turtle (*Pseudemys nelsoni*). Behav Processes 2007;75(2):225–30.
9. Chapple D. Ecology, life history, and behavior in the Australian scincid genus *Egernia*, with comments on the evolution of complex sociality in lizards. Herpetol Monogr 2003;17:145–80.
10. Cook EG, Murphy TG, Johnson MA. Colorful displays signal male quality in a tropical anole lizard. Naturwissenschaften 2013;100(10):993–6.
11. Durso AM, Maerz JC. Chapter 13: Natural behavior. In: Divers SJ, Stahl SJ, editors. Reptile and amphibian medicine and surgery. Saint Louis (MO): Elsevier; 2019. p. 90–9.
12. Lovern MB, Jenssen TA. Form emergence and fixation of head bobbing displays in the green anole lizard (*Anolis carolinensis*): a reptilian model of signal ontogeny. J Comp Psychol 2003;117(2):133–41.
13. Ligon RA, McGraw KJ. Chameleons communicate with complex colour changes during contests: different body regions convey different information. Biol Lett 2013;9(6):20130892.
14. McLean CA, Lutz A, Rankin KJ, et al. Red carotenoids and associated gene expression explain colour variation in frillneck lizards. Proc Biol Sci 2019; 286(1907):20191172.
15. Garcia JE, Rohr D, Dyer AG. Trade-off between camouflage and sexual dimorphism revealed by UV digital imaging: the case of Australian Mallee dragons (*Ctenophorus fordi*). J Exp Biol 2013;216(Pt 22):4290–8.
16. LeBas NR, Marshall NJ. The role of colour in signaling and male choice in the agamid lizard *Ctenophorus ornatus*. Proc Biol Sci 2000;267(1442):445–52.
17. Brumm H, Zollinger SA. Vocal plasticity in a reptile. Proc Biol Sci 2017;284(1855): 20170451.
18. Kaufmann JH. Stomping for earthworms by wood turtles, *Clemmys insculpta*: a newly discovered foraging technique. Copeia 1986;1986(4):1001–4.
19. Itescu Y, Schwarz R, Meiri S, et al. Intraspecific competition, not predation, drives lizard tail loss on islands. J Anim Ecol 2017;86(1):66–74.
20. Mayer J, Knoll J, Wrubel KM, et al. Chapter 3: reptile behavior. In: Bradley T, Lightfoot T, Mayer J, editors. Exotic pet behavior. Saint-Louis (MO): Elsevier; 2006. p. 103–62.
21. Gehrmann WH. Reptile lighting: a current perspective. Vivarium 1997;8(2):44–5.
22. Stoehr AM, McGraw K. Ultraviolet reflectance of color patches in male *Sceloporus undulatus* and *Anolis carolinensis*. J Herpetol 2001;35(1):168–71.
23. Edgehouse M, Latta LCt, Brodie ED 3rd, et al. Interspecific aggression and habitat partitioning in garter snakes. PLoS One 2014;9(1):e86208.
24. Brashears JA, Fokidis HB, DeNardo DF. Fear-based aggression and its relationship to corticosterone responsiveness in three species of python. Gen Comp Endocrinol 2019;289:113374.

25. Schoralkova T, Kratochvil L, Kubicka L. Female sexual attractiveness and sex recognition in leopard gecko: males are indiscriminate courters. Horm Behav 2018;99:57–61.

26. Sasa M, Curtis S. Field observations of mating behavior in the neck-banded snake *Scaphiodontophis annulatus* (Serpentes: Colubridae). Rev Biol Trop 2006;54(2):647–50.

27. Trnik M, Albrechtova J, Kratochvil L. Persistent effect of incubation temperature on stress-induced behavior in the Yucatan banded gecko (*Coleonyx elegans*). J Comp Psychol 2011;125(1):22–30.

28. Boyer T. Chapter 135: Differential diagnoses by clinical signs - Chelonians. In: Divers SJ, Stahl SJ, editors. Reptile and Amphibian medicine and surgery. Saint Louis (MO): Elsevier; 2019. p. 90–9.

29. Rose MP, Williams DL. Neurologic dysfunction in a ball python (*Python regius*) colour morph and implications for welfare. J Exot Pet Med 2014;23(3):234–9.

30. Hedley J, Eatwell K. Non-venomous colubrid snakes. In: Yeates J, editor. Companion animal care and welfare. Oxford (UK): UFAW, Wiley-Blackwell; 2019. p. 412–24.

31. James LE, Williams CJ, Bertelsen MF, et al. Evaluation of feeding behavior as an indicator of pain in snakes. J Zoo Wildl Med 2017;48(1):196–9.

32. Duncan A. Chapter 32: Reptile and Amphibian Analgesia. In: Miller RE, Fowler ME, editors. Fowler's zoo and wild animal medicine. 7th edition. Saint-Louis (MO): W.B. Saunders; 2012. p. 247–53.

33. Treede RD. The International Association for the Study of Pain definition of pain: as valid in 2018 as in 1979, but in need of regularly updated footnotes. Pain Rep 2018;3(2):e643.

34. Sladky KK. Analgesia. In: Mader DR, Divers SJ, editors. Current therapy in reptile medicine and surgery. Saint-Louis (MO): WB Saunders; 2014. p. 217–28.

35. Mosley C. Pain and nociception in reptiles. Vet Clin North Am Exot Anim Pract 2011;14(1):45–60.

36. Mosley C. Reptile-specific considerations. In: Muir WM, editor. Handbook of veterinary pain management. 3rd edition. Saint-Louis (MO): Elsevier; 2015. p. 555–66.

37. Desmarchelier M. Chapter 14 – A systematic approach in diagnosing behavior problems. In: Miller RE, Lamberski N, Calle PP, editors. Fowler's zoo and wild animal medicine current therapy. 9th edition. Saint-Louis (MO): Elsevier - Health Sciences Division; 2018. p. 76–91.

38. Flores D, Tousignant A, Crews D. Incubation temperature affects the behavior of adult leopard geckos (*Eublepharis macularius*). Physiol Behav 1994;55:1067–72.

39. Torrini L. Training snakes to voluntarily relocate. IAABC J 2019. Available at: https://spring2019.iaabcjournal.org/training-snakes-to-voluntarily-relocate/?fbclid=IwAR1ZxBDENYAZTOjlkwQIoeJzTRm5N_AAZgnHT9R6xqOh7iuo2AE0U7trMuk.

40. Hellmuth H, Augustine L, Watkins B, et al. Using operant conditioning and desensitization to facilitate veterinary care with captive reptiles. Vet Clin North Am Exot Anim Pract 2012;15(3):425–43.

41. Friedrichs KR, Harr KE, Freeman KP, et al. ASVCP reference interval guidelines: determination of de novo reference intervals in veterinary species and other related topics. Vet Clin Pathol 2012;41(4):441–53.

42. Skurski ML, Fleming GJ, Daneault A, et al. Behavioral training and enrichment of reptiles. In: Divers SJ, Stahl SJ, editors. Reptile and Amphibian medicine and surgery. Saint-Louis (MO): Elsevier - Health Sciences Division; 2018. p. 100–4.

43. Kanghae H, Thongprajukaew K, Jatupornpitukchat S, et al. Optimal-rearing density for head-starting green turtles (*Chelonia mydas* Linnaeus, 1758). Zoo Biol 2016;35(5):454–61.
44. Hunt CJG. Stress and Welfare. In: Divers SJ, Stahl SJ, editors. Reptile and amphibian medicine and surgery. Saint-Louis (MO): Elsevier - Health Sciences Division; 2018. p. 105–8.
45. Larson ET, Summers CH. Serotonin reverses dominant social status. Behav Brain Res 2001;121(1–2):95–102.
46. Deckel AW, Fuqua L. Effects of serotonergic drugs on lateralized aggression and aggressive displays in *Anolis carolinensis*. Behav Brain Res 1998;95(2):227–32.
47. Gollnski A, Kubicka L, John-Alder H, et al. Elevated testosterone is required for male copulatory behavior and aggression in Madagascar ground gecko (*Paroedura picta*). Gen Comp Endocrinol 2014;205:133–41.
48. Lock B, Bennett A. Changes in plasma testosterone and aggressive behavior in male green iguanas (*Iguana iguana*) following orchiectomy. J Herp Med Surg 2015;25:107–15.
49. Moore MC. Castration affects territorial and sexual behavior of free-living male lizards, *Sceloporus jarrovi*. Anim Behav 1987;35:1193–9.
50. Lock BA. Reproductive surgery in reptiles. Vet Clin North Am Exot Anim Pract 2000;3(3):733–52.
51. Innis CJ, Feinsod R, Hanlon J, et al. Coelioscopic orchiectomy can be effectively and safely accomplished in chelonians. Vet Rec 2013;172(20):526.
52. Kneidinger N, Knotek Z, Möstel E. Suppression of reproductive activity in green iguana females (*Iguana iguana*) caused by deslorelin implant. Paper presented at: Proceedings of the 7th EVSSAR Congress, May 14-15, 2010; Louvain-la-Neuve, Belgique.
53. Rowland MN. Use of a deslorelin implant to control aggression in a male bearded dragon (*Pogona vitticeps*). Vet Rec 2011;169(5):127.
54. Potier R, Monge E, Loucachevsky T, et al. Effects of deslorelin acetate on plasma testosterone concentrations in captive yellow-bellied sliders (*Trachemys scripta* sp.). Acta Vet Hung 2017;65:440–5.

Amphibian Behavior for the Exotic Pet Practitioner

Shannon T. Ferrell, DVM, DABVP (Avian), DACZM

KEYWORDS

- Amphibian • Behavior • Welfare • Captivity • Stress

KEY POINTS

- Evaluation of amphibian welfare is in its infancy due to numerous factors, but a lack of validated criteria is the most significant.
- Amphibian pain perception is a controversial subject and currently does not have regulatory or standard-of-care support for its implementation.
- Knowledge of the natural history of a species is crucial to proper management and will usually improve the health and welfare of any amphibian patient.
- Indirect and direct objective methods exist for measuring stress in amphibians.
- Relatively small environmental stressors can modify normal amphibian behavior with subtle, yet significant, impacts on reproduction and longevity in wild populations.

INTRODUCTION

There are 3 orders of amphibians: Anura (frogs), Caudata (salamanders), and Gymnophiona (caecilians). Approximately 8100 amphibian species have been identified, with the vast majority (7200 species) being frogs and toads. Together, newts, salamanders, and caecilians represent about 900 distinct species.[1] These facts are noted to highlight the incredible challenges in trying to provide any succinct and useful summary of behavioral repertoires in amphibians due to the complex differences in anatomy, physiology, and environment among this class. This review briefly examines the more salient facets of amphibian welfare, pain, and clinical behavior for the veterinary practitioner.

WELFARE

Before a specific examination of clinically relevant amphibian behaviors, a brief discussion of welfare is warranted, as this issue has a potentially large bearing on problematic behaviors for any animal. The definition of animal welfare currently used by the Association of Zoos & Aquariums (AZA) is that welfare refers to an animal's collective physical,

Zoo de Granby, 525, rue Saint-Hubert, Granby, Quebec J2G 5P3, Canada
E-mail address: sferrell@zoodegranby.com

Vet Clin Exot Anim 24 (2021) 197–210
https://doi.org/10.1016/j.cvex.2020.09.009
1094-9194/21/© 2020 Elsevier Inc. All rights reserved.

vetexotic.theclinics.com

mental, and emotional states over a period of time, and it is measured on a continuum from good to poor.[2] Unfortunately, assessment tools for amphibian and even reptile welfare are in their infancy. This realization is surprising given the long history of amphibian use in research and laboratory diagnostic settings.[3] A partial explanation for this discrepancy, at least in the United States, might be the intentional exclusion of ectotherms, farm animals, and some laboratory mammals from the federal regulatory requirements in the Animal Welfare Act.[4] To address this disparity, numerous groups such as the Detroit Zoo and the Zoologic Society of London (ZSL) have started to evaluate criteria for doing a welfare assessment and then attempting to validate these criteria. However, a recent workshop on this topic hosted by the ZSL found significant challenges to developing reliable and useful assessment tools for amphibians: diverse number of species kept in captivity with complex life stages, a lack of generally applicable husbandry and care guidelines, lack of communication and sharing in the research community about amphibian welfare, and a lack of viable and validated criteria of welfare in any amphibian species.[3] There is certainly a growing interest in responsible and humane care of captive animals, especially those used in a research or diagnostic setting, and the development of tools in this area would also be of benefit to the veterinary clinician in properly assessing amphibian health with clients.

For decades, the management of reptiles, and most likely amphibians, interpreted "…signs of 'good feeding', 'good bodyweight' and 'active reproduction' as positive indicators of welfare.[5] However, in isolation, these signs are poor indicators of welfare and may be highly misleading, and the presence of some "positive" signs does not override any concurrent negative health or welfare signs. Using the "Five Freedoms", developed in 1965, one can assess the conditions that animals should experience when under human control: freedom from hunger, malnutrition, and thirst; freedom from fear and distress; freedom from heat stress or physical discomfort; freedom from pain, injury, and disease; and freedom to express normal patterns of behavior.[6]

Pain

The subject of pain and analgesia has been a relatively contentious subject in ectotherms, which is surprising as most of the early research in neuroanatomy and neurophysiology was done in amphibians. Briefly, the nociceptive afferent pathways are present in amphibians as in other vertebrates, but due to the lack of cerebral and limbic cortices in amphibians, the perception of pain might be significantly different from mammals.[7] Recently, the National Institutes of Health included phrasing in their *Guidelines for Egg and Oocyte Harvesting in Xenopus Species* that analgesia could be provided in postoperative period, but that there was a paucity of well-researched analgesics for this amphibian species. Their use was considered discretionary.[8]

Most clinicians in academic facilities, zoologic institutions, and clinical practice routinely advocate the use of analgesics in amphibians if a potentially noxious procedure will be performed. Numerous reviews on this topic are available.[7]

Enrichment

Improving animal welfare through enrichment is a well-known concept; however, its application to amphibians is not well researched.[9] Concerns exist for a strong bias effect toward mammalian enrichment and a lack of criteria for measuring enhancements in welfare as mentioned earlier. In amphibians, the small number of enrichment studies, focusing primarily on *Xenopus* spp., has demonstrated that simple enrichment practices can reduce mortality and injury, improve growth rates and body conditions, and possibly prevent common diseases of captivity such as metabolic bone disease.[9] Finally, captive environments can select for less-fit progeny, with subsequent generations being less adaptable and less likely to survive in a natural environment or exposure to significant stressors (disease introduction, etc.). This lack of fitness can have profound deleterious effects on the genetic health of a captive population used for breeding and/or conservation. Enrichment practices in amphibians can help select for more robust animals and aid in breeding selection/management, having the potential to influence the fitness of future generations through both epigenetic and genetic effects.[9]

NATURAL HISTORY AND BEHAVIOR

Many times, medical problems in amphibians may seem to be solely a medical issue, but the underlying problem is inappropriate husbandry. Knowledge of the natural history of a species is crucial to proper management and will usually improve the health and welfare of any amphibian patient. As an example, the Panamanian golden frog (*Atelopus zeteki*) inhabits the Cordilleran cloud forests of west-central Panama. The temperature threshold of this species is a narrow 68 to 75°F (20–26°C) with exposure to temperatures outside of this range resulting in rapid morbidity and probable mortality.[10] As these animals are subjected to heat stress, they will congregate in the cooler regions in an enclosure and hide to escape the heat. Excessive hiding is not a typical behavior for this species and is an example of behavior signaling an underlying stressor. In addition, although salamanders and newts might seem similar and are classified under the family Salamandridae, there are many fundamental differences. The most important being that newts are almost exclusively aquatic, whereas salamanders can be aquatic, semiaquatic, or terrestrial.[11] Provision of the correct environment is imperative if the animal is to survive, and deficiencies in this area can result in aberrant, seemingly relentless searching behavior in the enclosure as the animal attempts to find the appropriate habitat.

PHYSIOLOGY AND BEHAVIOR IN AMPHIBIANS
Maintenance

Amphibians produce many physiologic behaviors related to routine maintenance, survival during environmental extremes, communication, and reproduction. A few of the more pertinent examples in each topic area will be explored, as they might be clinically relevant for the clinical veterinarian. For maintenance, many amphibians will shed their skin on a regular basis (intermoult interval from days to weeks) and then ingest the shed, which is considered a normal skin renewal process.[12] In addition, some species such as the waxy monkey frog (*Phyllomedusa sauvagii*) will also secrete a waxy substance from around the neck and then rubs this product all over its body to prevent dessication.[13] Retained sheds or loss of protective coatings strongly indicate something aberrant in the maintenance physiology for the animal and prompt further investigation into nutrition and environmental parameters. For personnel accustomed to working with other vertebrates, it is important to recall that amphibians obtain most of their fluid intake from cutaneous absorption and do not ingest water. In anurans, frogs will commonly place their caudoventral pelvis in a shallow basin of water and absorb water and electrolytes across a highly vascularized skin region known as "the drinking patch."[14]

Adaptation to Environmental Extremes

Even though the typical amphibian in a veterinary setting might not be subjected to obvious environmental extremes, the behavioral responses to environmental stressors should be briefly reviewed as animals might be accidently subjected to extreme conditions in captivity and yet still be alive. As environments alter drastically during seasons, amphibians might enter into estivation or hibernation. During cold periods with freezing, aquatic amphibians will bury themselves in mud or the bottom of a pond with simultaneous drops in metabolism, the use of transcutaneous gas exchanges, and the consumption of fat stores.[15] Terrestrial amphibians can bury themselves 1 to 3 feet below the freeze line in the soil to enter hibernation without the danger of freezing. However, some species such as the North American Wood Frog (*Rana sylvatica*) will only move into the superficial soil layers or even just leaf litter and allow itself to freeze. The animal will produce copious amounts of intracellular urea and glucose to increase cellular osmolarity to prevent cellular freezing; however, the extracellular water will freeze. Heart and respiratory function cease, and the animal will appear physically frozen. The species can even tolerate multiple freeze/thaw cycles. During spring, the reversal of this physiologic stasis ensues, but is still not fully understood.[16]

Similar to hibernation, but occurring during periods of prolonged heat and/or drought, is the process of estivation. Amphibians will burrow into the soil, secrete a mucus covering around their body, enter hypometabolism, and allow their serum osmolarity to increase up to around 487 mOsm/kg.[17] Similar to hibernation, some species will increase the production of intracellular urea to aid in water retention and absorption from the environment. The African clawed frog (*Xenopus laevis*) will tolerate dehydration up to 30% of total body water, and the duration of estivation has been documented up to 15 months in the cocooning frog (*Cyclorana platycephala*).[17,18]

Light

Light cycles are important for amphibians who must feed and reproduce, while avoiding predation.[15] Hunting success is likely to reflect both availability of prey and the ability to detect prey, both of which may be influenced by lunar light. Amphibians identify prey by primarily visual means and can do so at very low light intensities. Salamanders hunt at night to avoid predators, and one study demonstrated that exposure to excessive levels of light at night decreased their foraging activity.[19] Furthermore, tree frogs will decrease mating calls when exposed to artificial lights affecting reproductive success.[20] Finally, constant low levels of artificial light in a laboratory setting delayed metamorphosis in *X laevis* and resulted in fewer adults.[21]

Stress

Amphibian stress is regulated by the glucocorticoid, corticosterone (CTC).[22] CTC is involved in gluconeogenesis, regulation of ion and water balance, immune function, reproduction, and normal development.[23] Corticosterone also plays a substantial role in metamorphosis, increasing during late development, with peak levels developing toward the end of the process.[24] Acidic water, confinement, food deprivation, and crowding have resulted in elevated CTC in amphibian larvae.[22,25] Habitat fragmentation and pollution have caused similar CTC increases in adult amphibians.[22] Effects of some pollutants are not always straightforward as seen in experiments in tadpoles in which the herbicide atrazine, a proposed endocrine disruptor, seemed to dysregulate the production of CTC with likely significant effects on immunity, neurogenesis, and health.[26] Finally, exposure to population-limiting diseases such as *Batrachochytrium dendrobatidis* (Bd) also results in significant CTC levels. However, the long-term implications are difficult to predict, as much of the reported problems in growth associated with Bd infections do not seem to directly relate to the elevations in CTC. The direct effects of the pathogen are responsible for the induced morbidity and not the chronic immunosuppression from prolonged CTC secretion.[22]

Experimental application of CTC to larval tree frogs did increase the incidence of trematode infection, indicating the role of glucocorticoids in immunosuppression and subsequent reduced resistance to infection.[25] As expected, the level of stress, its duration, and the adaptive strategies of the animal influence the resulting effects on animal health (ie, sickness, interruption of normal behavior, etc.). As an example, exposure to stressors would usually interfere with successful reproduction, but species adapted to extreme environmental conditions with limited breeding seasons do not suppress with stress as seen in spotted salamanders (*Ambystoma maculatum*).[27]

Reproduction

In talking about reproductive physiology, it is important to recall the axiom that hormones influence behavior, but behavior also influences hormones through negative or positive feedback. In males, androgens, specifically testosterone and dihydrotestosterone, induce several anatomic changes related to production such as larger larynges, innervation, specific muscle development related to calling, and clasping females for reproduction.[28] In addition, androgens have a significant activating effect on male calling as well, which is the well-studied behavioral effect of these hormones. Interestingly, arginine vasotocin (AVT) is involved in reproductive behaviors in both anurans and salamanders. In salamanders, AVT facilitates amplexus, whereas in frog experiments, AVT stimulates courtship calling and aggression and also affects call patterns, call duration, and the use of multiple call types.[28]

In female American toads (*Bufo americanus*), a variety of peptide or steroid hormones, such as human chorionic gonadotropin (HCG) or prostaglandin, will stimulate a female to approach a conspecific mate signal. However, although estrogen and progesterone administration can induce receptivity in *Xenopus* females, maximal receptivity requires HCG administration.[28]

Finally, amphibians are either oviparous (laying eggs that mature outside the female), which is very common in frogs and toads, or viviparous (eggs mature inside the female with the embryo leaving the female after development).[15,29] There are no concrete delineations among the 3 orders of amphibians as to which aforementioned reproductive strategy is used and must be verified by examining the natural history of the species. In addition, variations within each strategy can exist such as the incubation of the larvae within the stomach of the female in the now extinct gastric brooding frogs (*Rheobatrachus* spp.) or the full maturation of larvae within the vocal sacs of the male Darwin's frog (*Rhinoderma* spp.).[30] Fertilization can be internal or external, depending on the species.[15]

Special Senses

Orientation within the environment is a useful skill for hunting, avoiding predation, and finding potential mates. Amphibians have a variety of adaptations to accomplish these tasks in their diverse habitats. Often unrecognized in importance, olfaction plays an important role in the identification of specific animals, familial relations, and suitable mates.[31] Chemical cues are used to recognize and choose habitat, denote a territory, and evaluate a location for ovipositioning. Amphibians are also capable of using celestial cues from star positions, have a time sense of day, and might be capable of detecting magnetic waves.[15]

BEHAVIOR AND CLINICAL PROBLEMS IN AMPHIBIANS

Although not often exhibiting typical mammalian behavioral problems such as separation anxiety, aberrant fear responses, inappropriate elimination, etc., amphibians can display many behaviors that might warrant further investigation. It is essential to highlight that aberrant behaviors in amphibians will likely have a medical condition as the underlying cause compared with other species due to the lack of brain complexity. This apparent fact would then make a diagnostic investigation (thorough medical history, examination, water quality, etc.) of paramount importance.[32,33] Common behavioral problems in amphibians include the following: anorexia, nasal rubbing, excessive activity/lethargy, aggression, cannibalism, and poor reproductive success.[32–35] This list is not exhaustive, but represents easily observed problems that are evident to owners or caregivers and would prompt consultation with a veterinarian.

Anorexia

Anorexia in amphibians can be a diagnostic challenge to ascertain the exact cause. In most endotherms provided the absolute minimum husbandry requirements, anorexia will usually indicate an underlying medical issue, unless the animal is significantly stressed. The following discussion explores reasons for anorexia in amphibians that are not related to a medical disease. The first step should be to determine if anorexia might be an appropriate response for the life stage of animal. Research into the natural history of species will help elicit if the anorexia might be a normal seasonal physiologic response related to environmental cues.[33] For example, amphibians engaged in reproduction might stop eating during mating. In amphibians, many times the anorexia is usually brought about by subtle, irritating, suboptimal environmental parameters such as excessive lighting, noise, temperature, etc. causing chronic stress.[36] In addition, the size of prey can induce anorexia if the animal is not capable of ingesting a prey item.[37] It is imperative to note that amphibians, especially terrestrial anurans, are visual hunters, and unmoving, dead prey items in their visual field will not be identified as food.[14] However, some aquatic species will eat inert prey items using olfaction. Of course, animals suffering from visual deficits such as corneal dystrophies or cataracts will be functionally blind and stop eating.[37] After evaluating the natural history of the animal, its environment, and the food and its presentation, a typical diagnostic regimen can be performed to elucidate a medical reason for the anorexia.

Nasal Rubbing

Three responses to stressors are common in any animal: (1) excessive activity to effect evasion, (2) hiding/severe lethargy, as the animal hopes to avoid interaction with the stressor, and (3) direct confrontation with possible aggression. Nasal rubbing can occur in exhibits with either completely opaque walls or within transparent aquaria and is often the result of escape or exploratory behaviors.[33,38] Within aquaria, nasal rubbing might be more related to ectotherms not appreciating a transparent boundary as a functional barrier combined with an excessive level of activity.[5] Usually adjustment of the environment (eg, improved water quality, larger enclosure, provision of appropriate of hiding spaces) will dramatically decrease nasal rubbing.[38] Furthermore, husbandry improvements will often replace the stress responses with more relaxed and appropriate behaviors.

Aggression

Aggression can be considered a normal behavior, but its intensity, focus, and duration can be heightened or inappropriate in captivity due to unwise husbandry selections.[15] For example, popular species such as the Pacman frogs (*Ceratophrys* spp.) are ambush predators and can attack other species in an attempt to eat them even if they might not be a suitable prey item. Other species use aggression as a form of defense against perceived threats such as Jimi's toads (*Rhinella jimi*) who engage in head butting behavior and secretion of parotid gland toxins onto the threat during the head butting.[39] Cannibalism could be considered a form of inappropriate aggression and is frequent in captive solitary species that are abnormally housed in group situations (eg, axolotls).[40] However, cannibalism can appear in the wild with tadpoles in ephemeral pools who rely on rapid development.[15] In wild cane toads (*Rhinella marina*), cannibalism frequency increases as encounter rates between large and small toads increase with low precipitation combined with a simultaneous reduction in alternative prey.[41] During the mating season, male anurans will often engage in territorial combats with wrestling, biting, kicking, and bumping.[15] Even females such as the Trinidadian stream frog (*Mannophryne trinitatis*) will engage in wrestling to gain access to the optimal streams for ovipositioning.[15]

Reproductive Problems

Reproductive problems in amphibians often are multifactorial, as so much of modern husbandry is still in its infancy as to the dietary and environmental requirements for many species.[29] Having said this, sometimes normal reproductive anatomy or behavior is misidentified as problematic. A commonly noted pseudoproblem is the development of "bilateral ulcers" on the forelimbs of breeding male frogs. These "ulcers" are in fact nuptial pads, which are hormonally stimulated mucous glands on the prepollex and the forearms that aid in gripping the female during amplexus.[14,29] Amplexus is a copulatory embrace in frogs and toads that can sometimes be mistaken for aggression if not witnessed before by a caregiver. There are generally 2 forms: inguinal with the male grasping the female around the waist and axillary with the male grasping the female closer to the axilla.[15] The behavioral objective is that the female will chose the optimal site for ovipositioning and that the male will be ready for immediate fertilization by semen distribution over the ova as they leave the cloaca. Amplexus can vary from a short period such as 11 minutes in the territorial olive frog (*Babina adenopleura*) to several weeks with species such as the Panamanian golden frog (*A zeteki*).[10,42] Nonamplexed male frogs will often try to displace an amplexed male from a female, and large groups of males can aggregate around a single female as a form of classic scramble competition creating a large mound of frogs.[15] Males in the midst of this frenzy will also attempt to amplex with inanimate objects.

Not all amphibian species use amplexus with some simply depositing semen over the ova after the departure of the female.[15] Salamanders will do the opposite, with the males placing a sperm packet called a spermatophore on a substrate in the water. The male will entice a female to the location who will then recover the sperm, internalize the packet in her cloaca, and store the sperm for future fertilization. The males engage in tail wagging and sometimes an elaborate dance to attract the females. The females will perform a reciprocal dance to indicate her interest.[29] The dance and the spermatophore can seem aberrant and represent potential pseudoproblems if the caregiver does not understand the ritual and the appearance of the spermatophore.

Egg care varies greatly in amphibians from none to near complete parental management of larvae with direct care. Two examples of direct parental care are the following: (1) dart frogs will carry the tadpoles to bromeliads and then lay nonfertile eggs for them to eat in a water trap in the plant or (2) the parent carrying the larvae during development (ie, eggs and tadpoles mature on the back of the Surinam toad, *Pipa pipa*).[15,29] The appearance of the gravid Surinam toad is remarkable and could appear to be a pathogenic cutaneous infection if not fully understood. Finally, amphibian larvae will often demonstrate aggregation behavior, as it improves the chances for foraging, appropriate thermoregulation, and antipredator defense.[15] These improvements will speed larval development especially in ephemeral environments.

Problems in reproduction can easily be related to issues in environmental quality in amphibians. It has been demonstrated that male anurans will attempt to attract mates with their calls in specific locations of a habitat.[40] However, the actual egg deposition sites can be significantly different in terms of water movement, light, seclusion, etc.[15] Therefore, a small aquarium habitat might not be able to provide the optimal sites for induction of calling and/or egg deposition. Separation of these locations spatially and the creation of microhabitats might be needed to successfully reproduce a species. Furthermore, something as fundamental as water temperature can simply shut down female egg laying as seen in bullfrogs who will not deposit their eggs if temperatures exceed 32°C.[43] In contrast to elevated temperatures, species that are late winter/early spring breeders are challenged by the lack of external heat to aid egg maturation. This challenge is overcome by egg deposition in shallow pools that allows for more rapid warming and the communal laying of eggs from several females in large masses that have significant thermal inertia.[44] Obviously, seasonal variations in light, humidity, water quality, and temperature are some of the main drivers of amphibian reproduction and should be researched thoroughly if problems with reproduction are occurring in captive animals to emulate the natural stimuli.[15,29]

Behavior During Clinical Examination

During presentation for a clinical problem, the veterinarian might be challenged by the variety of amphibian behaviors and their meaning, especially during a stressful event such as an examination. Potential clinical signs of amphibian stress, adapted from a welfare assessment for herpetofauna, might be the following: inflation, tail loss—autotomy, abnormal posture, flattening, cloacal evacuations, parotid gland secretions, and vocalizations.[5,34,38] For example, the Namaqua rain frog (Breviceps namaquensis) and the Malagasy rainbow frog (Scaphiophryne gottlebei) are reported to inflate themselves in front of a predator. Examination of the animal after inflation is often more difficult, as palpation can be obstructed with so much distention so care should be taken to be gentle, but efficient.[13] The Kihansi spray toad (Nectophrynoides asperginis) will feign death to avoid predation and demonstrate this behavior when stressed.[45] Somewhat related to cloacal evacuations is bladder voiding, which is exceedingly frequent and of a high volume during any amphibian restraint.[31] It is important to realize the bladder volume can represent a large proportion of the body weight, and fluctuations in weight might be simply related to weighing an animal before or after a bladder voiding event.[13]

Color changes might also occur but can be affected by light levels, color background, and stress such as in tree frogs (Hyla spp).[46] It has been determined that the catecholamines regulate rapid pigment change (within 5 minutes) in stony creek frogs.[47] In addition to color changes, tails are often used as a method of self-defense against predators. Salamanders will detach their tail before a predator, and as the tail continues to move even after detachment, the salamander will evade the predator or "play dead" to avoid attracting the predator.[15] Tiger salamanders (Ambystoma tigrinum) secrete toxin from pores onto their dorsum, arch their body, and then wave the tail to sling secretions onto the predator.[31] Many toads will also secrete a white substance from the cutaneous parotid glands, located on each side of the head, when stressed. The chemical composition of these bioactive secretions (bufotenins, bufalins, and bufotoxins) are typically bitter to the taste, sometimes capable of eliciting significant effects on cardiac activity, and can induce hallucinations and/or euphoria in humans who have ingested the secretions.[48]

Welfare and Behavior Diagnostics

After noting the type, frequency, and intensity of aberrant behaviors, an objective analysis should be performed to concretely define the behavior and its relation to external stimuli (environment, other animals, etc.). The basis of clinical behavior science is the ethogram, which is a list of species-specific behaviors describing the elements and function of each behavior.[49] Scheduled observations with a defined frequency and duration are done to help provide data about all behaviors and can be analyzed to see if one can detect potential causes for the problematic behavior. In reality, the task is relatively simple and requires patience and diligence on the part of the caregiver.

Actual small-scale behavioral studies with simple ethograms can be performed to improve amphibian welfare. One study using undergraduate students tested the hypotheses that enclosure design and complexity would affect both the extent of behavioral repertoires demonstrated and the overall activity levels in poison dart frogs (Dendrobates spp.). The study did demonstrate significant differences in frog activity levels and behavioral repertoires between the different enclosure types. Furthermore, as an additional benefit, the investigators commented that more active frogs would also enhance visitor experience, as the animals were more visible and not always hiding.[50]

Objective means to evaluate stress is always considered optimal when assessing animal welfare to reduce subjective opinion and bias. In amphibians, a slowly growing body of research is attempting to find noninvasive, but reliable, means to consistently evaluate the effects of certain stimuli (noise, light, chemical pollution, etc.) on animal health and welfare. As mentioned earlier, CTC is the stress hormone for amphibians and can be directly measured via numerous methods.[23] Researchers have detected CTC in urine via an enzyme immunoassay in both captive and wild amphibian populations, which was accomplished by collection of the urine doing routine handling when the animal voids.[23] One study evaluating the effects of road noise on wild frogs in Europe measured CTC in the saliva, and finally, skin swabs of captive frogs have been shown to contain a significant amount of CTC which could be useful in monitoring stress.[51,52] Similar to the skin swab study, CTC was also measured in wild and captive amphibians via assessing the CTC concentrations in a defined quantity of water surrounding amphibians who were in a water-filled container.[53,54] As immunosuppression is commonly linked to stress and high levels of glucocorticoids, the use of immune function tests should provide an indirect means to assess the global level of stress that an animal is experiencing. The phytohaemagglutinin (PHA) skin test is often performed as an assay of immuncompetence, involving the measurement of a cell-mediated immune response through the injection of an inflammatory protein into the skin or webbing. The resultant swelling is measured within 24 hours. The assay is preferred by wildlife biologists, as it is rapid, noninvasive, requires little equipment, and inexpensive.[55] The test has been used extensively in birds and is now being validated for frog species. Other indirect methods of assessing stress are elevations in the neutrophil/lymphocyte ratio, which entails having some reference ranges for the species and the measurement of immunoglobin X (IgX).[56] In mammals, diminution in secretory IgA, especially salivary, is associated with chronic stressors and increased susceptibility to infection. IgX is suspected to be a functional analogue of mammalian IgA in amphibians. Measurement of IgX in secretory fluids such as saliva or other secretions might afford a window into the stress levels in amphibians through the functional state of the immune system.[57]

Behavior Influencing Conservation

Amphibian conservation efforts commonly focus on the detrimental environmental factors causing direct physical injury or harm to wild populations and the possibility of using captive reproduction to augment wild populations. The morbidity and mortality effects of trauma and exposure to toxic compounds are obvious and easy to comprehend. More subtle, and yet significant, are the effects of smaller environmental factors that could affect behavior, influencing survival and/or reproduction. For example, light pollution, as mentioned earlier, can affect hunting, mate calling, and metamorphosis, whereas sound pollution has been linked to changes of coloration of the vocal sacs of optimal breeding males.[51,58] The latter would in turn decrease reproductive fitness of the affected males. Mitigation efforts to control light and noise pollution might have significant impacts in augmenting wild amphibian populations.

As stress increases in amphibians, many terrestrial species will spend increased time in water or humid environments as an attempt to avoid the underlying stressor, especially drought. As many population-limiting diseases, such as chytridiomycosis and ranavirus, are more easily transmitted by water, the increased additional periods in the focal bodies of water might make many terrestrial amphibians more likely to acquire an infection.[59] Thus, environmental stressors can simply modify normal behavior with potentially fatal consequences. Interestingly, studies have used evaluation of the neutrophil/lymphocyte (N/L) ratio to monitor the stress response in wild and domestic amphibians. In the frog (*Lithobates sphenocephalus*), there was no difference with baseline and stress episode sampling of the (N/L) ratio between wild and domestic specimens.[56] In salamanders (*Ambystoma opacum*), the magnitude of the stress response was similar between wild and captive animals, but the baseline N/L ratios were higher in captive salamanders due to some possible underlying issue such as elevated stocking density, which leads to cannibalism.

Many conservation programs in zoos and government programs focus on captive reproduction with the eventual goal of releasing progeny to augment wild populations. An important underlying reflection is whether captive-raised amphibian larvae reared in relatively stress-free environments will exhibit appropriate behaviors for normal activities such as feeding and also respond suitably to predation stress.[60] Captive-bred *Rana pipiens* metamorphs exhibited abnormal movement behavior after release, which could affect their ability to locate food sources when compared with native *R pipiens* in the same area.[61] Tadpoles, produced in a typical laboratory setting, have a higher likelihood of predation, and metamorphs are more susceptible to moving in a haphazard direction from a lack of familiarity with normal light cycles and the Y-axis orientation in nature.[60] The conclusions reached are that animal populations rapidly adapt to captivity, and captive breeding programs should recognize this problem. Prerelease training in amphibians is likely an important factor for improving survival.[62] Finally, as a positive behavior to assist in captive reproduction, studies have shown that anurans are capable of kin recognition, which should assist somewhat in the prevention of inbreeding.[63]

SUMMARY

Amphibian welfare and behavioral medicine are challenging areas for the veterinary and research communities. This class of animals has been a literal backbone of medical and scientific advancement for hundreds of years; however, the provision of evidence-based guidelines to support their welfare and care has not been of the same speed or quality. Recent research efforts highlight that subtle changes in the environment can have significant impacts on amphibian health through alterations in behavior, and it is imperative to address these issues to improve both individual animal and population welfare.

DISCLOSURE

The author has nothing to disclose.

REFERENCES

1. Amphibiaweb. Species By the Numbers. Available at: www.amphibiaweb.com. Accessed January 28, 2020.
2. Animal Welfare Committee. Available at: https://www.aza.org/animal_welfare_committee. Accessed January 28, 2020.
3. Brod S, Brookes L, Garner TWJ. Discussing the future of amphibians in research. Lab Anim 2019;48(1):16–8.
4. Bradfield JF, Bennett BT, Gillett CS. Oversight of research animal welfare in the United States. In: Guillén J, editor. Laboratory animals. 2nd edition. Cambridge (MA): Elsevier; 2018. p. 15–68.
5. Warwick C, Arena P, Lindley S, et al. Assessing reptile welfare using behavioural criteria. In Pract 2013;35(3):123–31.
6. Mäekivi N. Freedom in captivity: managing zoo animals according to the 'five freedoms. Biosemiotics 2018;11(1):7–25.
7. Stevens CW. Analgesia in amphibians: preclinical studies and clinical applications. Vet Clin North Am Exot Anim Pract 2011;14(1):33–44.
8. Animal Research Advisory Committee Guidelines | OACU. Available at: https://oacu.oir.nih.gov/animal-research-advisory-committee-guidelines.   Accessed February 2, 2020.
9. Michaels CJ, Downie JR, Campbell-Palmer R. The importance of enrichment for advancing amphibian welfare and conservation goals: A review of a neglected topic. Amphib Reptile Conserv 2014;8(1):7–23.
10. Poole V. Husbandry Manual Panamanian Golden frog (Atelopus zeteki). 2006. Available at: http://www.atelopus.com/uploads/pdf/HusbandryManual.pdf. Accessed January 29, 2020.
11. Amphibian Facts. Available at: https://amphibiaweb.org/amphibian/facts.html. Accessed January 29, 2020.
12. Cramp RL, McPhee RK, Meyer EA, et al. First line of defence: the role of sloughing in the regulation of cutaneous microbes in frogs. Conserv Physiol 2014;2(1): cou012.
13. Wright K, Whitaker B. Clinical techniques. In: Wright K, Whitaker B, editors. Amphibian Medicine and Captive Husbandry. Malabar (FL): Krieger; 2001. p. 89–110.
14. Pasmans F, Martel A. 12- Amphibian taxonomy, anatomy, and physiology. In: Divers SJ, Stahl SJ, editors. Mader's Reptile and Amphibian Medicine and Surgery. 3rd edition. St Louis (MO): Elsevier; 2019. p. 86–9.
15. Wells KD. The Ecology & Behavior of Amphibians. Chicago: University of Chicago; 2007.
16. Costanzo JP, Bayuk JM, Lee RE. Inoculative freezing by environmental ice nuclei in the freeze-tolerant wood frog, *Rana sylvatica*. J Exp Zool 1999;284(1):7–14.
17. Cartledge VA, Withers PC, Bradshaw SD. Water balance and arginine vasotocin in the cocooning frog *Cyclorana platycephala* (Hylidae). Physiol Biochem Zool 2008;81(1):43–53.

18. Romspert AP. Osmoregulation of the african clawed frog. *Xenopus laevis*, in hypersaline media. Comp Biochem Physiol A Mol Integr Physiol 1976;54(2):207–10.
19. Rohacek A, Buchanan B, Wise S. The effects of artificial night lighting on the nocturnal activity of the terrestrial red-backed salamander, *Plethodon cinereus*. 24th International Congress for Conservation Biology; Edmonton, Alberta, Canada, July 3-7, 2010.
20. Baker BJ, Richardson JML. The effect of artificial light on male breeding-season behaviour in green frogs, *Rana clamitans melanota*. Can J Zool 2006;84(10): 1528–32.
21. Buchanan B, Wise S, McCarthy T, et al. Effects of artificial night lighting on growth and development in aquatic snails and frog larvae. Symposium: Artificial lights and nature: challenges for dusk-to-dawn conservation management at the 24th International Congress for Conservation Biology; Edmonton, Alberta, Canada, July 3-7, 2010.
22. Searle CL, Belden LK, Du P, et al. Stress and chytridiomycosis: Exogenous exposure to corticosterone does not alter amphibian susceptibility to a fungal pathogen. J Exp Zool A Ecol Genet Physiol 2014;321(5):243–53.
23. Narayan EJ. Non-invasive reproductive and stress endocrinology in amphibian conservation physiology. Conserv Physiol 2013;1(1):cot011.
24. Denver RJ. 7 - neuroendocrinology of amphibian metamorphosis. In: Shi Y-B, editor. Current topics in developmental Biology, vol. 103. Waltham (MA): Elsevier; 2013. p. 195–227.
25. Belden LK, Kiesecker JM. Glucocorticosteroid hormone treatment of larval treefrogs increases infection by *Alaria* sp. trematode cercariae *Parasitology* 2005; 91(3):686–8.
26. McMahon TA, Boughton RK, Martin LB, et al. Exposure to the herbicide atrazine nonlinearly affects tadpole corticosterone levels. J Herpetol 2017;51(2):270–3.
27. Woodley S, Porter B. Handling stress increases expression of male sexual behaviour in an amphibian with an explosive mating strategy. J Zool 2015;298.
28. Wilczynski W, Lynch KS, O'Bryant EL. Current research in amphibians: Studies integrating endocrinology, behavior, and neurobiology. Horm Behav 2005;48(4): 440–50.
29. Whitaker B. Reproduction. In: Wright K, Whitaker B, editors. Amphibian Medicine and Captive Husbandry. Malabar (FL): Krieger; 2001. p. 285–99.
30. Wake MH. Fetal adaptations for viviparity in amphibians. J Morphol 2015;276(8): 941–60.
31. Durso AM, Maerz JC. 13 - Natural behavior. In: Divers SJ, Stahl SJ, editors. Mader's Reptile and Amphibian Medicine and Surgery. 3rd edition. St Louis (MO): Elsevier; 2019. p. 90–9.
32. Yaw T, Clayton L. 137 - Differential diagnoses by clinical signs—amphibians. In: Divers SJ, Stahl SJ, editors. Mader's Reptile and Amphibian Medicine and Surgery. 3rd ediiton. St Louis (MO): Elsevier; 2019. p. 1283–7.
33. Bays TB, Mattos de Souza Dantas L. 83 - Clinical behavioral medicine. In: Divers SJ, Stahl SJ, editors. Mader's Reptile and Amphibian Medicine and Surgery. 3rd edition. St Louis (MO): Elsevier; 2019. p. 922–31.
34. Arena PC, Steedman C, Warwick C. Amphibian and reptile Pet Markets in the EU: an investigation and assessment 2012. p. 1–53. Available at: www.apa.org.uk. Accessed December 15, 2019.
35. Wright K, Whitaker B, editors. Amphibian medicine and captive husbandry. Malabar (FL): Krieger; 2001.

36. Ferrie GM, Alford VC, Atkinson J, et al. Nutrition and health in amphibian husbandry: Ex Situ Amphibian Health and Nutrition. Zoo Biol 2014;33(6):485–501.

37. Hadfield CA, Clayton LA, Barnett SL. Nutritional Support of Amphibians. J Exot Pet Med 2006;15(4):255–63.

38. Clifford Warwick. Psychological and behavioural principles and problems. In: Frye FL, Murphy JB, editors. Health and welfare of captive reptiles. New York: Chapman & Hall; 1995. p. 205–38.

39. Jared C, Antoniazzi MM, Jordão AEC, et al. Parotoid macroglands in toad (*Rhinella jimi*): Their structure and functioning in passive defence. Toxicon 2009;54(3): 197–207.

40. Wright K. Idiopathic syndromes. In: Whitaker B, editor. Amphibian Medicine and Captive Husbandry. Malabar (FL): Krieger; 2001. p. 239–44.

41. Pizzatto L, Shine R. The behavioral ecology of cannibalism in cane toads (Bufo marinus). Behav Ecol Sociobiol 2008;63(1):123–33.

42. Chuang M-F, Bee MA, Kam Y-C. Short amplexus duration in a territorial anuran: a possible adaptation in response to male-male competition. PLoS One 2013;8(12): e83116.

43. Howard RD. The influence of male-defended oviposition sites on early embryo mortality in bullfrogs. Ecology 1978;59(4):789–98.

44. Waldman B, Ryan MJ. Thermal advantages of communal egg mass deposition in wood frogs (*Rana sylvatica*). J Herpetol 1983;17(1):70.

45. CBSG (IUCN/SSC). Kihansi spray toad (Nectophrynoides asperginis) population and habitat Viability assessment: Briefing Book. Bagamoyo (Tanzania): Conservation Breeding Specialist Group; 2007. p. 516. Available at: http://www.amphibianark.org/pdf/Kihansi%20Spray%20Toad%20Briefing%20Book.pdf. Accessed February 1, 2020.

46. King RB, Hauff S, Phillips JB. Physiological color change in the green treefrog: responses to background brightness and temperature. Copeia 1994;1994(2): 422–32.

47. Kindermann C, Narayan EJ, Wild F, et al. The effect of stress and stress hormones on dynamic colour-change in a sexually dichromatic Australian frog. Comp Biochem Physiol A Mol Integr Physiol 2013;165(2):223–7.

48. Meyer K, Linde H. Collection of toad venoms and chemistry of toad venom steroids. In: Bucherl W, Buckley E, editors. Venomous Animals and Their Venoms. New York: Academic Press; 1971. p. 521–56.

49. Watters JV, Margulis SW, Atsalis S. Behavioral monitoring in zoos and aquariums: a tool for guiding husbandry and directing research. Zoo Biol 2009;28(1):35–48.

50. Rose P, Evans C, Coffin R, et al. Using student-centred research to evidence-base exhibition of reptiles and amphibians: three species-specific case studies. J Zoo Aquar Res 2014;2(1):25–32.

51. Troïanowski M, Mondy N, Dumet A, et al. Effects of traffic noise on tree frog stress levels, immunity, and color signaling: Noise Consequences on Tree Frogs. Conserv Biol 2017;31(5):1132–40.

52. Santymire RM, Manjerovic MB, Sacerdote-Velat A. A novel method for the measurement of glucocorticoids in dermal secretions of amphibians. Conserv Physiol 2018;6(1):1–12.

53. Forsburg ZR, Goff CB, Perkins HR, et al. Validation of water-borne cortisol and corticosterone in tadpoles: Recovery rate from an acute stressor, repeatability, and evaluating rearing methods. Gen Comp Endocrinol 2019;281:145–52.

54. Baugh AT, Bastien B, Still MB, et al. Validation of water-borne steroid hormones in a tropical frog (*Physalaemus pustulosus*). Gen Comp Endocrinol 2018;261: 67–80.

55. Brown GP, Shilton CM, Shine R. Measuring amphibian immunocompetence: validation of the phytohemagglutinin skin-swelling assay in the cane toad, *Rhinella marina*. Methods Ecol Evol 2011;2(4):341–8.

56. Davis AK, Maerz JC. Assessing stress levels of captive-reared amphibians with hematological data: implications for conservation initiatives. J Herpetol 2011; 45(1):40–4.

57. Du CC, Mashoof SM, Criscitiello MF. Oral immunization of the African clawed frog (*Xenopus laevis*) upregulates the mucosal immunoglobulin IgX. Vet Immunol Immunopathol 2012;145(1–2):493–8.

58. Touzot M, Lengagne T, Secondi J, et al. Artificial light at night alters the sexual behaviour and fertilisation success of the common toad. Environ Pollut 2020; 259:1–6.

59. Longo A, Burrowes P, Joglar R. Seasonality of *Batrachochytrium dendrobatidis* infection in direct-developing frogs suggests a mechanism for persistence. Dis Aquat Organ 2009;92(3):253–60.

60. Mendelson JR III, Altig R. Tadpoles, froglets, and conservation: A discussion of basic principles of rearing and release procedures. Amphib Reptile Conserv 2016;10(1):20–7.

61. Fraser LD. Distribution characteristics of the eggs, tadpoles, and metamorphs of the Northern Leopard Frog (*Rana pipiens*) and their relation to conservation strategies. Thesis - University of Calgary Calgary, AB; 2008.

62. Griffiths RA, Pavajeau L. Captive breeding, reintroduction, and the conservation of amphibians: *Amphibian Captive Breeding*. Conserv Biol 2008;22(4):852–61.

63. Blaustein AR, Waldman B. Kin recognition in anuran amphibians. Anim Behav 1992;44:207–21.

Fish Behavior for the Exotic Pet Practitioner

Leigh Ann Clayton, DVM, DABVP (Avian, Reptile/Amphibian)[a],*,
Colin McDermott, VMD, CertAqV[b]

KEYWORDS

- Applied behavior analysis • Behavior • Chondrichthyes • Disease • Environment
- Fish • Osteichthyes • Natural history

KEY POINTS

- When evaluating fish behavior, veterinarians can use three models to categorize the possible cause of behavior—natural history (species typical modal action patterns), medical (disease state), and learning experience (classical and operant conditioning).
- Natural history model: The fish may be exhibiting normal, species-appropriate modal action patterns related to natural history. Common behaviors seen in pet fish are related to resource competition, breeding behavior, social interactions, and grooming (parasite removal).
- Medical model: The fish may be exhibiting behaviors in response to a medical condition. It is critical to consider water quality and other environmental factors as part of evaluating disease state. Common signs of disease include color change, pruritus, lethargy, erratic swimming, isolation, fin clamping, and tachypnea or dyspnea. Common causes include parasitic disease (particularly protozoal ectoparasites), buoyancy problems, poor nutritional condition, trauma, neoplasia, ocular changes, and poor water quality.
- Learning model: The fish may be exhibiting a learned behavior. Fish readily learn and this should be taken into account when evaluating fish behavior. Positive reinforcement training can be used to deliberately train behavior in fish. Although uncommon, fish may present for problem behaviors.
- These models are useful for ensuring clinicians take a holistic approach to fish behavior. They are not mutually exclusive and integrate naturally. Models help clinicians formulate appropriate differentials, ensuring they do not exclusively consider disease, particularly in unfamiliar species.

INTRODUCTION

There are over 28,000 species of fish; they are the oldest developed vertebrate and occupy a wide variety of environmental niches.[1] Veterinarians and fish caregivers must use behavior as part of assessing health and welfare. Many fish are housed in

[a] New England Aquarium, 1 Central Wharf, Boston, MA 02110, USA; [b] Zodiac Pet and Exotic Hospital, Shop 101A, 1/F, Victoria Centre, 15 Watson Road, Fortress Hill, Hong Kong
* Corresponding author.
E-mail address: leighannclayton@gmail.com

Vet Clin Exot Anim 24 (2021) 211–227
https://doi.org/10.1016/j.cvex.2020.09.010
1094-9194/21/© 2020 Elsevier Inc. All rights reserved.

groups of the same species, as well as within mixed-species habitats. This adds to the complexity of behavior interpretation. Veterinarians must move readily between individual animal and population management concepts and evaluate behavior not just of an individual animal but of species groups and mixed-species groups when evaluating for possible disease. Appropriately observing and interpreting behavior is a critical component of fish care.

Three behavioral frameworks can be utilized when evaluating fish health—natural history (species typical patterns), medical (disease state), and learning experience (classical and operant conditioning). (Susan Friedman, PhD, personal communication, 2010) All three models can be utilized for both individual animal and group behavior. The natural history model helps categorize behavior based on what might be normal for the species given its environmental niche—what it evolved to do. As with other taxa, fish demonstrate a wide range of typical behavior patterns that allow animals to thrive in specific environmental niches. These "modal action patterns" are important to understand, to provide appropriate habitats and interpret behavior. The medical model helps categorize behavior based on illness or major environmental problems (eg, inappropriate water quality). Understanding what healthy and unhealthy fish generally look like, as well as common differentials for certain behaviors, improves the veterinarian's ability to rapidly develop appropriate diagnostic and management plans across species. The operant conditioning model helps categorize behavior based on what fish might have learned. Although less frequently discussed in veterinary medicine, and even among some experienced caregivers, fish readily learn and learning history should be taken into account when evaluating behavior. As with other animals, fish learn to exhibit behaviors in relation to environmental cues.

These frames are not mutually exclusive, and in fact, integrate naturally. However, distinct frameworks allow veterinarians to rapidly group a broad range of possible etiologies to support holistic, critical thinking about health and welfare.

FISH CARE OVERVIEW

Fish are commonly kept under managed care in a wide variety of settings and for a range of purposes, from amateur casual pet to experienced home hobbyist, to professional public display aquaria, to captive assurance colonies, to intensive aquaculture. This article is primarily directed at veterinarians working with pet or hobbyist caregivers and those working in public display aquaria.

Veterinary fish medicine knowledge is growing, as are concerns for the general health of freshwater and saltwater environments. Climate change is driving rapid changes in water temperatures and water chemistry, and entire ecosystems are being rapidly affected. This is impacting species diversity and location, as well as animal numbers and health. In addition, there is a growing focus on animal welfare and rights, including in fish.[2] As with terrestrial species, veterinarians may find themselves on the forefront of integrating animal welfare practices, conservation needs, and animal-related ethics.

Fish are readily available for purchase in the United States by pet and home hobbyists, as well as public display aquaria, and are commonly available from general pet or specialty stores and local breeders. Compared with common pet mammal species, fish are more likely to be wild-caught, particularly saltwater species.[3] Some wild-caught fish readily adapt to aquaria and show marked resiliency through the major environmental changes associated with transportation and acclimation. However, there are significant species and individual fish differences in response; many fish end up severely stressed and ill. How fish are handled during and after capture impacts their health and welfare. Attentive care is important to ensure newly captured animals are adapting well. Fish caregivers should generally plan to quarantine new fish away from established communities to reduce infectious disease risk and give new fish time to acclimate and recover before integrating into a complex community.

Veterinarians work collaboratively with the client and when developing this relationship, it is critical to understand the motivation for veterinary care, as well as the client's knowledge base. Clients vary widely in their experience and expectations and understanding the client's needs improves the veterinarian's ability to balance a variety of options to reach optimal solutions. The motivation for the pet or hobbyist caregiver to have fish can vary quite a bit and this can impact both the quality of care the fishes receive and the purpose of the veterinary visit. Some examples include learning opportunity for children, enjoyment of individual fish, enjoyment of technical aspects of managing an aquatic system or having hard to find species, breeding animals, commercial ventures, and competition (eg, fish or aquarium shows). Owing to the technical challenges of managing a saltwater system, particularly a saltwater system with corals or other invertebrates, these hobbyists are frequently extremely knowledgeable about the water quality and species natural behavior, as well as potential disease conditions. There is often more variability in freshwater fish caregiver knowledge. Basic freshwater systems are much easier to set up and manage and it is more common for these clients to have limited knowledge.

BEHAVIOR AND NATURAL HISTORY

When evaluating the behavior of any animal, it is crucial to understand the normal or natural behavior pattern for that species. It is always important to consider that the fish may be in good health and displaying normal behavior and to understand normal when evaluating health and welfare concerns. One of the main challenges in evaluating fish behavior is in the reliability of information for a given species. FishBase is an online resource for basic species descriptions and information on 10s of thousands of species, and a starting point for clinicians and hobbyists for evaluating the natural history of a species.[4] There are references related to fish behavior generally and in specific groups and scientific and hobbyist publications can provide helpful information.[5,6]

Common behavioral categories to consider include food acquisition (eg, foraging, hunting, tool use), defense (eg, predator avoidance, cryptic matching, burying), territorial management (eg, hide structure defense, enclosure building), reproduction (eg, territorial, mate attraction, mating, nest building, egg protection), and social interactions (eg, dominance display, cleaner/client fish interactions, shoaling/schooling). Species have a range of standard behavior patterns related to their environmental niche. General behavioral patterns related to social grouping, feeding pattern, breeding behavior, aggression, and position in the water column for common pet fish are outlined in **Table 1** (freshwater) and **Table 2** (saltwater). As with other animals, there are both species and individual animal differences in personality, physiology, sociability, sensory perception, and learning and both individual and species levels should be taken into account when evaluating fish behavior.[2,4,6–15] A short list of specialized sensory abilities that impact basic fish care can be found in **Table 3**.

Fish are often kept in mixed-species groups and it is important to anticipate and integrate the behavioral needs of not only a single species and those individuals, but interactions between species. Common parameters caregivers should consider include the right mix of species and individuals for the system size and life support,

Table 1
Natural behavior patterns of commonly kept freshwater fish

Species	Scientific Name	Social Grouping	Feeding Pattern	Breeding Behavior	Aggression Pattern	Use of Water Column
Neon tetra	*Paracheirodon innesi*	Shoaling	Omnivorous, foraging	Uncommon in captivity	Nonaggressive, timid	Full water column, often upper water column
Black neon tetra	*Hyphessobrycon herbertaxelrodi*	Shoaling	Omnivorous	Egg scatter on plants	Nonaggressive	Upper water column
Cardinal tetra	*Paracheirodon axelrodi*	Shoaling	Carnivorous/ insectivorous	Uncommon in captivity	Nonaggressive	Full water column, often upper water column
Serpae tetra	*Hyphessobrycon serpae*	Shoaling	Omnivorous	Egg scatter, Uncommon in captivity	Nonaggressive, conspecific aggression in larger groups	Mid to upper water column, prefer shade
Ember tetra	*Hyphessobrycon amandae*	Shoaling	Omnivorous	Egg scatter on plants	Nonaggressive	Mid to upper water column
Glowlight tetra	*Hemigrammus erythrozonus*	Shoaling	Omnivorous	Egg scatter, uncommon in captivity	Nonaggressive	Mid to upper water column, prefers shade
Marbled hatchetfish	*Carnegiella strigata*	Shoaling	Omnivore, surface feeding	Egg scatter	Nonaggressive, timid	Upper water column at surface, can jump out of water
Zebra Danio	*Danio rerio*	Shoaling	Omnivorous, feed in water column	Egg scatter, common in captivity	Nonaggressive	Mid to upper water column
Guppy	*Poecilia reticulate*	Shoaling	Insectivorous, surface feeder	Internal fertilization, males chase females	Nonaggressive, male dominance displays	Upper water column, prefers vegetation for cover
Sailfin Molly	*Poecilia latipinna*	Shoaling, loose groupings	Omnivorous, predominantly plant matter	Internal fertilization, livebearers	Generally nonaggressive, male aggression and displays	Upper water column, utilizes hides or plant cover

Variable platy	Xiphophorus variatus	Shoaling, loose groupings	Omnivorous, predominantly plant matter	Internal fertilization, no parental care	Generally nonaggressive, timid, rare conspecific male aggression	Mid to upper water column, utilizes hides or plant cover
Betta fish	Betta splendens	Solitary	Primarily insectivorous, surface feeder	Male constructs bubble nests, male chases away female after breeding, paternal nest guarding	Highly aggressive, threat displays common	Upper water column
Dwarf gourami	Trichogaster lalius	Solitary or pairs	Omnivorous, slow feeder	Male constructs bubble nest, males court females, paternal nest guarding	Nonaggressive, timid	Mid to upper water column
Common pleco	Hypostomus plecostomus	Solitary, but tolerant of others with enough space	Algae eater, omnivorous	Uncommon, breed in caves or nests, paternal care of eggs and nest guarding	Conspecific aggression, aggression with other bottom dwelling fish	Substrate, hidden when not feeding
Bristlenose pleco	Ancistrus spp.	Solitary, but tolerant of conspecifics with enough space	Algae eater, hrbivorous, feed on bottom and tank surfaces	Breed in caves or nests, paternal care of eggs and nest guarding	Males territorial	Substrate, hidden when not feeding
Siamese algae eater	Crossocheilus oblongus	Solitary, can be tolerant of conspecifics	Primary herbivorous, omnivorous with age	Unlikely to breed in captivity	Conspecific aggression or aggression to similar species noted	Substrate or along tank walls
Corydoras catfish	Corydoras spp. (commonly C. aeneus)	Shoaling	Omnivorous, bottom feeder	Brood hider, fixes eggs to substrate	Nonaggressive, will feed on deceased fish	Substrate, uses hides

(continued on next page)

Table 1 (*continued*)

Species	Scientific Name	Social Grouping	Feeding Pattern	Breeding Behavior	Aggression Pattern	Use of Water Column
Tiger barb	*Puntius tetrazona*	Shoaling	Omnivorous	Egg scatter along plants, adults will eat eggs and fry	Semi-aggressive, conspecific aggression, target longer finned fish	Mid water column
Koi	*Cyprinus carpio*	Shoaling	Omnivorous, opportunistic	Common in ponds, egg scatter, males chase after females	Nonaggressive	Mid to upper water column, but can use whole water column
Goldfish (common)	*Carassius auratus*	Social groupings, gregarious	Omnivorous, opportunistic	Common in ponds, egg scatter, males chase females	Nonaggressive	Mid to upper water column, but can use whole water column
Rosy red, fathead minnow	*Pimephales promelas*	Shoaling	Omnivorous, benthic filter feeder	Eggs deposited in nests, paternal care of egg nest, males develop tubercles	Nonaggressive, territorial in smaller social groupings	Substrate or bottom of water column
Electric yellow cichlid	*Labidochromis caeruleus* (color morph)	Conspecific grouping	Omnivorous, opportunistic	Maternal mouthbrooder, eggs laid over sand before fertilization and mouthbrooding	Aggressive to more docile fish	Mid water column, active swimmer, will hide along rocks
Angelfish	*Pterophyllum scalare*	Small groups or male-female pairs	Carnivorous/ insectivorous	Common, eggs deposited along flat horizontal surfaces, mating pair guards nest	Territorial, conspecific and interspecies aggression, long fins commonly bitten	Mid to upper water column, uses plants for cover
Clown loach	*Chromobotia macracanthus*	Loose social grouping	Bottom feeders, omnivorous	Uncommon in captivity	Semi-aggressive, decreased aggression in larger groups	Substrate, hidden when not feeding, shade seeking

Table 2
Natural behavior patterns of commonly kept saltwater fish

Species	Scientific Name	Social Grouping	Feeding Pattern	Breeding Behavior	Aggression Pattern	Use of Water Column
Green chromis	*Chromis viridis*	Shoaling	Omnivorous, feeds in water column and off rocks	Oviparous, paternal nest guarding	Nonaggressive in larger groups, conspecific aggression possible	Shoal in groups around Acropora corals on reefs
Honey red talbot damsel	*Chrysiptera talboti*	Solitary, paired when breeding	Carnivorous, feeds on zooplankton	Oviparous, paternal nest guarding	Conspecific aggression, possibly other damsels	Close to rocks/ decorations along substrate, lower water column
Domino damsel	*Dascyllus trimaculatus*	Aggregates along coral heads/large rocks	Omnivorous	Oviparous, paternal nest guarding	Conspecific aggression in adults, can be aggressive to tank mates	Adults found along reefs, juveniles along small coral heads or anenome
Yellowtail blue damsel	*Chrysiptera parasema*	Small aggregates around coral patches	Omnivorous, feed toward bottom	Oviparous, breeding pairs, paternal nest guarding	Males territorial, minimal aggression to other tank mates	Aggregate around coral heads, feed toward bottom of water column
Ocellaris clownfish	*Amphiprion ocellaris*	Social hierarchy complex, dominant female and male	Omnivorous	Protandrous hermaphrodite, oviparous, paternal nest guarding	Territorial, conspecific aggression	Along reefs in association with anemone
Coral beauty angelfish	*Centropyge bispinosa*	Single or small aggregates	Primary herbivorous, feed on algae	Rare breeding in captivity	Conspecific aggression and with small angelfish	Along reefs, hide in crevices and caves

(continued on next page)

Table 2
(continued)

Species	Scientific Name	Social Grouping	Feeding Pattern	Breeding Behavior	Aggression Pattern	Use of Water Column
Yellow tang	*Zebrasoma flavescens*	Single or loosely associated groups	Primarily herbivorous, feed on algae	Paired spawning or group spawning observed, difficult to breed in captivity	Conspecific aggression, aggression with similar size fish and surgeonfish	Swims along reefs, common along most of the water column
Lyretail anthias	*Pseudanthias squamipinnis*	Shoaling	Carnivorous, feed on zooplankton	Protogynous hermaphrodite, pelagic spawner, breeding activity noted in captivity	Male conspecific aggression, territorial	Found in water column above reefs
Scooter blenny, ocellated dragonet	*Neosynchiropus ocellatus*	Loose aggregates of individuals	Carnivorous, bottom feeder	Breeding possible in captivity	Generally nonaggressive, males more aggressive than females	Found along substrate and rocks along substrate
Sixline wrasse	*Pseudocheilinus hexataenia*	Found in loose social groups	Carnivorous, feeds on small crustaceans, cleaner fish for larger species	Oviparous, distinct male-female paring, not bred in captivity	Conspecific aggression in smaller tanks, aggressive to other wrasses	Found in close association with reefs, rocks.
Firefish	*Nemateleotris magnifica*	Solitary or pairs, monogamous; Juveniles form loose social grouping	Carnivorous, feeds on small invertebrates	Monogamous pairing, breeding behavior noted in captivity	Conspecific aggression in smaller environments	Upper portion of reefs
Diamond sleeper goby, Maiden goby	*Valenciennea puellaris*	Often found in pairs, monogamous	Carnivorous bottom feeder, sand sifter	Monogamous pairing	Generally nonaggressive	Stays along substrate, forms shallow burrows in sand and gravel

Table 3
Major aspects of specialized sensory systems that impact basic fish care

Sensory System	Description	Environmental Considerations
Vision	Sensitivity to visual light, as well as UV and trichromatic light	Proper photoperiod for species. Provide adequate shade/hiding areas for sensitive species. Lighting source.
Olfaction/taste	Olfactory and taste receptors along nasal pits, oral cavity, and along epidermis in many species	Maintain proper water quality. Provide a proper diet.
Lateral Line	Sensitive to vibration and electrical current	Grounded circuits for all electric devices associated with habitat (eg, filtration, lighting). Proper padding along any vibrating filter components, proper padding below tank to absorb vibration from surrounding environment

the type of habitat complexity (eg, substrate, hides, plants, open space) needed to meet a wide range of behavioral needs, and the water chemistry, temperature, and lighting period needs of all species. Fish habitats lend themselves to creating "mini-ecosystems" with different species using various aspects of the enclosure (eg, substrate, different water column levels). Foresight and planning are needed to do this in a manner that optimizes the health, welfare, and longevity of all the fish, across the full lifespan. A wide variety of fish are available for purchase, often at a juvenile stage, and it is easy for those new to fish care to misjudge long-term or mixed-species needs. Common issues that come up include aggression to other fish, fish consuming other fish in the system, specialized feeding needs, large adult size or rapid growth, venomous species, and other dangers to people. **Table 4** reviews fish that may be readily available but should be avoided by all but the most dedicated fish caregiver. Purchasing them can perpetuate poor health and welfare outcomes for the fish.

Clinical Care Point: Freshwater species that may work well for the beginning aquarist.

The following species were selected for their relative hardiness, general availability, manageable adult size, and relative ease of care. Fish caregivers should be educated on the proper care and provide adequate husbandry for each species listed, not all species are appropriate for a community system.

Goldfish (*Carassius aratus*)
Betta fish (*Betta splendens*)
Zebra danios (*Danio rerio*)
Platys (*Xiphophorus variatus*)
Swordtails (*Xiphophorus helleri*)
Neon tetras (*Paracheirodon innesi*)
Guppies (*Poecilia reticulata*)
Corydoras catfish (*Corydoras spp.*)

Evaluation of tank size against the long-term growth potential of the species is critical. Unfortunately, many species are available when small and readily outgrow the original tank but cannot be placed. Misinformed caregivers may release them, causing invasive species concerns. The authors use a minimum of 1 "inch of fish" (2.5 cm) per gallon (3.8 L) for a rough estimate of basic tank size. This typically

Table 4
Fish species that are problematic for the casual hobbyist

Concern	Freshwater		Saltwater	
	Common Name	Scientific Name	Common	Scientific Name
Large adult size/ rapid growth	Red tail catfish	*Phractocephalus hemioliopterus*	Groupers (hinds)	*Cephallopholis* spp. typically
	Pacu, Tambaqui, Pirapitinga	Various species including *Colossoma macropomum, Piaractus brachypomus, P. mesopotamicus*	Moray eels (some)	Various
	Oscar	*Astronotus ocellatus*	Sharks (most)	
	Freshwater stingrays	Various	Rays	
	Arowana	Osteoglossidae		
	Bala shark	*Balantiocheilos melanopterus*		
	Mbu and other large pufferfish	*Tetraodon mbu*, various		
Potential aggression to other fish	Pufferfish (inter- and intraspecies common)	Various	Butterflyfish (particularly intraspecies)	Various
	Freshwater angelfish (interspecies and intraspecies common)	*Pterophyllum scalare*	Saltwater angelfish (particularly intraspecies)	Various
			Surgeonfish (particularly intraspecies)	Various
			Wrasses (interspecies and intraspecies common)	Various
Large carnivorous fish	Oscar	*A ocellatus*	Groupers (hinds)	*Cephallopholis* spp. typically
	Snakehead	*Channa* spp.	Moray eels	Various
	Pufferfish	Various		
Specialized feeding needs	Elephant nose fish	*Gnathonemus petersii*	Cleaner wrasse	*Labroides* spp.
			Seahorses	*Hippocampus* spp.
			Mandarinfish (dragonets)	*Synchiropus* spp.
Venomous species	Freshwater stingrays	Various	Rabbitfish	*Siganus* spp.
			Lionfish	*Pterois* spp.
Other danger to humans	Electric eel	*Electrophorus electricus*	Sharks	Various
	Electric catfish	Various	Moray eels	Various

matches nitrogen production/water volume to life support capacity, so that minimal water quality standards can be met. It is most appropriate for quarantine/temporary holding. Fish typically need more space (thus water volume) to meet long-term behavioral needs. For example, a 10-gallon (38 L) tank (a common size in pet stores) would hold 5 2" (5 cm) fish or 1 10" (25 cm) fish. In reality, although water quality might be adequate, a fish this size should generally have more space to meet minimal behavioral needs.

Basic social needs should also be considered. Shoaling/schooling species should be housed with others of the same species. Animals that are normally found isolated, are aggressive, or have large territories should be housed alone or with compatible different species. Although not necessarily aggressive, some predatory species readily eat other animals. As an example, a common freshwater species is the oscar cichlid (*Astronotus ocellatus*). They are a hardy and interactive fish, making them popular in the freshwater aquarium trade. They are routinely available when small, 2" (5 cm); however, they grow quickly, reaching up to 12" (30 cm). They will readily outcompete or consume other fish in the habitat and outgrow many "starter" habitats. Fish can benefit from environmental enrichment and a review for veterinarians is available.[16] Many fish caregivers strive to create aquaria with a wide diversity of animals and plants or microhabitats to mimic an ecosystem. In these systems, species may have a wide range of options to display normal behaviors. However, many items for sale in pet stores are not designed to promote natural fish behavior. As with other animals, enrichment activities can start by mimicking natural behavior opportunities, particularly around natural time budgets, and enhanced control/choice. Positive reinforcement training can be a source of enrichment and enhancing choice and control (Behavior and learning section).

In some cases, behavior may be normal but indicates an environment that does not support a range of natural behavior. These environments may not support good health and welfare and be excessively stressful (eg, inadequate/inappropriate hides, inappropriate stocking density, inappropriate sex ratio, inappropriate space, inadequate/inappropriate substrate) and should be corrected.

Natural behaviors of healthy fish can mimic behaviors related to disease and it is important for clinicians to consider both models when evaluating fish health.

Clinical Care Point: Common natural behaviors that can be mistaken for signs of illness.

- Flashing (quick rub of lateral body on substrate) and darting: Social displays, particularly in reproductively active males and with male-male aggression. Fish typically have bright, normal colors and good body condition. Often fish will be territorial and defending a specific area
- Listing on substrate/habitat items: Many species may rest laterally recumbent in rock caves, crevices, or along plants or the side of enclosures. They may rest directly at the bottom if no substrate or rock hides are available. Common in loaches (Cobitoidea) and some wrasses (Labridae).
- Isolation: Many species do not associate with a shoal or school and isolation is normal.
- Significant opercular movement/respiratory effort: Sedentary species exhibit significant opercular or siphon movement. Animals appear otherwise relaxed and exhibit full complement of normal behaviors. This is common in moray eels (Muraenidae).
- Piping/gulping at the surface: Certain species regularly exchange air at the surface of the water. Fish will come up for a breath but not remain at the surface and

otherwise have normal behavior. This is common in betta fish (*Betta splendens*), other gouramis (Osphronemidae), and bichirs (Polypteridae).

BEHAVIOR AND DISEASE OR WATER QUALITY ISSUES

Companion exotic animal veterinarians are accustomed to including a broad review of husbandry and habitat when evaluating patients and the approach is necessary with fish as well. The review should include water quality (testing program and results) and the life-support system, particularly when multiple individuals or species are impacted.[17–19] Water quality problems from inappropriately sized or broken life-support components can quickly become life threatening. Common water quality problems include inappropriate temperature, toxic levels of ammonia or nitrite, chlorine/chloramine presence, inappropriate pH, and inappropriate dissolved gas levels (eg, low dissolved oxygen, elevated carbon dioxide, elevated total gas). Home visits or a detailed set of photos showing the aquaria, its life-support components, and the general orientation in the room are helpful. Veterinarians should also specifically ask about any medications or "water conditioners" used. Fish antibiotic and antiparasitic medications are commonly available over the counter, options that are generally not available for other exotic pets. It is also helpful to specifically ask about new animal additions and quarantine protocols. Many fish caregivers appear to be motivated by ongoing additions of new fish to the habitat and this can be a source of infectious disease and social stress in a community system.

Healthy fish are typically in good body condition with smooth scales/skin, good fin condition, and normal body symmetry. They are attentive and responsive to the environment. Fish that actively swim generally constantly explore and interact with each other, frequently and calmly move their fins, and purposefully direct movement in relation to each other or to changes in the environment. Shoaling and schooling fish are loosely associated and will come together and move as a unit if startled. Some species, particularly those that rely on camouflage, are normally inactive and do not routinely move, but remain alert to the environment, such as through ocular movement. Opercular movement and mouth gap associated with respiration is relaxed and appropriate for the species. Speaking broadly, healthy, relaxed fish have a fairly loose body posture with some flexion as they position in the water or on substrate and the fins move independently with calm, short strokes to adjust position. A stressed fish will typically have a tense/rigid body posture with limited flexion and the fins are clamped or moving fully to direct movement through the water and schooling/shoaling species will gather tightly. The opercular rate may be elevated. Fish may hide more than usual or respond to environmental changes by freezing or with rapid, frantic motion and may run into walls or items in the habitat, in some cases fatally.

Animals that are ill may be darker or lighter than usual; they are often lethargic or weak and are isolated from the rest of the group (if shoaling or schooling species). The body may be rigid or too relaxed and the fins may be clamped or hanging. The fish is often less reactive to the environment. If a species that is normally swimming in the water column is on the substrate or at the surface, it is typically a sign of severe illness, particularly if combined with other signs. If a species that is normally on the substrate is free swimming, it can be a sign of environmental stress (eg, water quality, vibration, aggressors), although disease cannot be ruled out (eg, pruritus from external parasites). Fish in respiratory distress typically have tense/rigid body posture, rapidly moving and flaring operculum, and excessive oral gaping, and may be constantly at the surface or a turbulent area of water flow. In the early stages of an infectious disease outbreak, water quality problem, or other environmental issue, the case distribution is often uneven due to individual and species variability in physiology or preferred location in the habitat and these causes should not be ruled out.

Common diseases in pet fish include parasitic disease, particularly protozoan parasites (eg, freshwater and saltwater ich), which can quickly reach life-threatening levels, buoyancy problems, poor nutritional condition (particularly obesity), trauma, neoplasia, and ocular changes.

Certain species or breeds are commonly associated with specific disease. For example, in the pet trade, buoyancy issues in fancy goldfish (*Carassius auratus*) are common. Reports on causes and treatment are anecdotal. Animals are typically relaxed and otherwise appear normal. Feeding fresh or frozen peas has been recommended. In some cases, harnesses have been created to help position the fish in the water column.

Clinical Care Point: Behaviors frequently associated with illness and common general differentials.

- Flashing body on bottom or side of enclosure (pruritus): External parasitic infection, irritation from inappropriate water quality.
- Swimming slowly or isolated: Pain, parasitic or other infectious disease, organ disease.
- Dark coloration: Parasitic or other infectious disease, organ disease, inappropriate water quality.
- Fin clamping: Pain, parasitic disease, inappropriate water quality.
- Piping, gulping, time in areas of turbulent water flow often with flared operculum and tachypnea: Low dissolved oxygen, anemia, gill disease.
- Abnormal swim pattern: Infectious diseases, trauma, organ failure.
- Swimming at surface, particularly with some of the body out of the water: Over-inflated swim bladder, gastrointestinal gas. In early stages, fish may be able to maintain position in the water column but only with increased effort.

BEHAVIOR AND LEARNING

Fish readily learn as they interact with the environment and learning has been demonstrated in multiple species in both free-ranging and managed care habitats; training is used routinely in many public display aquariums to facilitate care.[2,6,11,13,14,20–29] Archerfish (*Toxotes chatareus*) have been shown to recognize human faces and, based on personal observations, the authors believe other species recognize individual people.[26] Clinicians should keep in mind that individual behavior in relation to specific environmental cues is often learned. For example, fish quickly learn to pair nets with captures and rapidly learn net avoidance. Conversely, fish quickly learn to predict feeding and can show a wide range of behaviors at feeding time, often unintentionally trained by the caregiver (eg, spitting water, frenetic swimming at the surface, aggressive interactions with other fish). As with other animals, fish are learning and adjusting behavior based on the results of that behavior.

The deliberate use of applied behavior analysis, the tools and technology to change behavior, is now routine in many care settings.[21] Within this context, positive reinforcement training is used to reduce aversive events and concurrent stress and facilitate care. For example, fish can be trained to approach and enter a net, stretcher, or other container for manual restraint or transportation. Deliberate training with positive reinforcement can be part of creating environments rich in positively reinforcing opportunities, choice, and control—ones that support good health and welfare and simplify veterinary care.[21]

Pet fish are rarely presented for "behavioral problems" although they can occur and the author (Clayton) has managed several cases around aggression between fish and maladaptive feeding responses. It is possible that with greater attention to fish welfare, behavior, and learning, behavioral problems may be avoided or noticed and managed productively.

Clinical Care Point: Husbandry behaviors commonly trained in managed care settings.

- Feeding in specific locations of habitat to reduce potentially aversive interactions between individuals or species.
- Positioning immediately near or with physical contact on an object inside or outside of the habitat (target training).
- Swimming into a transfer container (plastic cup, plastic bag, stretcher).
- Exercise activities such as going from one point to another, circling, moving objects in the enclosure.

A NOTE ON SOURCES OF FISH

In the United States, saltwater and freshwater fish are available through online vendors as well as in pet or hobbyist stores. It has been estimated that approximately 90% of saltwater fish are wild-caught and approximately 90% of freshwater fish are captive-reared, typically in ornamental fish aquaculture settings.[3]

The technology and techniques to support captive rearing of tropical, saltwater fishes are rapidly developing to support commercial and conservation needs.[28,29] The clownfish or anemonefish is the best-known saltwater species that is readily available from captive-reared sources. A list of saltwater fish successfully raised in captivity is available from CORAL magazine: https://www.reef2rainforest.com/2019/08/28/coral-magazines-captive-bred-marine-fish-species-list-for-2019/. Many freshwater species are routinely raised in aquaculture settings. Species that readily breed or have been bred for many years are often available in colors and patterns that vary form wild-type or with exaggerated morphology. Goldfish have the most exaggerated morphologic changes (eg, bubble eyes).

It can be challenging to understand the chain of custody for fish, particularly wild-caught fish, and there are concrete efforts to improve transparency and responsibility at all stages. Three major areas of focus include ensuring support for the local economy, preservation of the environment and ecosystems, and provision of appropriate fish care. As with many green marketing trends, it can be challenging to understand if company practices actually support this type of green and ethical sourcing and recent reviews are available.[3,29,30]

Clinical Care Point: Questions to consider when evaluating ethical sourcing of fish[3,29,30]

- Local Community and Economy
  - Does the collection provide meaningful employment for local people?
  - Do profits from the collection in the local community?
- Environmental Sustainability
  - Where was the fish collected? Are the fish populations sustainable in that location? Are other wildlife species impacted by the collection?
  - Is ancillary environmental damage mitigated, such as damage to coral structure or bycatch?

- ○ How does the holding and transportation process impact that environment? Is there excessive pollution from boats? Is runoff water managed to introduce infectious disease into new environments?
- ○ What is the large-scale carbon footprint/environmental impact of collecting and transporting the fish? Is there a large amount of waste (eg, plastic bags, styrofoam boxes) produced in the process of shipping and is this mitigated?
- Animal Health and Welfare
  - ○ How are the fish collected? Are they collected humanely using sustainable methods? Is cyanide capture avoided?
  - ○ How are animals handled after capture, such as during holding and transportation? Is the water quality managed well? Is the stocking density appropriate? Is stress mitigated appropriately?
  - ○ Are the husbandry considerations for the animal well understood to ensure survival when they reach their destination?

SUMMARY

Fish are an incredibly diverse group of animals with a wide range of natural behaviors, response to disease, and ability to learn. Many readily identify and interact with humans in the wild and under human care. By better understanding how natural history, disease, and learning interact, we can create better habitats for them and use our interactions to positively contribute to their welfare, no matter where they live.

ACKNOWLEDGMENTS

The authors would like to thank Dr Catherine A. Hadfield, Senior Veterinarian at Seattle Aquarium, and Ashleigh Clews, Curator of Animal Care and Rescue Center at National Aquarium, for their assistance in reviewing early drafts of the article. The authors also thank Dr Roy P. E. Yanong, Professor and Extension Veterinarian at the Tropical Aquaculture Laboratory at the University of Florida and Mr Alan Luken, Associate Brand Manager at Segrest Farms, for input into species common in the pet and hobbyist trade.

DISCLOSURE

The authors have nothing to disclose.

REFERENCES

1. Keat-Chuan Ng C, Aun-Chuan Ooi P, Wong WL, et al. A review of fish taxonomy conventions and species identification techniques. Surv Fish Sci 2017;4:54–93.
2. Brown C. Fish intelligence, sentience and ethics. Anim Cogn 2015;18:1–17.
3. King TA. Wild caught ornamental fish: a perspective from the UK ornamental aquatic industry on the sustainability of aquatic organisms and livelihoods. J Fish Biol 2019;94:925–36.
4. Froese R, Pauly D. FishBase. World Wide Web electronic publication. Available at: www.fishbase.org. Accessed December 2, 2019.
5. Deloach N. Reef fish behavior. 2nd ediiton. Jacksonville (FL): New World Publications; 2019.
6. Sloman KA, Wilson RW, Balshine S, editors. Behaviour and physiology of fish 24. Cambridge: Academic Press; 2005.
7. Brown C, Laland KN. Social learning in fishes: a review. Fish Fish 2003;4:280–8.

8. Budaev SV, Zworykin DD. Individuality in fish behavior: ecology and comparative psychology. Journal of Ichthyology Supplement 2002;42:S189–95.

9. Carleton KL, Hárosi FI, Kocher TD. Visual pigments of African cichlid fishes: evidence for ultraviolet vision from microspectrophotometry and DNA sequences. Vis Res 2000;40:879–90.

10. Jacobs GH. Ultraviolet vision in vertebrates. Am Zoologist 1992;32:544–54.

11. Lucon-Xiccato T, Bisazaa. Individual differences in cognition among teleost fishes. Behav Processes 2017;141:184–95.

12. Marshall NJ, Vorobyev M. The design of color signals and color vision in fishes. In: Collin SP, Marshal NJ, editors. Sensory processing in aquatic environments. New York: Springer; 2003. p. 194–222.

13. Mourier J, Brown C, Planes S. Learning and robustness to catch-and-release fishing in a shark social network. Biol Lett 2017. https://doi.org/10.1098/rsbl.2016.0824.

14. Tebbich S, Bshary R, Grutter AS. Cleaner fish *Labroides dimidiatus* recognise familiar clients. Anim Cogn 2002;5:139–45.

15. Toms CN, Echevarria DJ, Jouandot DJ. A methodological review or personality-related studies in fish: focus on the shy-bold axis of behavior. Int J Comp Psychol 2010;23:1–25.

16. Corcoran M. Environmental enrichment for aquatic animals. Vet Clin North Am Exot Anim 2018;18:305–21.

17. Stamper MA, Semmen KJ. Basic water quality evaluation for zoo veterinarians. In: Miller RE, Fowler M, editors. Fowler's zoo and wild animal medicine current therapy, Vol. 7. Missouri: Elsevier Sunders; 2012. p. 177–86.

18. Stamper MA, Semmen KJ. The mechanisms of aquarium water conditioning. In: Miller RE, Fowler M, editors. Fowler's zoo and wild animal medicine current therapy, Vol. 7. Missouri: Elsevier Sunders; 2012. p. 187–94.

19. Stamper MA, Semmen KJ. Advanced water quality evaluation for zoo veterinarians. In: Miller RE, Fowler M, editors. Fowler's zoo and wild animal medicine current therapy, Vol. 7. Missouri: Elsevier Sunders; 2012. p. 195–201.

20. Braithwaite VA. Cognitive ability in fish. In: Sloman KA, Wilson RW, Balshine S, editors. Behavior and physiology of fish 24. Cambridge: Academic Press; 2005. p. 1–37.

21. Corwin AL. Training fish and aquatic invertebrates for husbandry and medical behaviors. Vet Clin North Am Exot Anim 2012;15:455–67.

22. Häderer IK, Michiels NK. Successful operant conditioning of marine fish in their natural environments. Copeia 2016;104:380–6.

23. Kuba MJ, Byrne RA, Burghardt GM. A new method for studying problem solving and tool use in stingrays (*Potamotrygon castexi*). Anim Cogn 2010;13:507–13.

24. Newport C, Wallis G, Reshitnyk Y, et al. Discrimination of human faces by archerfish (*Toxotes chatareus*). Sci Rep 2016;6. https://doi.org/10.1036/srep27523.

25. Petrazzini MEM, Bisazza A, Agrillo C, et al. Sex differences in discrimination reversal learning in the guppy. Anim Cogn 2017;20:1081–91.

26. Schluessel V, Blackmann H. Spatial learning and memory retention in the grey bamboo shark (*Chiloscyllium griseum*). Zoology 2012;115:346–53.

27. Siebeck UE, Litherland L, Wallis GM. Shape learning and discrimination in reef fish. J Exp Biol 2009;212:2113–9.

28. Pouil S, Tlusty MF, Rhyne AL, et al. Aquaculture of marine ornamental fish: overview of the production trends and the role of academia in research progress. Rev Aquaculture 2019;12:1–14.

29. Tlusty M. The benefits and risks of aquaculture production for the aquarium trade. Aquaculture 2002;205(3–4):203–19.
30. Mini Sekharan N, Ramachandran A, eds Proceedings of the International Conference on Sustainable Ornamental Fisheries - Way Forward SOFI-WF:2012; March 23-25, 2012; Cochin, India. Available at: https://www.researchgate.net/publication/301364614_Sustainable_Ornamental_Fisheries_-_Way_Forward. Accessed February 13, 2020.

Invertebrate Behavior for the Exotic Pet Practitioner

Gregory A. Lewbart, MS, VMD, DACZM, DECZM (ZHM)[a,*], Laurie Bergmann, VMD, DACVB[b]

KEYWORDS

- Invertebrates • Behavior • Coelenterate • Mollusks • Chelicerates • Crustaceans
- Echinoderms

KEY POINTS

- Invertebrates represent more than 95% of animal species, and aside from lacking a backbone, many taxa have little in common and are frequently not closely related.
- This review provides a short survey of each taxon's natural history, highlighting key and unique aspects of anatomy, physiology, and importance to humans.
- For certain groups, like the cephalopods and insects, entire books have been dedicated to the topic of behavior.
- We have tried to focus on the aspects of behavior and pertinent literature that might be of benefit and interest to the veterinary practitioner.

COELENTERATES

Taxonomic Overview

This large phylum includes the comb jellies (Ctenophores), Hydrozoans (hydras, fire coral, Portuguese Man-O-War), Scyphozoans (jellyfishes), and Anthozoans (stony corals, soft corals, sea anemones). This is an economically important group for environmental monitoring, public and private display, research, and tourism. Jellyfish exhibits are now some of the most popular displays in public aquariums, upscale restaurants, and even private homes throughout the world. Coral reefs collectively are one of the most beautiful, diverse, and fragile ecosystems on the planet. Investigations on the diseases of corals are some of the most active areas of research for any aquatic animal group.

It is beyond the scope of this article to include details of taxonomy, anatomy, and physiology, but some basics are worthy of inclusion. Most coelenterates are marine and there are individual and colonial forms. They have a single opening to their gastrointestinal tract and most use stinging nematocysts, contained in cnidocytes, for defense and prey capture.

[a] Department of Clinical Sciences, NC State University College of Veterinary Medicine, 1060 William Moore Drive, Raleigh, NC 27607, USA; [b] NorthStar VETS, 315 Robbinsville-Allentown Road, Robbinsville, NJ 08691, USA
* Corresponding author.
E-mail address: greg_lewbart@ncsu.edu

Vet Clin Exot Anim 24 (2021) 229–251
https://doi.org/10.1016/j.cvex.2020.09.011
1094-9194/21/© 2020 Elsevier Inc. All rights reserved.
vetexotic.theclinics.com

Coelenterates lack a distinct central neural ganglion (brain), although all have a "nerve net" that is used for sensory and motor transmissions. This nerve net was described in detail 85 years ago in 3 important papers.[1–4] In the 1950s, slow motion photography was used to prove that anemones not only move using their pedal disc but also contract, sway, and display other movements without apparent stimulation.[4,5]

Although the goal of most veterinarians or veterinary health professionals reading this article would be to improve the health and welfare of coelenterates, it should be kept in mind that coelenterate behavior and ecology are also important with regard to the welfare of other marine animals and humans.[6,7] There are numerous instances in which interactions with coelenterates, especially pelagic forms, are detrimental to hosts, prey, or inadvertent victims.[6–8] Although human fatalities are rare, they do occur, and most are attributed to the tropical multitentacled box jelly, *Chironex fleckeri*.[7] Jellyfish, especially large jellyfish blooms, can have detrimental economic consequences, mostly with regard to negative impacts on tourism and fisheries.[7] **Fig. 1** illustrates this in graphic form.

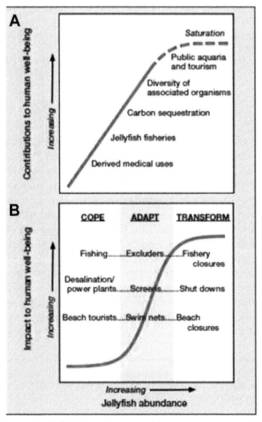

Fig. 1. The relationships of jellyfish abundance and human economics. (*A*) Jellyfish contributions to human well being. (*B*) Impacts of jellyfish on human well being. (*From* Graham WM, Gelcich S, Robinson KL, et al. Linking human well-being and jellyfish: ecosystem services, impacts, and societal responses. Front Ecol Environ. 2014; 12(9): 515-523; with permission.)

Jellies

Albert[9] provides a fascinating review of the moon jellyfish (*Aurelia* sp) behavior in his article entitled, "What's on the mind of a jellyfish? A review of behavioral observations on *Aurelia* sp. jellyfish." The investigator describes how many people think jellyfish simply drift about the oceans subject to wind, tides, and currents; this could not be further from the truth. Jellyfish have an elaborate sensory system rich with nerves, chemoreceptors, gravity sensors, hydrostatic pressure receptors, photoreceptors, pressure sensors, and the ability to sense direction.[9] At least 10 different behaviors have been attributed to *Aurelia* sp, and these are summarized in **Fig. 2**. Virtually all of these behaviors rely on the 8 rhopalia (**Figs. 3** and **4**), which are equally spaced sensory clusters located at the bell's margin.[10–12] Jellies, at least *Aurelia aurita* (the moon jelly), can use "taste" to discriminate between agar pellets with edible brine shrimp and those without. The nonfood agar pellets were secured by the tentacles, tasted, and then discarded into the currents produced by bell pulsations while the edible pellets were transferred via ciliary movement to the mouth.[13,14]

One of the most interesting jellies, and one that has been extensively studied, is the upside-down jellyfish, *Cassiopeia* spp.[15,16] These subtropical and tropical marine jellies are unusual in that they rest upside-down with the dorsal surface of the bell on the bottom and their manubria and tentacles reaching toward the surface.[16] In addition, these jellies are host to photosynthetic dinoflagellates, similar to the corals, which provide the jelly with supplemental nutrition. This animal's unique behaviors, anatomy, physiology, and life history make an important research animal for many biological and biomedical disciplines. **Fig. 5** highlights the importance of various life stages to a variety of scientific disciplines.

Corals and Anemones

The anemones and corals belong to the most evolutionarily advanced group of coelenterates, the Anthozoa. Anemones are typically solitary whereas corals, both hard (or stony) and soft (gorgonians), are colonial.[17] In recent years, numerous studies have been published looking at the impact of climate change on coral reefs, other anthropogenic impacts on corals, and coral diseases in general.[18–24] Although a disease and health review is beyond the scope of this article, it is important to recognize the global importance of corals, and the many efforts under way to understand and protect them from a veterinary standpoint.

A very interesting study is one of the few examining "personality" in an invertebrate.[25] The investigators defined "animal personality" as the way *individuals differ from one another in either single behaviors or suites of related behaviors in a way that is consistent over time.*[25] They found that individual anemones (*Actinia equina*) had their own startle responses and behavior patterns.

Nearly all anemones and corals capture prey using cnidocyte-armed tentacles. One exception is the scleractinian coral *Mycetophyllia reesi*, which inhabits coral reefs of the Caribbean and Gulf of Mexico.[26] This unusual coral lacks tentacles and uses mucus strands to entangle prey that can then be ingested.[26]

GASTROPODS
Taxonomic Overview

The gastropods are a class in the phylum Mollusca and include more than 80,000 marine, fresh water, and terrestrial species. The group includes abalone, conchs, nudibranchs, sea hares, slipper shells, slugs, snails, and whelks, among many others. All gastropods have a ventrally flattened foot that provides locomotion along the

A
Species typical behaviours of *Aurelia* sp.

Behaviour	Category
Swim up following somatosensory stimulation	Swim away, up
Swim up when encountering low oxygen	Swim away, up
Swim down when encountering low salinity	Swim away, down
Swim down when touching the surface	Swim away, down
Swim down at top 2 m of column water during day	Swim away, down
Swim down and out of turbulence	Swim away, down
Staying away from rocks walls	Swim away
Staying below turbulence	Response inhibition
Horizontal directional swimming	Directional swimming
Remain in areas with the scent of conspecifics	Aggregation
Accumulate in vertical circles	Aggregation
Remain in areas containing the scent of prey	Foraging
Swim faster after capturing prey	Foraging
Swim more variable pattern after capturing prey	Foraging
Swim slower after catching several prey	Foraging

B

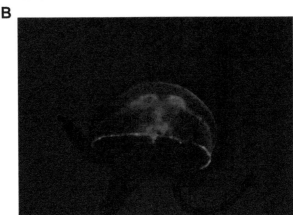

Fig. 2. (*A*) Some typical behaviors that have been documented in the moon jellyfish, *Aurelia* sp, (*B*) along with a photograph of a captive animal. ([*A*] *Adapted from* Albert DJ. What's on the mind of a jellyfish? A review of behavioral observations on *Aurelia* sp. jellyfish. Neurosci Biobehav Rev. 2011; 35: 474-82; with permission.)

various surfaces of their habitats. Most are aquatic and have a well-developed head with sensory organs, an external shell, a muscular foot, and a respiratory chamber containing gills. As the molluscan class with the most species, and morphologic variety, it is hard to make generalizations for the entire group. One need only examine a common garden slug (lacking gills, a shell, and terrestrial), to appreciate the exceptions to the norm and diversity within the taxon. Gastropod reproductive and feeding behaviors cover a wide spectrum. Many gastropods are dioecious (separate sexes), but, most terrestrial pulmonates (snails and slugs) are hermaphrodites.[27] Although many gastropods are carnivorous, especially marine snails,[28] there are examples of herbivores, omnivores, parasites, and even a large group that displays kleptoplasty,

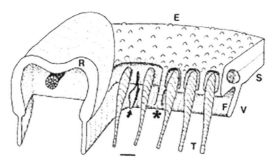

Fig. 3. This drawing represents the side view of the bell's rim from the moon jellyfish, *Aurelia aurita*. The (*) represents an extension of the intertentacular partition. The arrow indicates a variably shaped sessile protuberance of the pseudovelarium in the pararhopalial region. (*From* Chapman DM. Microanatomy of the bell rim of Aurelia aurita (Cnidaria: Scyphozoa). Can J Zool. 1999; 77(1): 34-46; with permission.)

where plant material is consumed and the chloroplasts are retained with the gastropod's tissues and provide the slug with nourishment via photosynthesis.[28] One area of gastropod feeding behavior that has received a lot of attention is the shell-boring ability of certain gastropods, like the oyster-drill (*Urosalpinx cinerea*), to drill through the shell of a prey mollusk and consume the animal's soft tissues.[29]

A recent paper summarized learning and memory of gastropods and reviews the pertinent literature of the past century.[30] The article summarizes, in graphic form, the various behaviors, mostly shared with vertebrates, associated with the appropriate significant taxonomic groups. Nargeot and Bédécarrats[30] begin their article with a review of the various types of learning and behavior that apply to nearly all animal species. Behaviorists categorize learning into associative and nonassociative, and, either of these can affect behavior.[30] A single stimulus that causes habituation or sensitization is a form of nonassociative learning.[31,32] Gastropods learn through nonassociative means but also can learn through association. Associative learning is either instrumental (operant) conditioning or Pavlovian conditioning.[30] With operant conditioning, an animal develops a predictable relationship between a particular behavior and a negative or positive result. With Pavlovian conditioning, the animal develops a

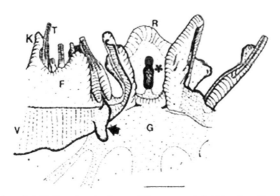

Fig. 4. This drawing details the rhophalium of the moon jellyfish, *Aurelia aurita*. The (*) represents the rhopalium, which is covered by the rhopalial hood. The arrow indicates the sessile protuberance of the pseudovelarium. (*From* Chapman DM. Microanatomy of the bell rim of Aurelia aurita (Cnidaria: Scyphozoa). Can J Zool. 1999; 77(1): 34-46; with permission.)

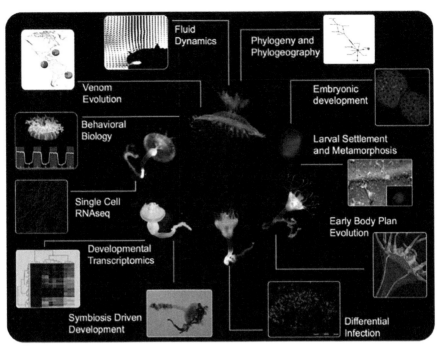

Fig. 5. The "*Cassiopea* system" in schematic form, showing the various disciplines that benefit from this unique, upside-down jellyfish. These disciplines include behavioral ecology. (*From* Ohdera AH et al. Upside-down but headed in the right direction: Review of the highly versatile Cassiopea xamachana system. Front Ecol Evol. 2018; 6(35); with permission.)

predictable relationship between different stimuli.[30] Gastropods provide excellent models to study learning and behavior because their systems are relatively simple compared with vertebrates. For example, the sea hare (*Aplysia californica*) brain has 20,000 neurons whereas the mammal brain may have a trillion. In addition, the brain cells of *Aplysia* are quite large (**Fig. 6**), and can individually be mapped and worked with. In fact, in 2000, Eric Kandel received a Nobel Prize in Physiology or Medicine for his work related to nonassociative learning in the sea hare.[33] **Fig. 7** illustrates how a marine snail learns and converts short-term memory to long-term memory.

CEPHALOPODS
Taxonomic Overview

There are approximately 800 species of cephalopods, a group that includes the octopuses, squids, cuttlefish, and the chambered nautilus,[34] yet detailed science has only been published on approximately 60 of these species.[35] This is a very important group of animals in that they serve as a food source for humans and other animals, have been frequently used in a variety of research projects, and are popular display animals.[35] Their excellent vision, dexterity, closed circulatory system, and intelligence make them fascinating animals to observe and study. Most species are short-lived in the wild and captivity (the exception being the chambered nautilus, which can live 20 years). Common problems in captivity include trauma, anorexia, microbial infections, and water quality problems. Anesthetic and surgical protocols have been established for some species. In Great Britain and Canada, an Institutional Animal Care and Use Committee equivalent protocol is required to perform research on cephalopods.

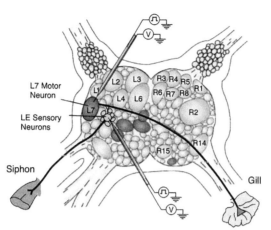

Fig. 6. This is a dorsal representation of the *Aplysia* (sea hare) abdominal ganglion (brain). The 7 sensory gill neurons are blue and the 6 motor neurons are brown. Small electrodes are being used to stimulate and record responses. (*From* Kandel ER. The molecular biology of memory storage: A dialogue between genes and synapses. Science. 2001; 294(5544): 1030-1038; with permission.)

Virtually all species are predatory carnivores; **Table 1** summarizes their behaviors and adaptations for this lifestyle.[36] Of interest to the readers of this article should be that in the 10 years between 2006 and 2015. there were nearly 500 research papers published on cephalopod behavior, far outpacing a number of other areas including aquaculture, climate change, cognition, genetics, neuroscience, and welfare.[35] **Fig. 8** illustrates this information as well as the number of publications in these specific areas between 1985 and 2005. It is also worth noting that the number of cephalopod behavior studies has been greater than all of the other research areas each year for the 1985 to 2015 period.[35] Recent years have also included a push to perform and publish

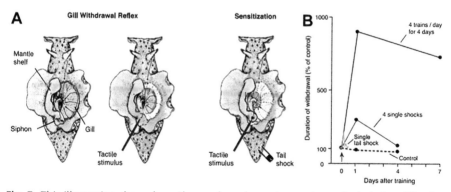

Fig. 7. This illustration shows how the sea hare (a marine gastropod), *Aplysia californica*, learns and converts short-term memory to long-term memory. (*A*) These three images show how the gill withdrawal reflex can become reduced with sensitization. (*B*) This graph shows how the duration of gill withdrawal becomes shorter over time as the sea hare becomes sensitized to the stimulus. (*From* Kandel ER. The molecular biology of memory storage: A dialogue between genes and synapses. Science. 2001; 294(5544): 1030-1038; with permission.)

Table 1
Biological and behavioral adaptations used by cephalopods for the sake of their predatory behavior

Predatory Adaptations		Activities
Senses	Eyes and vision; epidermal hair cells; equilibrium receptor organs for linear and angular accelerations; epidermal tactile receptors; contact and distance chemoreceptors; vibration receptors and hearing	Searching for prey
Respiratory, circulatory and nervous systems	Efficient branchial ventilation; closed circulatory system; central nervous system; giant fiber system	Catching prey
Physical features	Arms and tentacle; suckers; beaks; jet propulsion; skin color change	Catching and handling prey
Cognitive capabilities	Learning and memory abilities	Searching, recognition and catching prey
Hunting strategies[a]	Ambushing, luring, pursuit, stalking, speculative and cooperative hunting	Catching prey

Morphologic, physiologic, sensory, neural and behavioral adaptations and corresponding behavioral outcomes (Activities) are listed here as deduced from several reviews (Packard, 1972[105]; Young, 1977[106]; Hanlon, 1988[107]; Hanlon and Messenger, 1996[108]; Borrelli et al., 2006[109]; Borrelli and Fiorito, 2008[110]).

This table illustrates some of the behaviors used by cephalopods to enhance their predatory success.

[a] See also **Table 2**.

From Villanueva R, Perricone V, Fiorito G. Cephalopods as predators: A short journey among behavioral flexibilities, adaptions, and feeding habits. Front Physiol. 2017;8:598.; with permission.

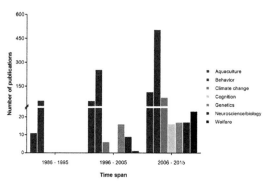

Fig. 8. This bar graph illustrates the number of cephalopod papers published by time and topic. (*From* O'Brien CE, Roumbedakis K, Winkelmann IE. The current state of cephalopod science and perspectives on the most critical challenges ahead from three early-career researchers. Front Physiol. 2018; 9: 700; with permission.)

genomics research on cephalopods.[37] **Table 2** summarizes this work and the research attributes of each cephalopod taxonomic group. No cephalopod has received more attention in the area of behavior and neurobiology than the octopus. **Table 3** summarizes the various behaviors attributed to cephalopods, and of the 17 listed, only 2 do not include octopus.[38]

Much of the research conducted in cephalopods can be applied to captive husbandry. As with other intelligent animals, cephalopods, especially octopuses, should be provided with a wide variety of enrichment. Recent research shows that octopuses use chemical cues more than visual ones in prey selection. Enrichment could be built on studies like this by providing food in opaque jars and allowing the animal to use chemical cues to find prey.[39]

Cephalopods also display a variety of complex reproductive behaviors.[40] Nearly all are sexually dimorphic and polygamy is the norm. There is also female selection of males and inter-male aggression. These traits make cephalopods interesting models to study vertebrate sexuality.[40]

CRUSTACEANS
Taxonomic Overview

The crustaceans are a highly successful class of the Phylum Arthropoda. Estimates vary but there are probably between 35,000 and 55,000 species.[17] Pechenik[41] presents the number as 42,000. Crustaceans are defined by 5 pairs of head appendages that include 2 pair of antennae and a larval stage called a nauplius that possesses 3 body segments and a lone medial eye.[41] This class includes the well-known barnacles, crabs, crayfish, hermit crabs, lobsters, and shrimp, as well as numerous other taxa, including amphipods, brine shrimp, and isopods, among others. Economically, this is one of the most important groups of invertebrates. Its members are important as food for humans and other species, many are maintained as display animals, and large numbers are used in research. In recent years, more attention is being paid to crustacean welfare, perhaps more than any other invertebrate group excluding the cephalopods. Diggles provides a good review of the subject.[42] Decapod crustaceans are known for their cannibalistic behavior, especially the lobsters and crabs, and this behavior makes many species unsuitable for aquaculture.[43]

There is a wealth of published information to support the fact that decapod crustaceans have a nervous system analogous to the autonomic nervous system of

Table 2
Commonly studied cephalopod species

Clade	Species	Genome Published (Genome Size)	Closed Life Cycle	Length of Life Cycle	Main Areas of Research
Nautiloidea	Nautilus sp	No	No	20 y	Evolution
Decapodiformes	Doryteuthis pealeii	No (4.5 Gb)	No	2 y	Evolution, development, neurobiology
	Euprymna scolopes, Euprymna berryi	Yes (5 Gb)	Yes	3–7 mo	Symbiosis, evolution, genomics, development, neurobiology
	Sepia officinalis, Sepia bandensis	No	Yes	~2 y (S officinalis), ~9 mo (S bandensis)	Behavior, neurobiology, development
	Sepioteuthis lessoniana	No	Yes	6–12 mo	Population genetics
	Idiosepius paradoxus	No (2 Gb) (111)	No	4 mo	Neurobiology, development
	Architeuthis dux	No	No	2.5 y	Evolution, population genetics
Octopodiformes	Octopus bimaculoides	Yes (2.7 Gb)	Yes	1–1.5 y	Evolution, development, neurobiology, genomics
	Octopus vulgaris	Yes (3 Gb)	No	1–2 y	Neurobiology, behavior, regeneration
	Callistoctopus minor	Yes (5 Gb)	No	1 y	Evolution, plasticity
	Hapalochlaena maculosa (blue ring octopus)	No	No	1 y	Venom evolution, toxicity

Many species of cephalopods are used in a variety of research venues. This table summarizes this information.
Features of commonly studied cephalopod species, with a focus on attributes that are important for developing a model system. Numbers provided are estimates; for more details on species, genomes, culturing successes, and references, please see the text.
From Albertin CB, Simakov O. Cephalopod biology: At the intersection between genomic and organismal novelties. Annu Rev Anim Biosci. 2020; 8: 71-90; with permission.

Table 3
Examples of cephalopod cognitive behaviors

Examples	Situation	Groups
Flexibility (same and different actions modified or selected to attain it)		
Activity change to casual not common predators[71]	Facultative predation	Octopus
Skin background matching (pattern texture)[48]	Immediate visual feedback	All groups
Arm use allocation try body movement direction[28]	Goal direction	Octopus
Home construction by modification[48]	Learned kinesthetic feedback	Octopus
Causal reasoning (actions selected or modified by feedback about attaining a specific end)		
Deimatic skin display use[55,56]	Predator action or choices	All groups
Passing cloud skin display[53]	Previous prey startle	Octopus
Change-combination of actions to predators[48,72]	Previous attack	Al groups
Learning characteristics of potential prey[39]	Previous attack success	Cuttlefish
'Theory of mind' about predator actions[57]	Previous evasions success	Squid
Prospection (selecting actions broadly for a category of desired ends)		
Head bob to get motion parallax information[26]	Ambiguous situation	Octopus
Coconut carrying to a location with no shelter[70]	Need for future shelter	Octopus
Manipulation of sexual skin displays[65,66]	Avoidance of competition	Cuttlefish, Squid
Navigation, especially after displacement[20]	Cognitive map	Octo, Cuttlefish
Imagination (actions selected from a new/modified category in a novel situation)		
Arm/tentacle tip wiggle[43]	Prey capture	All groups
'Pain' behavior[14]	Mitigate body damage	Octopus
Moving item through hole[23]	Manipulation tor reward	Octopus
Play by water jet or arms[33,34]	Boredom relief	Octopus

Example of categories of cognitive operation in cephalopods.
Cephalopods display a variety of cognitive behaviors. This table outlines and summarizes these behaviors.
From Mather JA, Dickel L. Cephalopod complex cognition. Current Opinion in Behavioral Science. 2017;16: 131-137; with permission.

vertebrates.[44] The 2 main ganglia that are involved in this crustacean autonomic system are the cardiac ganglion and the stomatogastric ganglion.[44] These ganglia are connected to nerve nets that innervate the major organs of the animal. For a detailed review of this topic, including informative tables and diagrams, the reader is encouraged to review the article by Suranova and colleagues.[44] It is well known and even obvious from gross inspection that decapod crustaceans are well equipped with elaborate sense organs in the form of eyes, antennae, and sensory mouth parts.[41] There is also evidence that crustaceans are able to hear, or sense vibrations, and this acoustic ability can alter their behavior.[45]

Most of the behavior research has focused on the decapod crustaceans, an order in the Class Malacostraca that contains approximately 14,500 species.[46] This group includes all of the crabs, crayfish, hermit crabs, lobsters, prawns, and shrimp. Although most are marine, there are freshwater and terrestrial members.

Much of the research has been centered on crustacean aggression, as these behaviors are easily observed and crustaceans make an appealing model for aggression in vertebrates.[47] Another area of behavioral research with much attention is the escape response, which in crayfish (*Procambarus clarkii*), involves a series of rapid tail flips that are controlled by giant afferent and efferent neurons, which bypass the central nervous system.[48,49]

When considering the vast number of species and the huge variety within the decapods, behaviors are not consistent between groups. For example, a number of workers have tested the effects of isolation on aggressive behavior and memory. When crayfish (*Cherax destructor*) are isolated for 30 days, and then exposed to a conspecific that was not isolated, the isolated individual usually loses a territorial battle.[47] On the contrary, when the hermit crab *Pagurus samuelis* is isolated for 30 days, the isolate is usually the winner.[50]

Even though the literature is rich with crustacean behavior studies, very few of these papers focus on animal personality.[51] In fact, as of 2012, animal personality had been studied in only a handful of decapod species (**Fig. 9**). A species of hermit crab (*Pagurus bernhardus*) has been an important model for studying animal behavior in invertebrates.[52–54]

A recent study found that crayfish (*P clarkii*) exhibit the behavioral satiety sequence (BSS) after feeding, similar to other species, including many vertebrates.[55] The BSS generally includes exploration, grooming, and resting in rodents and pigeons.[56,57] Crayfish exhibit all of these behaviors after eating as well as leg waving.[55] Crayfish (and crustaceans) are not alone in exhibiting behavioral satiety among the invertebrates. In 2008, a research team published their work on the nematode, *Caenorhabditis elegans*, where they identify this important research species as a model for satiety in higher animals.[58]

CHELICERATES
Taxonomic Overview

The chelicerates are an arthropod subphylum with approximately 75,000 species.[41] There are 3 classes: Merostomata (horseshoe crabs and the extinct water scorpions), Arachnida (scorpions, spiders, pseudoscorpions, ticks, and mites), and Pycnogonida (sea spiders). More than 90% of the 75,000 species are arachnids; this article focuses on horseshoe crabs, spiders, and scorpions.

Limulus polyphemus, the American horseshoe crab, is actually not a crab at all, because it is a member of the order Xiphosura. This is the only species that occurs on our coast (western Atlantic) but there are 3 species of horseshoe crabs that occur

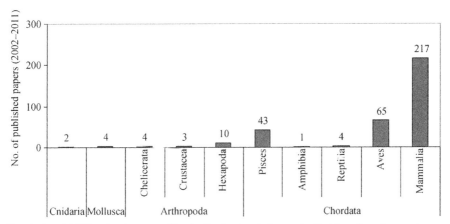

Fig. 9. As of 2012 animal personality studies had only been studied in a few decapod crustacean species. There were more than 3 times as many studies in this area published on insects compared with more than 200 for mammals. (*From* Gherardi F, Aquiloni L, Tricarico E. Behavioral plasticity, behavioral syndromes and animal personality in crustacean decapods: An imperfect map is better than no map. Curr Zool. 2012; 58(4): 567-579; with permission.)

in Asia. *Limulus* is a very important animal for biomedical research, is used as bait for the blue crab and eel fisheries, has been ground up for fertilizer (controversial), and is an important display and "touch tank" animal in public aquaria and science museums. In addition to its value for producing millions of dollars' worth of *Limulus* lysate per year, investigators examining vision and the *Limulus* lateral eye were awarded the Nobel Prize for medicine or physiology in 1967.

There are numerous detailed accounts of horseshoe crab biology, natural history, and conservation,[59–63] as well as work dealing with health and veterinary techniques.[64–66] Entire books and symposia have been devoted to *L polyphemus*. Like many animals, horseshoe crab behavior is largely impacted by circadian rhythms, but in the case of these marine chelicerates, tides play a huge role, with animals more active during high tides and less active at low tide.[67]

Approximately 500,000 American horseshoe crabs are captured for hemolymph extraction to produce *Limulus* lysate every year.[68] Normally, 30% of the animal's hemolymph is removed via cardiocentesis.[68] Based on a number of studies, the mortality rate from this process ranges from 10% to 30%.[69,70] Much less research has focused on morbidity and nonlethal effects of the process on behavior and reproductive fitness. One study found that surviving crabs were less mobile, possessed decreased hemocyanin, and females were less fecund.[68]

Horseshoe crabs are unusual, as they appear to be the only marine arthropods that have external fertilization and do not brood or care for their eggs and young.[71] There is good evidence that population density affects reproductive success in both Asian and the North American species.[71] With fewer crabs one finds less polygamy (resulting in less genetic diversity) and more single females.[71] Mating horseshoe crabs are a common site in the spring months along the northern hemisphere western Atlantic and Gulf of Mexico beaches. It has been known that visual cues are very important for males to find and track females, but a 2010 study found that male horseshoe crabs also use olfactory (chemoreception) cues to find females.[72]

Scorpions are famous, or at least infamous, for their ability to deliver a toxic sting when threatened. In fact, this can be such a problem in some areas of the world that governmental and military units have formally addressed the problem. In Iran, more than 40,000 scorpion stings occur annually, and a large number of these require medical treatment.[73] Most of the published research on scorpion behavior focuses on stinging and prey capture.[74–76] Scorpions are also able to control the potency of venom they release according to the perceived threat level[77] and at least one scorpion (*Parabuthus transvaalicus*) is able to spray venom when grasped by the telson (tail).[78] This same species will use its stinger to inject venom when its body (metastoma) is touched.

The order Amblypygi is an interesting group of arachnids called whip spiders or false whip scorpions. Social behavior is rare among arachnids and only a handful of cases have been reported. Although maternal care of eggs and young is common, this generally dissipates once the young are independent.[79] **Fig. 10** illustrates maternal protection by *Damon diadema* when 6-week-old young are threatened.

Spiders are certainly the most numerous and well recognized of the arachnids. Their ability to weave intricate webs, and their complex and varied feeding strategies have been the focus of behavioral research for many decades.[80] Vollrath and Selden[81] have written a detailed article examining web types and evolution (**Fig. 11** illustrates these varying web morphologies in a metaphorical evolutionary tree). Like many invertebrates, spider welfare and captive enrichment is starting to get some attention, especially when it comes to laboratory and public display species. Theraphosid spiders (tarantulas) provided with an enriched environment were less aggressive and displayed a diminished flight response compared with their unenriched cohorts.[82] **Table 4** shows the variety of behaviors documented and observed in this study.

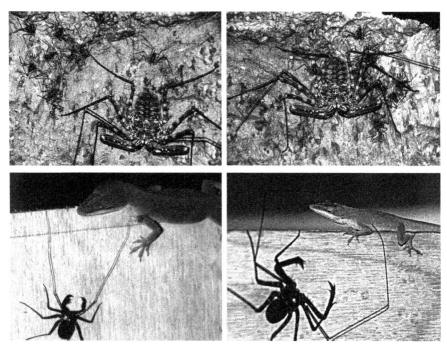

Fig. 10. Amblypygids (false scorpions) behave differently depending on their age, size, and stimuli. (*Courtsey of* L.S. Raynor, PhD, Ithaca, NY.)

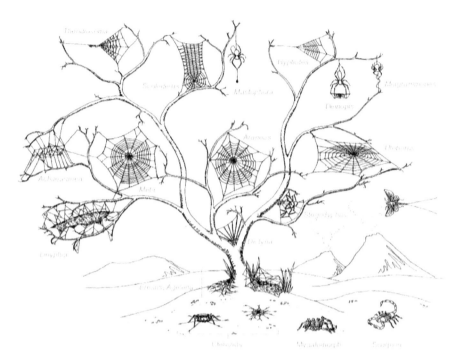

Fig. 11. This schematic tree illustrates the evolution of spider webs in a graphic and visually appealing way. (*From* Vollrath F, Selden P. The role of behavior in the evolution of spiders, silks, and webs. Annu Rev Ecol Evol Syst. 2007; 38: 819-846; with permission.)

Some tarantulas exhibit a defensive behavior in which they shake irritating hairs from their body, primarily their dorsal abdomen, that become airborne and can strike a potential predator. These smaller than 1.0 mm barbed projectiles are termed urticating hairs and are unique to New World tarantulas.[83] Old world tarantulas (Africa and Asia) do not possess urticating hairs and instead are much more likely to strike or bite than their American counterparts.[84] Spiders are not restricted to aggression for defense and can display a variety of protective behaviors including anachoresis (hiding), barrier webs, communal web-building, crypsis (camouflage), flight (running away), mimicry, phenology (cyclical behavior patterns based on weather or light), and warning coloration/ornamentation.[85]

One area of spider behavior that has received a fair amount of attention is mating and copulation. Tarantulas in the genus *Grammostola* display a number of pre-copulatory behaviors including body vibrations, drumming with the appendages, and leg tapping.[86] Tarantulas are somewhat famous for post-copulatory cannibalization, in which the female will kill and consume the male if the male does not safely escape. Although this does occur, it does not appear to be the norm, and in some cases the female will kill the male before copulation.[86,87]

Although not as large or commonly kept in captivity, the largest family of spiders, the salticids (jumping spiders), have been widely studied for their behavior and vision.[88,89] Jumping spiders have a number of strategies to capture prey, including mimicry (typically mimicking ants), and also have shown the ability to display behavioral flexibility when it comes to finding prey.[89] Jumping spiders are not the only spiders with a close association with ants, and in fact, hundreds of spider species consume ants and/or

Table 4
Behavioral ethogram exhibited by the arboreal tarantula

Behavior	Definition
Rest	Legs I and II pulled tightly together outstretched in front of spider and legs III and IV pulled tightly together outstretched behind spider
Alert	All legs splayed
Leg raise[a]	Raises pedipalps and legs 1 and II off ground, elevates the prosoma, pushes chelicerae forward and exposes fangs
Ground tap[a]	Leg raise followed by rapidly tapping legs 1 and II down on the ground
Lunge[a]	Jumping forward, grabbing threat with pedipalps, legs 1 and II, and biting
Flinch[a]	Legs twitch and body jerks away from ground briefly, raises limb(s) briefly before placing them back on ground, jerk backwards/forwards but then settles
Saltate[a]	Jumping and running away
Hide[a]	Moving underneath, into or behind something, or retreating into web
Chase	Pursues prey around enclosure
Pounce	Pounces forward at prey and grabs hold of it with pedipalps and legs 1 and II
Feed	Prey grasped between pedipalps and held up in chelicerae to mouth
Climb	Vertical ascent or descent using the enclosure sides or items in enclosure
Walk	Forward movement at slow to moderate pace
Run[a]	Forward movement at fast pace

This behavioral ethogram applies to the arboreal tarantula, *Psalmopoeus cambridgei*.
[a] Indicates a negative behavior.
From Bennie M, Loaring C, Trim S. Laboratory husbandry of arboreal tarantulas (Theraphosidae) and evaluation of environmental enrichment. Anim Technol: J Inst AnimTechnicians. 2011;10(3):163-69; with permission.

have developed complex relationships with ants that include a type of Batesian mimicry in which the spider myrmecomorphs blend in with the ant colony and receive protection from predators as well as a ready food supply.[90] Cushing's review lists 180 references and is rich with tables and images.[90]

INSECTS

The insects (Ectognatha) are a class of the superclass Hexapoda that include more than 1 million species and likely many times that number yet to be described.[17] In fact, the group is so expansive, and important, that it warrants its own field of scientific study, entomology. As such, most invertebrate zoology courses devote only a small amount of time to insects because they would overwhelm the course and displace the other phyla based on the number of taxa and scientific publications. Various books and review articles adequately cover this expansive topic.[91–94] For perspective, one insect species, the honey bee (*Apis mellifera*), has numerous books and review articles written just about it, including very thorough behavior and disease studies.[95–99]

ECHINODERMS

The echinoderms are a phylum of exclusively marine animals, that like vertebrates, are deuterostomes (the first embryonic opening becomes the anus). There are more than 6500 species in 5 classes that possess in common a water vascular system, pentamerous radial symmetry, and mesodermal calcareous ossicles that form the endoskeleton.[17] Members include the brittle stars, feather stars, sand dollars, sea bis-cuits, sea cucumbers, and sea stars. They do not have either a true brain or distinct ganglia and their nervous system consists of 3 distinct networks.[17] The ectoneural system is circumoral and receives impulses from the animal's surface. The motor hyponeural network is also circumoral and is most developed in the ophuroids (brittle stars). The crinoids (feather stars) use an aboral entoneural system that is either very reduced or entirely absent in the other echinoderm classes.[17]

Echinoderms display some interesting behaviors. Covering (securing items like algae, shells, debris with tube feet) is commonly used by echinoids (sea urchins) to hide or camouflage themselves.[100–102] In the laboratory, urchins exposed to increased water temperature were less likely to cover, and when they did, the process was pro-longed.[102] These investigators also investigated 2 other urchin behaviors: sheltering and righting. Urchins (*Strongylocentrotus intermedius*) acclimated to warm water shel-tered more than those in the normal temperature water, yet righting reflex times did not vary between the temperature groups.[102]

Perhaps one of the most interesting behaviors exhibited by echinoderms, and by any animal for that matter, is the process of evisceration. Many species of sea cucum-bers are able expel parts of or entire internal organs when threatened or attacked.[17,103] This is not a uniform process, and different species (there are approx-imately 1200) display different levels of evisceration, and subsequently, regeneration. Some species simply expel Cuvierian tubules, which are sticky noodlelike projections from the respiratory tree. These regrow within a few weeks.[17] Other species may expel their entire visceral mass, including the gastrointestinal tract, gonads, and respiratory tree. Amazingly, these animals can regenerate all of the lost organs.[17] For more details on echinoderm behavior, there is an entire volume devoted to cephalopods and echinoderms.[104]

CLINIC CARE POINTS

- While it's unlikely a private client will seek your assistance with an invertebrate behavior problem, understanding normal invertebrate behavior is important in maintaining their health in captivity.
- While an upside-down tarantula may appear like a major problem, this is normal behavior for a tarantual preparing to molt.
- Of all invertebrates we probably know the most about honey bee (Apis mellifera) behavior. Understanding this species various means of communication and in-hive actions are key to understanding the health and disease prevention of the colony.
- When a possible abnormal or unusual behavior is observed in an invertebrate, the first thing a clinician should do is investigate normal behaviors in the taxon. This may involve learning about behavior changes related age, sex, life stage, or time of year.

DISCLOSURE

The authors have nothing to disclose.

REFERENCES

1. Pantin CFA. The nerve net of the Actinozoa. I. Facilitation. J Exp Biol 1935a;12:
119–38.

2. Pantin CFA. The nerve net of the Actinozoa. II. Plan of the nerve net. J Exp Biol 1935b;12:139–55.

3. Pantin CFA. The nerve net of the Actinozoa. III. Polarity and after-discharge. J Exp Biol 1935c;12:156–64.

4. Josephson R. The neural control of behavior in sea anemones. J Exp Biol 2004; 207(14):2371–2.

5. Pantin CFA. The elementary nervous system. Proc R Soc Lond B 1952;140: 147–68.

6. Thakiruea L, Siriariyaporn P, Wutthanarungsan R, et al. Review of fatal and severe cases of box jellyfish envenomation in Thailand. Asia-pacific J Public Health 2015;27(2):1639–51.

7. Graham WM, Gelcich S, Robinson KL, et al. Linking human well-being and jellyfish: ecosystem services, impacts, and societal responses. Front Ecol Environ 2014;12(9):515–23.

8. Purcell JE, Arai MN. Interactions of pelagic cnidarians and ctenophores with fish: a review. Hydrobiologia 2001;451:27–44.

9. Albert DJ. What's on the mind of a jellyfish? A review of behavioral observations on *Aurelia* sp. jellyfish. Neurosci Biobehav Rev 2011;35:474–82.

10. Spangenberg DB. Rhopalium development in *Aurelia aurita* ephyrae. Hydrobiologia 1991;(216/217):45–9.

11. Nakanishi N, Hartenstein V, Jacobs DK. Development of the rhopalial nervous system in *Aurelia* sp.1 (Cnidaria, Scyphozoa). Dev Genes Evol 2009;219: 301–17.

12. Chapman DM. Microanatomy of the bell rim of *Aurelia aurita* (Cnidaria: Scyphozoa). Can J Zool 1999;77:34–46.

13. Archdale MV, Yamanouchi T, Anraku K. Feeding behavior of *Aurelia aurita* towards Artemia and artificial pellets. Jpn J Taste Smell Res 2002;9:747–50.

14. Archdale MV, Anraku K. Feeding behavior in Scyphozoa, Crustacea, and Cephalopoda. Chem Senses 2005;30(1):i303–4.

15. Nath RD, Bedbrook CN, Abrams MJ, et al. The jellyfish *Cassiopea* exhibits a sleep-like state. Curr Biol 2017;27:2984–90.e3.

16. Ohdera AH, Abrams MJ, Ames CL, et al. Upside-down but headed in the right direction: review of the highly versatile *Cassiopea xamachana* system. Front Ecol Evol 2018;6(35). https://doi.org/10.3389/fevo.2018.00035.

17. Ruppert EE, Fox RS, Barnes RD. Invertebrate zoology: a functional evolutionary approach. 7th edition. Belmont (CA): Brooks/Cole — Thomson Learning; 2004.

18. Negri AP, Smith LD, Webster NS, et al. Understanding ship-grounding impacts on a coral reef: potential effects of antifoulant paint contamination on coral recruitment. Mar Pollut Bull 2002;44:111–7.

19. Bielmyer-Fraser GK, Patel P, Capo T, et al. Physiological responses of corals to ocean acidification and copper exposure. Mar Poll Bull 2018;133:781–90.

20. Jafarabadi AR, Bakhtiari AR, Spanó N, et al. First report of geochemical fractionation distribution, bioavailability and risk assessment of potentially toxic inorganic elements in sediments of coral reef islands of the Persian Gulf, Iran. Mar Poll Bull 2018;137:185–97.

21. Lamb JB, Willis BL, Fiorneza EA, et al. Plastic waste associated with disease on coral reefs. Science 2018;359:460–2.

22. Muller EM, Bartels E, Barums IB. Bleaching causes loss of disease resistance within the threatened coral species *Acropora cervicornis*. eLife 2018;7:e35066.

23. Gintert BE, Precht WF, Fura R, et al. Regional coral disease outbreak over-whelms impacts from a local dredge project. Environ Monit Assess 2019; 191:630.

24. Mohamed AR, Sweet M. Current knowledge of coral diseases present within the red sea. In: Rasul N, Stewart I, editors. Oceanographic and biological aspects of the red sea. Cham (Switzerland): Springer Oceanography. Springer; 2019. p. 387–400.

25. Briffa M, Greenway J. High in situ repeatability of behaviour indicates animal personality in the beadlet anemone *Actinia equina* (Cnidaria). PLoS ONE 2011;6:e21963.

26. Goldberg WM. Feeding behavior, epidermal structure and mucus cytochemistry of the scleractinian *Mycetophyllia reesi*, a coral without tentacles. Tissue & Cell 2002;34(4):232–45.

27. Delgado GA, Glazer RA, Stewart NJ. Predator-induced behavioral and morpho-logical plasticity in the tropical marine gastropod *Strombus gigas*. Biol Bull 2002;203(1):112–20.

28. Middlebrooks ML, Pierce SK, Bell SS. Foraging behavior under starvation con-ditions is altered via photosynthesis by the marine gastropod, *Elysia clarki*. PLoS ONE 2011;6(7):e22162.

29. Carriker MR, Van Zandt D. Predatory behavior of a shell-boring muricid gastropod. In: Winn HE, Olla BL, editors. Behavior of marine animals. New York: Plenum Press; 1972. p. 157–244.

30. Nargeot N, Bédécarrats A. Gastropod learning and memory (Aplysia, Hermis-senda, Lymnea, and others). Invert Neuros 2020. Available at: https://doi.org/10.1093/acrefore/9780190264086.013.086.

31. Thompson RF, Spencer WA. Habituation: A model phenomenon for the study of neuronal substrates of behavior. Psychol Rev 1966;73(1):16–43.

32. Byrne JH, Hawkins RD. Nonassociative learning in invertebrates. Cold Spring Harbor Perspect Biol 2015;7:a021675.

33. Kandel ER. The molecular biology of memory storage: a dialogue between genes and synapses. Science 2001;294(5544):1030–8.

34. Norman M, Finn J, Hochberg F, et al. Cephalopods of the world. An annotated and illustrated catalogue of cephalopod species known to date. Volume 3. Oc-topods and vampire squids. In: Jereb P, Roper CFE, Norman MD, et al, editors. FAO species Catalogue for Fishery purposes. Rome (Italy): FAO); 2014. p. 370.

35. O'Brien CE, Roumbedakis K, Winkelmann IE. The current state of cephalopod science and perspectives on the most critical challenges ahead from three early-career researchers. Front Physiol 2018;9:700.

36. Villanueva R, Perricone V, Fiorito G. Cephalopods as predators: a short journey among behavioral flexibilities, adaptions, and feeding habits. Front Physiol 2017;8:598.

37. Albertin CB, Simakov O. Cephalopod biology: At the intersection between genomic and organismal novelties. Annu Rev Anim Biosci 2020;8:71–90.

38. Mather JA, Dickel L. Cephalopod complex cognition. Curr Opin Behav Sci 2017; 16:131–7.

39. Maselli V, Al-Soudy A, Buglione M, et al. Sensorial hierarchy in *Octopus vulgar-is's* food choice: Chemical vs. visual. Animals (Basel) 2020;10(3):457.

40. Apostólic LH, Marian JEAR. Cephalopod mating systems as models for the study of sexual selection and alternative reproductive tactics: a review. Bull Mar Sci 2019. https://doi.org/10.5343/bms.2019.0045.

41. Pechenik JA. Biology of the invertebrates. 6th edition. New York: McGraw-Hill; 2010. p. 606.

42. Diggles BK. Review of some scientific issues related to crustacean welfare. ICES J Mar Sci 2019;76(1):66–81. https://doi.org/10.1093/icesjms/fsy058.

43. Romano N, Zeng C. Cannibalism of decapod crustaceans and implications for their aquaculture: a review of its prevalence, influencing factors, and mitigating methods. Rev Fish Sci Aquacult 2016;25(1):42–69.

44. Shuranova ZP, Burmistrov YM, Strawn JR, et al. Evidence for an autonomic nervous system in decapod crustaceans. Intl J Zool Res 2006;2(3):252–83.

45. Popper AN, Salmon M, Horch KW. Acoustic detection and communication by decapod crustaceans. J Comp Physiol A 2001;187:83–9.

46. De Grave S, Pentcheff ND, Ahyong ST, et al. A classification of living and fossil genera of decapod crustaceans. Raffles Bull Zool 2009;21:1–109.

47. Hemsworth R, Villareal W, Patullo BW, et al. Crustacean social behavioral changes in response to isolation. Biol Bull 2007;213:187–95.

48. Edwards DH, Heitler WJ, Krasne FB. Fifty years of a command neuron: the neurobiology of escape behavior in the crayfish. Trends Neurosci 1999;22: 153–60.

49. Faulkes Z. Turning loss into opportunity: the key deletion of an escape circuit in decapod crustaceans. Bran Behav Evol 2008;72:251–61.

50. Courchesne E, Barlow GW. Effect of isolation on components of aggressive and other behaviour in the hermit crab, *Pagurus samuelis*. Z Vgl Physiol 1971;74: 32–48.

51. Gherardi F, Aquiloni L, Tricarico E. Behavioral plasticity, behavioral syndromes and animal personality in crustacean decapods: an imperfect map is better than no map. Curr Zool 2012;58(4):567–79.

52. Briffa M, Elwood RW. Motivational change during shell fights in the hermit crab *Pagurus bernhardus*. Anim Behav 2001;62:505–10.

53. Briffa M, Rundle SD, Fryer A. Comparing the strength of behavioural plasticity and consistency across situations: animal personalities in the hermit crab *Pagurus bernhardus*. Proc R Soc B 2008;275:1305–11.

54. Briffa M, Twyman C. Do I stand or blend in? Conspicuousness awareness and consistent behavioural differences in hermit crabs. Biol Lett 2011;7:330–2.

55. Tierney AJ, MacKillop I, Rosenbloom T, et al. Post-feeding behavior in crayfish (Procambarus clarkii): Description of an invertebrate behavioral satiety sequence. Physiol Behav 2020. https://doi.org/10.1016/j.physbeh.2019.112720.

56. López-Alonso VE, Mancilla-Díaz JM, Rito-Domingo M, et al. The effects of 5-HT1A and 5-HT2C receptor agonists on behavioral satiety sequence in rats. Neurosci Lett 2007;416(3):285–8.

57. Spudeit WA, Sulzbach NS, Bittencourt M de A, et al. The behavioral satiety sequence in pigeons (*Columba livia*). Description and development of a method for quantitative analysis. Physiol Behav 2013;122:62–71.

58. You Y, Kim J, Raizen DM, et al. Insulin, cGMP, and TGF-beta signals regulate food intake and quiescence in *C. elegans*: a model for satiety. Cell Metab 2008;7(3):249–57.

59. Shuster CN, Brockmann JH, Barlow RB, editors. The American horseshoe crab. Cambridge (MA): Harvard University Press; 2003.

60. Carmichael RH, Botton ML, Shin PKS, et al, editors. Changing global perspectives on horseshoe crab biology, conservation and management. Cham, Switzerland: Springer; 2015. p. 619.

61. Kenny NJ, Chan KW, Nong W, et al. Ancestral whole-genome duplication in the marine chelicerate horseshoe crabs. Heredity 2015;116(2):190–9.
62. Smith DR, Brockmann HJ, Beekey MA, et al. Conservation status of the American horseshoe crab (*Limulus polyphemus*): a regional assessment. Rev Fish Biol Fish 2017;27(1):135–75.
63. Krisfalusi-Gannon J, Ali W, Dellinger K, et al. The role of horseshoe crabs in the biomedical industry and recent trends impacting species sustainability. Front Mar Sci 2018;5:185.
64. Spotswood T, Smith SA. Cardiovascular and gastrointestinal radiographic contrast studies in the horseshoe crab (*Limulus polyphemus*). Vet Rad Ultras 2007;48(1):14–20.
65. Nolan MW, Smith SA. Clinical evaluation, common diseases, and veterinary care of the horseshoe crab, *Limulus polyphemus*. In: Tanacredi JT, Botton ML, Smith DR, editors. Biology and conservation of horseshoe crabs. Cham, Switzerland: Springer; 2009. p. 479–99.
66. Archibald KE, Scott GN, Bailey KM, et al. 2-phenoxyethanol (2-PE) and tricaine methanesulfonate (MS-222) immersion anesthesia of American horseshoe crabs (*Limulus polyphemus*). J Zoo Wild Med 2019;50(1):96–106.
67. Chabot CC, Watson WH. Circatidal rhythms of locomotion in the American horseshoe crab *Limulus polyphemus*: underlying mechanisms and cues that influence them. Curr Zool 2010;56(5):499–517.
68. Anderson RL, Watson WH III, Chabot CC. Sublethal behavioral and physiological effects of the biomedical bleeding process on the American horseshoe crab, *Limulus polyphemus*. Biol Bull 2013;225:137–51.
69. Hurton L, Berkson J. Potential causes of mortality for horseshoe crabs (*Limulus polyphemus*) during the biomedical bleeding process. Fish Bull 2006;104(2):293–8.
70. Leschen AS, Correia SJ. Mortality in female horseshoe crabs (*Limulus polyphemus*) from biomedical bleeding and handling: implications for fisheries management. Mar Freshw Behav Physiol 2010;43:135–47.
71. Mattei JH, Bekey MA, Rudman A, et al. Reproductive behavior in horseshoe crabs: does density matter? Curr Zool 2010;56(5):634–42.
72. Saunders KS, Brockmann HJ, Watson WH, et al. Male horseshoe crabs *Limulus polyphemus* use multiple sensory cues to locate mates. Curr Zool 2010;56(5):486–98.
73. Dehghani R, Khoobdel M, Sobati H. Scorpion control in military units: a review study. J Mil Med 2018;20(1):3–13.
74. Casper GS. Prey capture and stinging behavior in the emperor scorpion, *Pandinus imperator* (Koch) (Scorpiones, Scorpionidae). J Arachnol 1985;13(3):277–83.
75. Rein JO. Prey capture behavior in the East African scorpions *Parabuthus leiosoma* (Ehrenberg, 1828) and *P. pallidus* Pocock, 1895 (Scorpiones: Buthidae). Euscorpius 2003;6:1–8.
76. Edmunds C, Sibly RM. Optimal sting use in the feeding behavior of the scorpion *Hadrurus spadix*. J Arachnol 2010;38:123–5.
77. Lira AFA, Santos AB, Silva NA, et al. Threat level influences the use of venom in a scorpion species, *Tityus stigmurus* (Scorpiones, Buthidae). Acta Ethol 2017;20:291–5.
78. Nisani Z, Hayes WK. Venom-spraying behavior of the scorpion *Parabuthus transvaalicus* (Arachnida: Buthidae). Behav Process 2015. https://doi.org/10.1016/j.beproc.2015.03.002.

79. Rayor LS, Taylor LA. Social behavior in amblypygids, and a reassessment of arachnid social patterns. J Arachnol 2006;34(2):399–421.

80. Heselberg T. Exploration behaviour and behavioural flexibility in orb-web spiders: a review. Curr Zool 2015;61(2):313–27.

81. Vollrath F, Selden P. The role of behavior in the evolution of spiders, silks, and webs. Annu Rev Ecol Evol Syst 2007;38:819–46.

82. Bennie M, Loaring C, Trim S. Laboratory husbandry of arboreal tarantulas (Theraphosidae) and evaluation of environmental enrichment. Anim Technol J Inst Animtechnicians 2011;10(3):163–9.

83. Bertani R, Marques OAV. Defensive behaviors in Mygalomorph spiders: release of urticating hairs by some Aviculariinae (Araneae, Theraphosidae). Zool Anz 1996;234:161–5.

84. Blatchford R, Walker S, Marshall S. A phylogeny-based comparison of tarantula spider anti-predator behavior reveals correlation of morphology and behavior. Ethol 2011;117:473–9.

85. Cloudsley-Thompson JL. A review of the anti-predator devices of spiders. Bull Br Arachnol Soc 1995;10(3):81–96.

86. Ferretti NE, Ferrero AA. Courtship and mating behavior of *Grammostola schulzei* (Schmidt 1994) (Araneae, Theraphosidae), a burrowing tarantula from Argentina. J Arachnol 2008;36:480–3.

87. Costa FG, Pérez-Miles F. Reproductive biology of Uruguayan theraphosids (Araneae, Theraphosidae). J Arachnol 2002;30:571–87.

88. Richman DB, Jackson RR. A review of the ethology of jumping spiders (Araneae, Salticidae). Bull Br Arachnol Soc 1992;9(2):33–7.

89. Jackson RR, Pollard SD. Predatory behavior of jumping spiders. Annu Rev Entomol 1996;41:287–308.

90. Cushing PE. Spider-ant associations: an updated review of myrmecomorphy, myrmecophily, and myrmecophagy in spiders. Psyche 2012. https://doi.org/10.1155/2012/151989.

91. Mullen GR, Durden LA. Medical and veterinary entomology. Cambridge, Massachusetts: Academic Press; 2009. p. 637.

92. Matthews RW, Matthews JR. Insect behavior. 2nd edition. Cham, Switzerland: Springer; 2010. p. 527.

93. Price PW, Denno RF, Eubanks MD, et al. Insect ecology, behavior, populations and communities. Cambridge, United Kingdom: Cambridge University Press; 2011. p. 801.

94. Pedigo LP, Rice ME. Entomology and pest management. 6th edition. Long Grove, Illinois: Waveland Press; 2014. p. 784.

95. Galizia CG, Eisenhardt D, Giurfa M, editors. Honeybee neurobiology and behavior: a tribute to Randolph Menzel. Cham, Switzerland: Springer; 2012. p. 512.

96. Morse RA, Flottum K. Honey bee pests, predators, and diseases. 3rd edition. United Kingdom: Northern Bee Books; 2013. p. 732.

97. Vidal-Naquet N. Honeybee veterinary medicine: *Apis mellifera* L. Great Easton, Essex, England: 5 M Publishing; 2016.

98. Seeley TD. Honeybee ecology: a study of adaptation in social life. Princeton, New Jersey: Princeton University Press; 2014. p. 212.

99. Seeley TD. The lives of bees: the untold story of the honey bee in the wild. Princeton, New Jersey: Princeton University Press; 2019. p. 371.

100. Dumont CP, Drolet D, Himmelman I, et al. Multiple factors explain the covering behaviour in the green sea urchin, *Strongylocentrotus droebachiensis*. Anim Behav 2007;73(6):979–86.

101. Pawson DL, Pawson DJ. Bathyal sea urchins of the Bahamas, with notes on covering behavior in deep sea echinoids (Echinodermata: Echinoidea). *Deep Sea Research Part II*. Topical Stud In Oceanography 2013;92:207–13.

102. Zhang L, Zhang L, Shi D, et al. Effects of long-term elevated temperature on covering, sheltering and righting behaviors of the sea urchin *Strongylocentrotus intermedius*. PeerJ 2017. https://doi.org/10.7717/peerj.3122.

103. García-Arrarás JE, Greenberg MJ. Visceral regeneration in holothurians. Micros Res Tech 2001;55:438–51.

104. Corning WC, Dyal JA, Willows AOD, editors. Invertebrate learning: volume 3 cephalopods and echinoderms. Springer; 2013. p. 236.

105. Packard A. Cephalopods and fish: the limits of convergence. Biol Rev 1972;47: 241–307.

106. Young JZ. Brain, behaviour and evolution of cephalopods. Symp. Zool. Soc. Lond 1977;38:377–434.

107. Hanlon RT. Behavioral and body patterning characters useful in taxonomy and field identification of cephalopods. Malacologia 1988;29:247–64.

108. Hanlon RT, Messenger JB. Cephalopod behaviour. Cambridge: Cambridge University Press; 1996.

109. Borrelli L, Gherardi, F, Fiorito G. A catalogue of body patterning in cephalopoda. Napoli: Stazione Zoologica A. Dohrn; Firenze University Press; 2006.

110. Borrelli L, Fiorito G. Behavioral analysis of learning and memory in cephalopods," in Learning and Memory: a comprehensive reference, Byrne JJ, editor. (Oxford: Academic Press), 2008. p. 605–627.

Diagnostic and Therapeutic Guidelines to Abnormal Behavior in Captive Nonhuman Primates

Maya Kummrow, DMV, DVSc, FTA Wildtiere (ZB Zootiere), DACZM, DECZM (ZHM)

KEYWORDS

- Abnormal behavior • Functional analysis • Nonhuman primates
- Operant conditioning • Psychopathology

KEY POINTS

- Abnormal behavior must be regarded as a symptom of disturbances in the neuronal structures of the brain (ie, underlying psychopathological disease).
- A diagnostic procedure consisting of behavioral and functional analyses, medical examination, and life history research is necessary for the identification of triggering factors and underlying psychopathology.
- Treatment approaches must be individually tailored combinations of changes in husbandry and social structure, medical treatment of underlying diseases, supporting psychopharmacological treatment, and operant conditioning.
- Genetic selection in regard to mental health and stability may offer a viable strategy for captive breeding programs of nonhuman primates.
- Interdisciplinary cooperation between veterinary clinicians, primatologists, veterinary behavior specialists, and human psychiatrists is recommended.

INTRODUCTION

Animal well-being is not only important for any institution or private person holding animals in captivity, but has also attracted increased attention of the public perception in the past decades. It is well acknowledged that behavior constitutes an important indicator of welfare.[1] However, common misconceptions of behavior serving as a direct measure of psychological welfare, and erroneous direct inference of suboptimal environmental conditions from abnormal behaviors are largely ignoring the underlying pathophysiological processes in the brain. Mental illness is often prematurely blamed on certain conditions, in the case of captive animals, readily so on their husbandry.

Clinic for Zoo Animals, Exotic Pets and Wildlife, Vetsuisse Faculty, University of Zurich, Winterthurerstrasse 260, Zurich 8057, Switzerland
E-mail address: mkummrow@vetclinics.uzh.ch

Vet Clin Exot Anim 24 (2021) 253–266
https://doi.org/10.1016/j.cvex.2020.09.012
vetexotic.theclinics.com
1094-9194/21/© 2020 The Author. Published by Elsevier Inc.

Additionally, mental illness, or psychopathology, is often not regarded as a neutral construct but laden with negative valorization.[2] Nonhuman primates (NHPs) and people share an array of qualities and neural substrates (including consciousness, self-awareness, social bonding mechanisms, memory, compassion, strategic thinking, and humor), and NHPs' social functioning closely approximates that in people.[3] This proximity provokes subjectively biased interpretations of behavior even more than with other taxa. Consequently, unfavorable reactions of visitors to captive animals demonstrating conspicuous behavior quickly result in undue public pressure on the holding institution, calling for immediate action to reduce or eliminate the behavior rather than carefully diagnosing and treating underlying etiologies. Detailed and evidence-based diagnostic approaches, imperative for sustainable treatment success in any disease, are oftentimes not feasible, accepted, or granted in the case of overt abnormal behavior in captive NHPs.

The present article is intended to promote and increase the understanding of conspicuous behavior as a sign of a malfunctioning and/or diseased organ (ie, brain disorders) and provide guidelines for a structured and comprehensive diagnostic and therapeutic approach for the veterinary clinician faced with a case of abnormal behavior in a captive NHP. The guidelines revolve around a proposed scheme of etiology, pathogenesis, diagnostic and therapeutic approaches. Although any model scheme presents with limitations due to simplification of complex connections, it is useful as a communication tool to illustrate the complex situation and necessary diagnostic and therapeutic procedures to involved stakeholders. The components of the scheme are supported by a large body of literature about psychopathologies in NHP used as model species in human medicine. The full dimensions of the topic of trans-species psychology are beyond the scope of this article; therefore, only certain aspects were selected to substantiate the proposed working scheme. For more detailed background information, the reader is referred to a recent review publication.[4]

THE PSYCHOPATHOLOGY SCHEME

The proposed scheme for etiology, pathogenesis, diagnostic, and therapeutic approaches for abnormal behavior in captive NHPs is depicted in **Fig. 1** and consists of 3 layers. The inner, red core represents the pathogenesis of psychopathologies leading to abnormal behavior; the middle blue counter-clockwise arrow represents the diagnostic pathway, and the outer, green circle indicates therapeutic approaches.

PATHOGENESIS OF ABNORMAL BEHAVIOR

The pathogenesis of abnormal behavior is depicted with 3 different entities: predisposition, psychopathological disorders and triggers, and resulting abnormal behavior (see **Fig. 1**). Importantly, the relationships of the factors of these 3 entities are nonspecific, resulting in a diversity of manifestations of psychopathologies, impeding direct deduction from known predispositions, observed behaviors or triggers to underlying psychopathologies.[5]

Predisposition

In analogy to other pathologic processes, such as infectious diseases, predisposition in the context of psychopathology may be regarded as susceptibility, rendering the individual vulnerable or resistant to developing a psychopathological condition.

Despite interspecific differences in neuroanatomy and physiology, mechanisms of psychopathologies are believed to be shared among all vertebrates.[6] Experience of early onset, repeated, sustained, or highly invasive events or trauma lead to

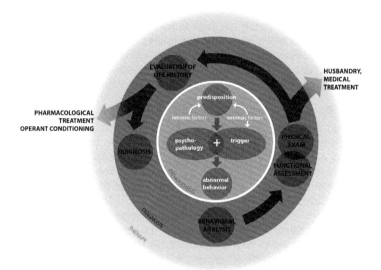

Fig. 1. Scheme for etiology, pathogenesis, diagnostic, and therapeutic approaches for abnormal behavior in captive NHP. The inner, red core represents the pathogenesis of psychopathologies leading to abnormal behavior; the middle blue counter-clockwise arrow represents the diagnostic pathway, and the outer, green circle indicates therapeutic approaches.

dysregulation of the neuroendocrine system and its central control, both on the level of the activation and feedback control by neurotransmitters (eg, serotonin, monoamine oxidase MAO-A, dopamine, norepinephrine), as well as the downstream stress hormones axes, (ie, the sympathetic-adrenomedullary system, hypothalamic-pituitary-adrenal axis, and the endogenous opioid system).[4]

Research into human personality psychology indicates a hereditary basis for temperament and personality, and allelic variations have been demonstrated in people as potential contributors to the development of a wide range of psychiatric disorders.[5,7] Similarly, numerous studies claim evidence for inherent expression of personality factors in various animal taxa.[8,9] In rhesus macaques (*Macaca mulatta*), an active personality was positively related to the animals' predisposition for stereotypic behavior.[10] Additionally, sex and age were identified as intrinsic risk factors for the development of behavioral irregularities in several studies.[11–15] The interplay of environment and genes (ie, epigenetics) results in amalgamation of intrinsic and extrinsic factors in the process of shaping predisposition. Genetically fixed, intrinsic factors (eg, sex and endocrinology or neuroanatomy and physiology) and hereditary traits for development of personality and temperament are influenced by the interaction with extrinsic factors, such as environmental conditions or events or diseases, in particular those affecting the brain (eg, infections, neoplasm, neurodegenerative or autoimmune diseases) and pain.[3] Hence, each brain is a unique construct, resulting from the inputs of an individual life history, constantly being shaped by intrinsic and extrinsic factors.

One of the most important predisposing factors for psychopathologies in primatology are social deprivation and in particular early maternal separation. These factors have served as 2 of the most studied and dramatic strategies to experimentally alter early neurobiological development in NHPs in order to use them as models for the understanding of developmentally based vulnerability to adult depression in people.[3,16,17] In rhesus macaques, early social separations, maternal neglect, and abuse have been demonstrated to result in severe long-term effects in behavioral and cognitive, but also physiologic (eg, differences in thermoregulation, or immune and endocrine responses), neurochemical (eg, differences in neurotransmitter levels and altered responses to neuroactive drugs), and neuroanatomical domains, such as alterations in gross morphology and functional microstructure of the brain.[18]

Psychopathology

Psychopathological processes need to be considered as underlying diseases of abnormal behavior.[19] When applied to nonhuman vertebrates, psychopathology may be considered a controversial term. Bearing the imprint of suppositions, world views, general beliefs and values exemplified in science, history, and general culture of human societies, the attribution of a mind and mental illness to animals has long been considered anthropomorphism and speciescism.[2] The shift to a more clinical and physicalist approach, considering psychopathologies as manifestation of aberrant behavior as consequence of a damaged phenotype, has opened doors to cross-species psychology. In view of the psycho-socio-biological continuity between NHPs and people, dysfunctions of homologous brain structures must be expected to result in psychopathologies in people and NHPs alike.[5,6]

Trigger

Psychopathological disorders and neuroendocrine imbalances remain subclinical until proximal triggers cause the disease to manifest. Triggers are usually acute, extrinsic factors, events, situations, or conditions that can be different from those that first triggered the behavior. Multiple triggers may result in presentation of the same clinical symptoms (ie, abnormal behavior). To complicated the issue, triggers do not only activate clinical symptoms but also continue to shape predisposition for development of psychopathological disorders.

Abnormal Behavior

Abnormal behavior must be regarded as the outward expression or – in analogy to other diseases – symptom of disturbances in the neuronal structures of the brain (ie, underlying psychopathological disease) that is activated by the trigger event or situation.[20] Although at the end of the causative sequence of the pathogenesis, the abnormal behavior, as the component manifesting the underlying disease process, naturally serves as the starting point for the diagnostic procedure (see **Fig. 1**).

DIAGNOSTIC APPROACH TO ABNORMAL BEHAVIOR
Behavior: What Is Normal?

In a first step, any reported abnormal behavior should be scrutinized regarding the normality of the behavior and reference standards used (**Box 1**). Generally, comparisons with behavioral patterns of conspecifics in the same group, wild counterparts, and - inevitably - people are self-evident, but all pose risks and limitations. Behavior not only serves to cope with environmental circumstances, but is also subject to cultural differences and traditions in groups of great apes and therefore is expected to differ between individuals in different social settings and situations.[31,32] The interdisciplinary approach between human and primate behavior raises conceptual dilemmas termed speciescism and anthropomorphism, concerning differences in behavioral ecology, expressions of emotions, and in gene expression in the brain, not unlike those encountered in comparative human studies across cultures and historic periods.[2] The following general criteria of cross-cultural approaches may therefore serve

Box 1
Abnormal behaviors reported in primates

- Self-directed behaviors: automutilation/bite-hit-lick, eye-/ear-poking, hair-plucking/self-depilation, thumb-sucking, overgrooming
- Stereotypies
  - Oral: suckling, lip pursing, raspberry vocalization, sticking out tongue
  - Motor: pacing, rocking/bouncing, somersaulting, head tossing, clapping
- Sleep-disturbance
- Eating behaviors: coprophagy, urine drinking, saliva eating, regurgitation, and reingestion (R&R)
- Social behaviors: aggression, withdrawal, indifference, decreased play behavior
- Sexual behaviors: masturbation
- Maternal behaviors: infanticide, abuse, overly protective
- Dissociative and displacement behaviors: inactivity, catatonia, trance-like stares, floating limbs, twirl/rotate torso, vacuum behaviors (chewing, displaying)

Data from Refs.[5,6,13,16,18,19,21–30]

as a pragmatic approach to identification of abnormal behavior: persistence and exclusion of any given context, disruption of the flow in an individuals life, and psychological and/or somatic distress (**Table 1**).[2,6]

Stereotypies and regurgitation and reingestion (R&R) qualify as abnormal behaviors because of their repetitive nature without obvious function.[13,22,23,30] Antisocial behaviors interfere with the individual's social life, and automutilative behavior obviously causes physical harm.[19,27] The classification of other behaviors must be individually scrutinized. Coprophagy, for example, was also observed in wild primates and did not seem to interfere with the individual's flow of life; on the contrary, it was identified as a learned, cultural behavior and was associated with positive social behaviors, such as grooming.[23,31] In view of the possibly natural background and lack of detrimental effects on the affected individuals, terms like disagreeably normal or natural and not preferred have been proposed for such behaviors.[31]

Care should be taken when behavioral alterations are classified abnormal relative to an understood social and cultural space; the existence of shame and guilt, prerequisites for ethical standards, are controversially discussed in NHPs, challenging the

Table 1
Application of cross-cultural behavior criteria: selected behaviors tested for normality

The Behavior...	...Shows Persistence and Exclusion of any Given Context	...Causes Disruption of the Flow of Individual's Life	...Is Associated with Psychological and/or Somatic Distress
R&R[13,22,23,30,33,34]	Yes	No	Potentially
Automutilation[19,27]	Potentially	Potentially	Yes
Stereotypies[35]	Yes	Potentially	Potentially
Infanticide[5]	No	No	No
Aggression[36,37]	Potentially	Potentially	Potentially

Data from Refs.[5,13,19,22,23,27,30,33–37]

pathologic nature of for example, female infanticide.[2,5] Hair-pulling (trichotillomania) and skin-picking (excoriation) behavior are classified as obsessive-compulsive disorders in people[38]; however, in primates, they would have to be scrutinized in regard to species-specific grooming behavior.[28,39] Similarly, aggression must be carefully interpreted in view of the individual's social hierarchical status, social competence and interactions of the other group members, and species-specific social dominance behavior.[37] For example, aggressive behavior of a silverback gorilla toward a female may have to be classified as normal, if the female does not show socially competent, submissive integration into the patriarchic 1-male group structure.[36]

Behavioral Analysis

A structured, comprehensive behavioral analysis and the answering of the question "what is the animal doing when, how often and how much?" is a prerequisite for the therapeutic approach of a potentially abnormal behavior.[40] Consultation with biologists and veterinary behavioral specialists is encouraged to ensure standardized and objectively documented ethological studies. Examples of behavioral profiles in NHPs can be drawn from the literature.[25,39,41] In theory, observations need to encompass 24-hour observations and may have to take seasonality and reproduction into account. Ideally, behavioral observations are performed by remote video recording to exclude the influence of observers. Although resource investment for professional ethological studies can be prohibitive for some institutions, behavioral observations naturally take place during each interaction of daily husbandry by keeping staff. These are self-evident to be included in the behavioral analysis; however, they are particularly vulnerable to preconceptions and bias. Therefore, training of primate caregivers in observation techniques, structured documentation, and sensitizing caregivers about the impact of their own interactions on the behavior are important to attain objectively exploitable information during the daily husbandry routine.[19]

Functional Analysis: What Triggers and Maintains the Behavior?

Most reports of abnormal behavior (see **Box 1**) are mere descriptions of the behavioral patterns. The ABC of Behavior proposes a differentiation of the

Antecedent - the preceding stimulus, event or condition
Behavior - anything the animal does
Consequence - the outcome immediately following the behavior and potentially impacting antecedents via a feedback mechanism[40]

Although behavioral analyses primarily describe the behavior itself, functional analysis serves to identify the triggering and maintaining events and conditions.[19] In this respect, the analysis considers environmental conditions and events, social interactions, and physical health status, including a medical examination to exclude chronic pain, discomfort, or underlying disease (eg, primary neurologic disorders [eg, age-related degenerative diseases], neoplasia or infectious diseases, osteoarthrosis and degenerative joint disease, metabolic disease [eg, diabetes in older primates], or dental disease (**Box 2**).[27,42–46] Special attention is warranted to abiotic factors, predictability of husbandry measures, and possibility of individual control of environmental or social factors.[4] Once identified, testing functional significance of the assumed maintaining/triggering condition in controlling the occurrence of the target behavior by providing and withholding the assumed trigger is necessary to demonstrate the contingent relationship of trigger and behavior.[19]

Box 2
Examples of potential triggers and maintaining factors for abnormal behavior

- Disease-related: discomfort, pain, disfunction, medical interventions
- Socially related: social/human attention seeking, social separation, social incompatibility/ entrapment, change in social structure
- Husbandry-related: translocations/relocation, resocialization; novel objects, change in abiotic environmental factors (eg, light), presence of nearby predators, feeding schedules, restraint practices, recurrent medical interventions, space limitations, suboptimal levels of stimulation, lack of environmental control
- Miscellaneous: anticipation, boredom

Data from Refs.[6,14,19,27,30,40,47]

Life History

In order to understand the individual's background, research about its life history is helpful (see **Fig. 1**). In some situations, the past history of an individual may be more predictive of abnormal behavior patterns than its present environmental conditions.[48] Factors such as rearing history, sex, age, reproductive history, social history, and chronic disease processes are important, and should be routinely available from the holding institution's documentation. If that is not the case, a standardized survey may be helpful to gather information from previous holding institutions.

Diagnosis of Psychopathology

The diagnosis of psychopathologies and the use of proper terminology are not part of a standard veterinary training, and most veterinarians will feel at a loss trying to put a name to the clinical picture observed in their patient. For the inexperienced veterinarian, staying at the purely descriptive level of behavioral irregularities may prove far more constructive than attempting to associate the observed behavior with a defined disorder in human medicine (**Box 3**).

However, a thorough comparison of symptoms observed in NHPs with symptoms found in people may help generate testable hypotheses regarding the underlying disturbed psychological mechanisms and identify suitable treatment approaches.[5] For this process, collaboration with a human psychiatrist is encouraged; while veterinarians and/or biologists provide descriptive observations of the behavioral pattern in

Box 3
Selection of terms for the description of abnormal behavior in nonhuman primates

- Hyperactive, impulsive, irritable, unpredictable, outbursting, aggressive
- Lethargic, withdrawn, indifferent, distrustful, suspicious, depressive
- Anxious, tense, restless, fearful, (selectively) phobic
- Exaggerated startle response, hypervigilant, reckless, self-destructive
- Uncoordinated, clumsy, slow, stereotypic
- Dominant, submissive, impertinent, playful
- Severe, moderate, mild, frequent, occasional, rare

Data from American Psychiatric Association. Diagnostic and Statistical Manual of Mental Disorders. 5th ed. Washington D.C.: 2013.

regard to species-specific bio-social norms, human psychiatrists can compare these descriptions to defined human psychopathological diagnoses (see **Fig. 1**). The Diagnostic and Statistical Manual of Mental Disorders (DSM-5)[38] has been used to diagnose human mental disorders; it offers a list of categories of mental disorders and associated symptoms, such as neurodevelopmental, depressive, anxiety, trauma- and stress-related, dissociative, feeding/eating, and impulse-control disorders, all of which have been recognized in NHPs also.[5,6,11,25] Naturally, the description and diagnosis of other disorders like schizophrenia, bipolar disorder, somatic symptom disorder, and personality disorders are also based on verbally reported symptoms and closely linked to human personality traits and cultural norms, and may therefore be less useful in the context of NHP medicine.

TREATMENT APPROACHES TO ABNORMAL BEHAVIOR

Various therapeutic approaches can be deduced from the counter-clockwise diagnostic procedure proposed by the scheme: environmental/husbandry changes, medical treatment, psychopharmacological treatment, and behavioral therapy (see **Fig. 1**). All factors of the pathogenesis considered, the combination of several therapeutic options will provide an individually tailored approach.[27,49]

Abnormal behavior itself cannot be treated, but merely managed or prevented. Attempts to treat abnormal behavior must be considered analogous to symptom control in other diseases, without sustainably addressing the underlying disease. In urgent cases, such as automutilation, prevention of further injury or automatically reinforcing consequences may, however, require immediate action and symptom control, such as with special constraints and protective equipment (eg, cast bandages) or negative reinforcing techniques.[19] Treatment goals need to be individually tailored, realistically formulated, and clearly defined in consultation with all stakeholders. Working stepwise toward smaller goals (eg, temporary social integration for a few hours per day, reducing the frequency of abnormal behavior by 50%) may be necessary to appreciate treatment progress and avoid frustrations. Depending on the severity of disease, certain goals may never be attained, and the affected animal may remain susceptible to manifestation of abnormal behavior and require life-long management; for example, social integration and breeding may be attained, but maternal care may never be reached.[18]

Environmental/Husbandry Changes and Medical Treatment

If a functional analysis has identified reinforcing factors, changes in husbandry and management routine, nutrition, social group composition, and medical attention to chronic, painful conditions (eg, dental treatment, analgesia, physiotherapy) may already be efficient to reduce the frequency of abnormal behavior significantly.[19,50] The reader is referred to the large body of literature available on enrichment techniques for NHPs (food-based, sensory, animate and inanimate, cognitive).[21,23,26,51,52] If the enrichment is not carefully chosen to address identified reinforcing factors, the effect will likely prove inconsistent and oftentimes unsustainable in alleviating abnormal behavior.[4]

Behavioral Training/Operant Conditioning

Positive reinforcement training (PRT) can be applied to train and increase affiliative behaviors in asocial animals,[53] and it is generally used to habituate the animal to random medical and husbandry measures to alleviate or avoid associated stressors; yet, it only shows inconsistent success to sustainably treat established abnormal behaviors.[54–56] Operant conditioning as specific behavioral therapy can only be sustainably effective if 2 principles are respected; the behavioral therapy must address the individual pathogenesis of the abnormal behavior, and it must be aimed at not only reducing the aberrant behavior but simultaneously introducing more desirable, alternative behaviors (differential reinforcement of alternative behavior).[19,50] Specific operant behavioral therapy procedures are used in human medicine and have shown an overall effectiveness of more than 80% reduction in frequency of stereotyped and automutilative behavior.[57] The implementation of these procedures bears great potential in NHPs with abnormal behaviors, but the detailed description of these procedures (eg, non-contingent reinforcement, differential-reinforcement-of-other-behavior, functional communication) goes beyond the scope of this article. The reader is referred to a review article, and cooperation with veterinary behavioral specialists and human psychiatrists for an individually tailored operant conditioning training is encouraged.[19]

Pharmacologic Treatment

If the diagnostic procedure leads to the conclusion of an underlying psychopathological disorder, pharmacologic treatment must be considered, not as a last resort but as valuable flanking measure, as psychopathologically affected patients may not always be able to benefit from behavioral therapy or environmental changes without psychopharmacological support.[5] Sedation is not a target effect but may occur as side effect, and should be avoided or minimized so as to not interfere with social interactions and the learning process from operant conditioning. Therefore, the commonly used benzodiazepines are not recommended as a first-line choice. Although they may be helpful to control acute episodes of abnormal behavior, particularly with imminent risk of harm, inconsistent and unsustainable long-term effects are likely, because the sole GABAergic effect of benzodiazepines fails to address the complex neuroendocrine imbalances of most psychopathologies.[58]

The major categories of drugs used for pharmacologic interventions in psychopathologies target the opiate (eg, opiate antagonists), serotonergic (eg, selective serotonin reuptake inhibitors [SSRIs]), dual-serotonin-norepinephrine uptake inhibitors (SNRIs), serotonin-receptor agonists or antagonists (MAO-A inhibitors, tryptophan supplements), and dopaminergic (eg, dopamine receptor blocker) systems.[11] Consultation with a veterinary behavioral specialists or human psychiatrists is recommended to appropriately attune the drug therapy to specific features of the psychopathological disease (eg, hyperactivity, anxiety, or motor stereotypy) and to control potential undesirable effects. Whereas most reports of psychopharmacological drug use in NHPs originate from experimental research with NHPs as models for human psychopathologies,[11,27,59–69] reports about the use and effect of psychopharmacological drugs in captive NHPs in zoologic institutions are rare.[49,70,71]

Genetic Selection

Given the genetic influence on personality traits and susceptibility to psychopathological disorders, genetic selection may offer a viable strategy, as it has been successfully used to reduce stereotypic behavior in poultry and farmed minks.[48] This approach is currently not of major relevance to zoos but the inclusion of not only physical but also mental health may have to be increasingly included as a criterion for captive breeding programs (**Box 4**).

Box 4
Case report

The patient, life history, and behavior

Western lowland gorilla (*Gorilla gorilla gorilla*), female, 39 years, nulliparous, living in a group of 3 adult females and one silverback gorilla in a zoologic institution in Western Europe.

The animal was born in captivity and handraised for unknown reasons. At the age of 2 years, she was placed in a family group at another zoologic institution, but resocialization failed, whereupon she was sent back to the institution of origin. At the age of 3 years, another attempt failed to introduce her to a family group in a zoologic institution, whereupon she was sent on to her final destination, where she was tolerated into a group of 3 other handraised females and 1 silverback but remained the lowest-ranking member of the group.

According to anecdotal reports, the animal started showing automutilation of hands and feet at the age of 5 years, prompting several invasive, surgical, and preventative (cast bandages) measures and various medical treatments, including administration of alcoholic beverages for tranquilization. Detailed medical history started at the age of 24 years, documenting at least 3 severe episodes of self-injurious mutilation to hand and feet within the following 15 years, crippling her right foot and hand significantly. During this time, the animal underwent approximately 88 documented anesthestic procedures for surgical and medical wound treatments, bandage changes, and diagnostic procedures (general health examinations, imaging diagnostics, and virologic and bacteriologic screenings), went through many months of social isolation for treatments, countless drug treatments (analgesics, antibiotics, psychopharmacological treatment, homeopathy, and nutritional supplementations) and was exposed to a myriad of enrichment procedures. None of the diagnostic screenings provided any coherent evidence for etiology, nor were any of the treatment approaches sustainably effective. Therefore, interdisciplinary consultation with veterinarians, human psychiatrists, and biologists was chosen for a comprehensive approach.

Diagnostic procedure and results

1. Behavioral analysis: the self-injurious behavior as described was considered abnormal because of significant physical harm.

2. Functional analysis: remote video recording revealed purposeful display of automutilative behavior in presence of keeping staff, in order to attract attention from keepers, particularly during cleaning routine, when interaction with the animals was limited. Medical examination revealed a chronic subluxation of the right elbow and coxarthrosis.

3. Life history: early maternal separation, handraising, and several placements in 3 social groups were likely to result in altered development and dysregulation of the neuroendocrine system.

4. Diagnosis of psychopathology:
   a. Descriptive terminology: little patience, low frustration threshold, sudden mood changes, irritable, aggressive bouts against keepers, anxiety
   b. Suspect diagnosis by human psychiatrist: borderline-like syndrome

Therapeutic approaches:

1. Withdrawal of attention in regard to self-injurious behavior: keepers were instructed to strictly ignore any self-injurious behavior. In fact, during separation of the animals in the background of the exhibit during cleaning routine, keepers had to first observe the animals on a remote video screen before approaching their enclosures. If any self-injurious behavior or even intentions for such were evident, keepers had to turn away and leave the animals alone.

2. Operant conditioning: several elements of training were introduced as targets for keepers' attention. Because of the impatient and irritable personality of the animal, training goals

had to be carefully chosen not to elicit any frustrations, such as assuming positions for physical examination or trading of objects.

3. Physiotherapy and analgesia: chronic pain was addressed by long-term analgesia (primarily nonsteroidal anti-inflammatory drugs), and part of the training elements consisted of physiotherapeutic exercises, such as reaching for targets out of immediate reach, prompting the animal to stretch and mobilize her disabled elbow and stiff joints.

4. Psychopharmacological drugs: not considered necessary in this case.

Outcome

Only a few months after implementation of strict disregard of the self-injurious behavior and training of alternative behaviors to seek attention, the previously chronic wounds on hand and feet healed up without medical treatment. About a year later, inadvertent testing of the hypothesis of human attention as maintaining factor happened when a new keeper, who had missed respective instructions regarding the interaction with this animal, triggered a new episode of self-injurious wound manipulations by paying attention and reporting small skin wounds well-meaningly. Correction of the keeper's behavior resulted in wound healing within a few weeks.

DISCLOSURE

The author has nothing to disclose.

REFERENCES

1. Broom DM. Animal welfare: concepts and measurement. J Anim Sci 1991;69: 4167–75.

2. Fabrega H Jr. Making sense of behavioral irregularities of great apes. Neurosci Biobehav Rev 2006;30:1260–73.

3. Barr CS, Newman TK, Becker ML, et al. The utility of the non-human primate model for studying gene by environment interactions in behavioral research. Genes Brain Behav 2003;2:336–40.

4. Kummrow MS, Brüne M. Psychopathologies in captive nonhuman primates and approaches to diagnosis and treatment. J Zoo Wildl Med 2018;49:259–71.

5. Brüne M, Brüne-Cohrs U, McGrew WC, et al. Psychopathology in great apes: concepts, treatment options and possible homologies to human psychiatric disorders. Neurosci Biobehav Rev 2006;30:1246–59.

6. Bradshaw GA, Capaldo T, Lindner L, et al. Building an inner sanctuary: complex PTSD in chimpanzees. J Trauma Dissociation 2008;9:9–34.

7. Munafo MR, Clark TG, Moore LR, et al. Genetic polymorphisms and personality in healthy adults: a systematic review and meta-analysis. Mol Psychiatry 2003;8: 471–84.

8. Gosling SD, John OP. Personality dimensions in nonhuman animals: a cross-species review. Curr Dir Psychol Sci 1999;8:69–75.

9. Uher J, Asendorpf JB. Personality assessment in the great apes: comparing ecologically valid behavior measures, behavior ratings, and adjective ratings. J Res Pers 2008;42:821–38.

10. Gottlieb DH, Capitanio JP, McCowan B. Risk factors for stereotypic behavior and self-biting in rhesus macaques (*Macaca mulatta*): animal's history, current environment, and personality. Am J Primatol 2013;75:995–1008.

11. Beaudoin-Gobert M, Sgambato-Faure V. Serotonergic pharmacology in animal models: from behavioral disorders to dyskinesia. Neuropharmacology 2014;81: 15–30.
12. Camus SM, Rochais C, Blois-Heulin C, et al. Birth origin differentially affects depressive-like behaviours: are captive-born cynomolgus monkeys more vulnerable to depression than their wild-born counterparts? PLoS One 2013;8:e67711.
13. Crast J, Bloomsmith MA, Perlman JE, et al. Abnormal behaviour in captive sooty mangabeys. Anim Welf 2014;23:167–77.
14. Lutz C, Well A, Novak M. Stereotypic and self-injurious behavior in rhesus macaques: a survey and retrospective analysis of environment and early experience. Am J Primatol 2003;60:1–15.
15. Novak MA. Self-injurious behavior in rhesus monkeys: new insights into its etiology, physiology, and treatment. Am J Primatol 2003;59:3–19.
16. Bellanca RU, Crockett CM. Factors predicting increased incidence of abnormal behavior in male pigtailed macaques. Am J Primatol 2002;58:57–69.
17. Gilmer WS, McKinney WT. Early experience and depressive disorders: human and non-human primate studies. J Affect Disord 2003;75:97–113.
18. Arling GL, Harlow HF. Effects of social deprivation on maternal behavior of rhesus monkeys. J Comp Physiol Psychol 1967;64:371–7.
19. Bloomsmith MA, Marr MJ, Maple TL. Addressing nonhuman primate behavioral problems through the application of operant conditioning: is the human treatment approach a useful model? Appl Anim Behav Sci 2007;102:205–22.
20. Dantzer R. Stress, stereotypies and welfare. Behav Process 1991;25:95–102.
21. Bayne K, Mainzer H, Dexter S, et al. The reduction of abnormal behaviors in individually housed rhesus monkeys (Macaca mulatta) with a foraging/grooming board. Am J Primatol 1991;23:23–35.
22. Baker KC, Easley SP. An analysis of regurgitation and reingestion in captive chimpanzees. Appl Anim Behav Sci 1996;49:403–15.
23. Akers JS, Schildkraut DS. Regurgitation/reingestion and coprophagy in captive gorillas. Zoo Biol 1985;4:99–109.
24. Birkett LP, Newton-Fisher NE. How abnormal is the behaviour of captive, zoo-living chimpanzees? PLoS One 2011;6:e20101.
25. Botero M, Macdonald SE, Miller RS. Anxiety-related behavior of orphan chimpanzees (Pan troglodytes schweinfurthii) at Gombe National Park, Tanzania. Primates 2013;54:21–6.
26. Bourgeois SR, Brent L. Modifying the behaviour of singly caged baboons: evaluating the effectiveness of four enrichment techniques. Anim Welf 2005;14: 71–81.
27. Bourgeois SR, Vazquez M, Brasky K. Combination therapy reduces self-injurious behavior in a chimpanzee (Pan Troglodytes Troglodytes): a case report. J Appl Anim Welf Sci 2007;10:123–40.
28. Brand CM, Marchant LF. Hair plucking in captive bonobos (Pan paniscus). Appl Anim Behav Sci 2015;171:192–6.
29. Brent L, Koban T, Ramirez S. Abnormal, abusive, and stress-related behaviors in baboon mothers. Biol Psychiatry 2002;52:1047–56.
30. Cassella CM, Mills A, Lukas KE. Prevalence of regurgitation and reingestion in orangutans housed in North American zoos and an examination of factors influencing its occurrence in a single group of Bornean orangutans. Zoo Biol 2012; 31:609–20.
31. Hopper LM, Freeman HD, Ross SR. Reconsidering coprophagy as an indicator of negative welfare for captive chimpanzees. Appl Anim Behav Sci 2016;176:112–9.

32. Whiten A, Goodall J, McGrew WC, et al. Cultures in chimpanzees. Nature 1999; 399:682–5.

33. Hill SP. Do gorillas regurgitate potentially-injurious stomach acid during 'regurgitation and reingestion? Anim Welf 2009;18:123–7.

34. Miller LJ, Tobey JR. Regurgitation and reingestion in bonobos (*Pan paniscus*): Relationships between abnormal and social behavior. Appl Anim Behav Sci 2012;141:65–70.

35. Mason GJ, Latham N. Can't stop, won't stop: is stereotypy a reliable animal welfare indicator? Anim Welf 2004;13:S57–69.

36. Robbins MM. Male aggression against females in mountain gorillas: courtship or coercion. In: Muller MN, Wrangham RW, editors. Sexual coercion in primates and humans. An evolutionary perspective on male aggression against females. Cambridge (MA): Harvard University Press; 2009. p. 112–27.

37. Sousa C, Casanova C. Are great apes aggressive? A cross-species comparison. Antropologia Portuguesa 2006;22:71–118.

38. American Psychiatric Association. Diagnostic and statistical manual of mental disorders. 5th edition. Washington, DC: American Psychiatric Association; 2013.

39. Judge PG, Evans DW, Schroepfer KK, et al. Perseveration on a reversal-learning task correlates with rates of self-directed behavior in nonhuman primates. Behav Brain Res 2011;222:57–65.

40. Desmarchelier MR. A systematic approach in diagnosing behavior problems. In: Miller RE, Lamberski N, Calle PP, editors. Fowler's zoo and wild animal medicine. St. Louis (MO): Elsevier; 2019. p. 76–82.

41. Hansen EW. The development of maternal and infant behavior in the rhesus monkey. Behaviour 1966;27:107–49.

42. Adkesson MJ, Rubin DA. Degenerative skeletal diseases of primates. In: Miller RE,, Fowler M, editors. Fowler's zoo and wild animal medicine current therapy. St. Louis (MO): Elsevier Saunders; 2012. p. 396–407.

43. Johnson-Delaney CA. Nonhuman primate dental care. J Exot Pet Med 2008;17: 138–43.

44. Tigno XT, Gerzanich G, Hansen BC. Age-related changes in metabolic parameters of nonhuman primates. J Gerontol A Biol Sci Med Sci 2004;59:1081–8.

45. Price DL, Martin LJ, Sisodia SS, et al. Aged non-human primates: an animal model of age-associated neurodegenerative disease. Brain Pathol 1991;1:287–96.

46. Capitanio JP, Emborg ME. Contributions of non-human primates to neuroscience research. Lancet 2008;371:1126–35.

47. Davenport MD, Lutz CK, Tiefenbacher S, et al. A rhesus monkey model of self-injury: effects of relocation stress on behavior and neuroendocrine function. Biol Psychiatry 2008;63:990–6.

48. Mason G, Clubb R, Latham N, et al. Why and how should we use environmental enrichment to tackle stereotypic behaviour? Appl Anim Behav Sci 2007;102: 163–88.

49. Prosen H, Bell B. A psychiatrist consulting at the zoo (the therapy of Brian bonobo). Conference proceedings of The Apes Challenges for 21st Century, Brookfield Zoo, USA, May 10-13, 2000. p. 161–4.

50. Dorey NR, Rosales-Ruiz J, Smith R, et al. Functional analysis and treatment of self-injury in a captive olive baboon. J Appl Behav Anal 2009;42:785–94.

51. Lutz CK, Novak MA. Environmental enrichment for nonhuman primates: theory and application. ILAR J 2005;46:178–91.

52. Clark FE. Great ape cognition and captive care: Can cognitive challenges enhance well-being? Appl Anim Behav Sci 2011;135:1–12.

53. Schapiro SJ, Perlman JE, Boudreau BA. Manipulating the affiliative interactions of group-housed rhesus macaques using positive reinforcement training techniques. Am J Primatol 2001;55:137–49.
54. Bloomsmith M, Lambeth S, Stone A, et al. Comparing two types of human interaction as enrichment for chimpanzees. Am J Primatol 1997;42:96.
55. Morgan L, Howell SM, Fritz J. Regurgitation and reingestion in a captive chimpanzee (Pan troglodytes). Lab Anim 1993;22:42–5.
56. Coleman K, Maier A. The use of positive reinforcement training to reduce stereotypic behavior in rhesus macaques. Appl Anim Behav Sci 2010;124:142–8.
57. Kahng S, Iwata BA, Lewin AB. Behavioral treatment of self-injury, 1964 to 2000. Am J Ment Retard 2002;107:212–21.
58. Tiefenbacher S, Fahey MA, Rowlett JK, et al. The efficacy of diazepam treatment for the management of acute wounding episodes in captive rhesus macaques. Comp Med 2005;55:387–92.
59. Fontenot MB, Padgett EE, Dupuy AM, et al. The effects of fluoxetine and buspirone on self-injurious and stereotypic behavior in adult male rhesus macaques. Comp Med 2005;55:67–74.
60. Fontenot MB, Musso MW, McFatter RM, et al. Dose-finding study of fluoxetine and venlafaxine for the treatment of self-injurious and stereotypic behavior in rhesus macaques (Macaca mulatta). J Am Assoc Lab Anim 2009;48:176–84.
61. Hugo C, Seier J, Mdhluli C, et al. Fluoxetine decreases stereotypic behavior in primates. Progr Neuropsychopharmacol Biol Psychiatry 2003;27:639–43.
62. Weld KP, Mench JA, Woodward RA, et al. Effect of tryptophan treatment on self-biting and central nervous system serotonin metabolism in rhesus monkeys (Macaca mulatta). Neuropsychopharmacology 1998;19:314–21.
63. Eaton GG, Worlein JM, Kelley ST, et al. Self-injurious behavior is decreased by cyproterone acetate in adult male rhesus (Macaca mulatta). Horm Behav 1999; 35:195–203.
64. Fam SD, Tan YS, Waitt C. Stereotypies in captive primates and the use of inositol: lessons from obsessive–compulsive disorder in humans. Int J Primatol 2012;33: 830–44.
65. Kempf DJ, Baker KC, Gilbert MH, et al. Effects of extended-release injectable naltrexone on self-injurious behavior in rhesus macaques (Macaca mulatta). Comp Med 2012;62:209–17.
66. Lee KM, Chiu KB, Didier PJ, et al. Naltrexone treatment reverses astrocyte atrophy and immune dysfunction in self-harming macaques. Brain Behav Immun 2015;50:288–97.
67. Macy JD, Beattie TA, Morgenstern SE, et al. Use of guanfacine to control self-injurious behavior in two rhesus macaques (Macaca mulatta) and one baboon (Papio anubis). Comp Med 2000;50:410–25.
68. McKinney WT, Young LD, Suomi SJ, et al. Chlorpromazine treatment of disturbed monkeys. Arch Gen Psychiatry 1973;29:490–4.
69. Pond CL, Rush HG. Self-aggression in macaques: five case studies. Primates 1983;24:127–34.
70. Espinosa-Avilés D, Elizondo G, Morales-Martínez M, et al. Treatment of acute self-aggressive behaviour in a captive gorilla (Gorilla gorilla gorilla). Vet Rec 2004; 154:401–2.
71. Redrobe SP. Neuroleptics in great apes, with specific reference to modification of aggressive behavior in a male gorilla. In: Fowler ME, Miller RE, editors. Zoo and wild animal medicine, current therapy. St. Louis (MO): Saunders Elsevier; 2008. p. 243–50.

Printed and bound by CPI Group (UK) Ltd, Croydon, CR0 4YY

03/10/2024

01040407-0009